BI■MECHANICAL
SYSTEMS TECHN■L■GY

COMPUTATIONAL METHODS

BIOMECHANICAL SYSTEMS TECHNOLOGY
A 4-Volume Set
Editor: Cornelius T Leondes *(University of California, Los Angeles, USA)*

Computational Methods
ISBN-13 978-981-270-981-3
ISBN-10 981-270-981-9

Cardiovascular Systems
ISBN-13 978-981-270-982-0
ISBN-10 981-270-982-7

Muscular Skeletal Systems
ISBN-13 978-981-270-983-7
ISBN-10 981-270-983-5

General Anatomy
ISBN-13 978-981-270-984-4
ISBN-10 981-270-984-3

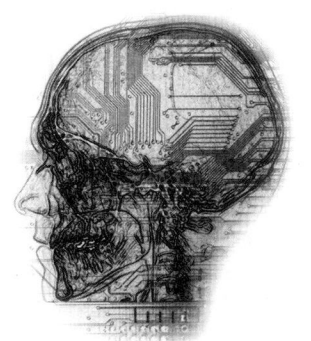

A 4-VOLUME SET

BI■MECHANICAL
SYSTEMS TECHN■L■GY

COMPUTATIONAL METHODS

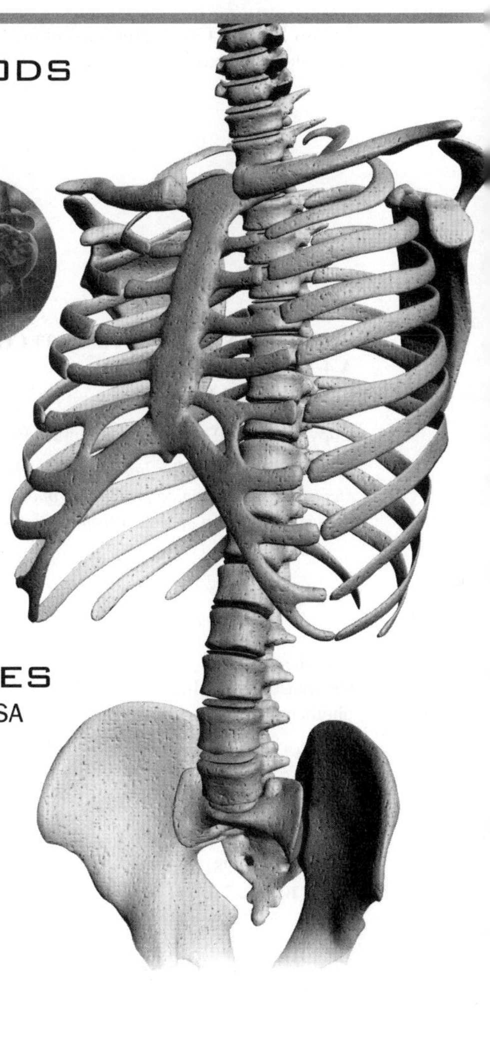

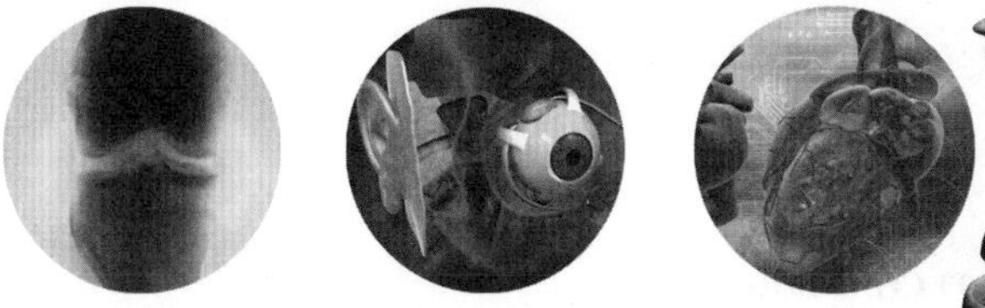

EDITOR

CORNELIUS T LEONDES
University of California, Los Angeles, USA

World Scientific

NEW JERSEY · LONDON · SINGAPORE · BEIJING· · SHANGHAI · HONG KONG · TAIPEI · CHENNAI

Published by

World Scientific Publishing Co. Pte. Ltd.

5 Toh Tuck Link, Singapore 596224

USA office: 27 Warren Street, Suite 401-402, Hackensack, NJ 07601

UK office: 57 Shelton Street, Covent Garden, London WC2H 9HE

British Library Cataloguing-in-Publication Data
A catalogue record for this book is available from the British Library.

BIOMECHANICAL SYSTEMS TECHNOLOGY
A 4-Volume Set
Computational Methods

ISBN-13 978-981-270-798-7   (Set)
ISBN-10 981-270-798-0   (Set)

ISBN-13 978-981-270-981-3
ISBN-10 981-270-981-9

Typeset by Stallion Press
Email: enquiries@stallionpress.com

Printed in Singapore by World Scientific Printers (S) Pte Ltd

PREFACE

Because of rapid developments in computer technology and computational techniques, advances in a wide spectrum of technologies, and other advances coupled with cross-disciplinary pursuits between technology and its applications to human body processes, the field of biomechanics continues to evolve. Many areas of significant progress can be noted. These include dynamics of musculosketal systems, mechanics of hard and soft tissues, mechanics of bone remodeling, mechanics of implant-tissue interfaces, cardiovascular and respiratory biomechanics, mechanics of blood and air flow, flow-prosthesis interfaces, mechanics of impact, dynamics of man-machine interaction, and many more. This is the first of a set of four volumes and it treats the area of Computational Methods in biomechanics.

The four volumes constitute an integrated set. The titles for each of the volumes are:

- Biomechanical Systems Technology: Computational Methods
- Biomechanical Systems Technology: Cardiovascular Systems
- Biomechanical Systems Technology: Muscular Skeletal Systems
- Biomechanical Systems Technology: General Anatomy

Collectively they constitute an MRW (Major Reference Work). An MRW is a comprehensive treatment of a subject area requiring multiple authors and a number of distinctly titled and well integrated volumes. Each volume treats a specific but broad subject area of fundamental importance to biomechanical systems technology.

Each volume is self-contained and stands alone for those interested in a specific volume. However, collectively, this 4-volume set evidently constitutes the first comprehensive major reference work dedicated to the multi-discipline area of biomechanical systems technology.

There are over 120 coauthors from 18 countries of this notable MRW. The chapters are clearly written, self contained, readable and comprehensive with helpful guides including introduction, summary, extensive figures and examples with comprehensive reference lists. Perhaps the most valuable feature of this work is the breadth and depth of the topics covered by leading contributors on the international scene.

The contributors of this volume clearly reveal the effectiveness of the techniques available and the essential role that they will play in the future. I hope that practitioners, research workers, computer scientists, and students will find this set of volumes to be a unique and significant reference source for years to come.

CONTENTS

DEFORMABLE IMAGE REGISTRATION FOR RADIATION THERAPY PLANNING: ALGORITHMS AND APPLICATIONS

MICHAEL R. KAUS

Philips Radiation Oncology Systems, Madison, WI, USA
michael.kaus@philips.com

KRISTY K. BROCK

Medical Physics Department
Princess Margaret Hospital, Toronto, Ontario, Canada
kristy.brock@rmp.uhn.on.ca

Approximately 60% of cancer patients are treated with external beam radiotherapy at some point during disease management. Despite the extended time frame of fractionated therapy (4–6 weeks), radiation therapy planning is carried out based on information that is currently limited to a single 3D anatomical computed tomography scan at the onset of treatment. This concept may result in severe treatment uncertainties, including the irradiation of risk organs and reduced tumor coverage. Repeat 3D single or multi-modality imaging acquired at various time intervals during and after a radiation course provides the opportunity to increase treatment accuracy and precision by optimizing treatment in response to anatomical changes; to improve target delineation through modality-specific complementary tumor representations, and to assess treatment response. Integration of multiple imaging sources into a single patient model requires compensation of geometric differences while maintaining modality-specific differences in information content. Deformable image registration aims to reduce such uncertainties by estimating the spatial relationship between the volume elements of corresponding structures across image data. This paper reviews the algorithmic components of deformation algorithms, and their application to treatment sites with evident geometric changes, including mono- and multi-modal image registration for cancer of the head and neck, lung, liver, and prostate.

Keywords: Cancer; external beam radiotherapy; treatment planning; deformable image registration.

1. Introduction

Cancer is the second leading cause of death in the industrialized countries and the only major disease for which death rates are increasing. The demand for cancer care will increase over the decade as the aging of the baby boomer population drives a dramatic increase in the incidence of many cancers.

Approximately 60% of cancer patients are treated with external beam radiotherapy (EBRT) at some point during management of their disease. The main goal of radiation therapy (RT) is to maximize the dose to the target while limiting the dose to nearby healthy organs ("risk organs"), in order to improve control of tumor growth and limit side effects.

Radiation therapy is primarily used to treat cancer by locally targeting radiation to the diseased tissue. Radiation beams are produced by medical linear accelerators (Fig. 1). These devices are mounted on a gantry with a rotating couch to allow for many beam directions to be focused on the target volume. Sparing of normal tissues is accomplished in two fundamental ways: geometric avoidance of normal tissues is accomplished by directing multiple beams at the target, thus delivering a high dose where the beams intersect at the target, and a relatively lower dose outside of the intersection. Biological sparing of normal tissue is accomplished by fractionating the therapy over several weeks, irradiating daily. The tumor tissue lacks repair mechanisms to repair DNA damage from the radiation, whereas normal tissues can repair minor DNA damage. Therefore, by fractionating the treatment, normal tissues are provided time to repair, thus biologically sparing the normal tissue.

Despite the extended time frame of fractionated radiotherapy (4–6 weeks), RT planning is carried out based on information that is currently limited to a single 3D anatomical computed tomography (CT) image data set acquired at the onset of treatment design (Fig. 2). The patient is marked for repeated alignment with localization lasers in the treatment room. The treatment planning is then performed on the CT scan where beam geometries, energies, and collimation are determined, and the resultant dose distribution is computed. This concept may result in severe treatment uncertainties, resulting in irradiation of risk organs and reduced tumor coverage.[1,2]

Natural processes in the body and response of normal and target tissue to the treatment result in significant inter- and intra-fractional geometrical changes. Intra-fractional (during a single treatment fraction) geometric change occurs during

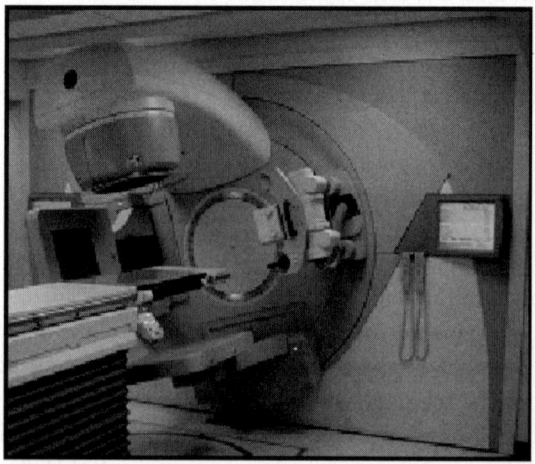

Fig. 1.   Linear accelerator with on-board kV cone-beam CT imaging unit. The device enables therapeutic irradiation and soft-tissue imaging while the patient is on the treatment unit.

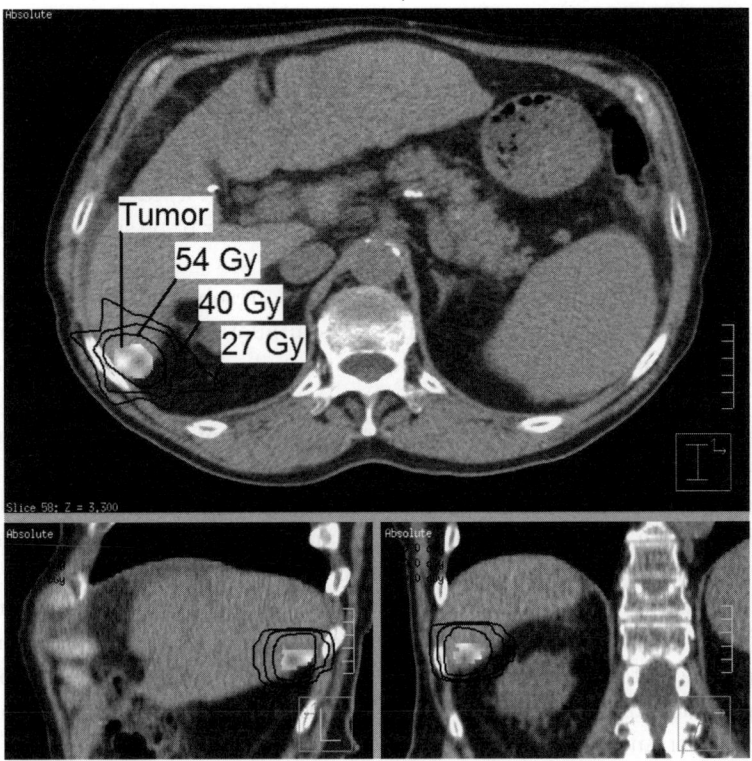

Fig. 2. Example of a radiation treatment plan of a patient with liver cancer treated in 6 fractions with 36 Gy. Displayed are orthogonal cuts through the 3D CT, and target contours, and iso-dose lines. Images courtesy Radiation Medicine Program, Princess Margaret Hospital (L. Dawson).

radiation delivery due to breathing, cardiac motion, rectal peristalsis and bladder filling. Inter-fractional (day-to-day) geometric change occurs over the weeks of therapy, due to digestive processes, change of breathing patterns, difference in patient setup, and treatment response like growth or shrinkage of the tumor or nearby risk organs (e.g., the parotids in head and neck treatment). These changes are taken into account by population-based "uncertainty" margins around the target area, which may be excessive or conservative and are applied to the structures identified before the therapy begins.

Repeat 3D imaging with single or multiple imaging modalities acquired at various time intervals during and after a radiation course provides the opportunity to increase treatment accuracy and precision by optimizing treatment in response to anatomical changes; to improve target delineation through modality-specific complementary tumor representations, to quantify patient specific physiological motion, and to assess treatment response. The exploitation of integrated imagery may allow both dose escalation to the tumor and reduction of dose given to organs at risk. This has the potential to allow for dose escalation using larger fractions size hypo-fractionated regimes increasing the chance of local control without increasing toxicity.

The concepts of adaptive radiotherapy (ART) and image-guided radiotherapy (IGRT) provide methods to monitor and adjust the treatments to accommodate the changing patient. ART is an off-line approach where the anatomical and biological changes are monitored over the course of treatment, and the treatment is modified when significant changes are identified. IGRT is typically an on-line concept where the patient or treatment plan is shifted or modified for each treatment. Both concepts require advanced image processing tools in order to be successful in clinical practice.

The goal of deformable image registration is to resolve differences in geometry while maintaining modality-specific differences in information content by means of estimating the spatial relationship between the volume elements (i.e., the image voxels) of corresponding structures across image data sets. The solution of this task in turn allows for the geometrically corrected transfer of target and organ at risk contours (or regions of interest, ROI) between images, quantitative description of physiological motion patterns, measurement of image-based surrogates of treatment response, and the design of dose patterns and determination of their effect in deforming anatomy on a patient-specific basis.

The remainder of this chapter reviews the basic algorithmic components of deformable image registration techniques commonly used in RT planning, and their applications to treatment sites where geometric changes are most prominent, including mono- and multi-modal image registration for cancer of the head and neck, lung, liver and prostate.

2. Algorithmic Components of Deformable Image Registration Techniques

Deformable image registration has been studied since the early 80s and for many years, brain surgery and neurosciences have been the driving applications for developing an abundant number of techniques.[3,4] Despite the significant progress that has been made, deformable registration is still not clinically accepted and remains a challenging problem.

In the following sections we will describe the core components of a deformable registration algorithm — similarity measures, deformation models, and commonly used optimization methods. This section does not intend to provide a complete literature overview, but to give a flavor of methods applied to radiation therapy problems, and to provide a basis for the subsequent discussion of application to the various treatment sites.

2.1. *Similarity measures*

2.1.1. *Intensity-based similarity measures*

Registration methods that use voxel similarity measures determine the registration transformation by optimizing the similarity function directly from the voxel values rather than from points or surfaces derived from the image.[4]

One of the simplest voxel similarity measures between a transformed image I_2 and a fixed image I_1 is the sum of squared grey value differences

$$SSD = \sum_{i \in M} (I_1(i) - I_2(i))^2,$$

where M is the region of overlap of the images I_2 and I_1. SSD is very sensitive to voxels with large intensity differences (outliers) which makes SSD only applicable in single-modality registration contexts, or more precisely, in cases where the images to be registered only differ by noise when registered. The least-squares form of SSD makes the measure computationally very attractive since fast optimization schemes such as Gauss–Newton or Levenberg–Marquardt can be applied.[5]

If a linear relationship between the grey values of the images can be assumed, correlation-based similarity measures such as the cross-correlation

$$CC = \frac{\sum (I_1(i) - \bar{I}_1)(I_2(i) - \bar{I}_2)}{\sqrt{\sum (I_1(i) - \bar{I}_1)^2} \sqrt{\sum (I_2(i) - \bar{I}_2)^2}}$$

can be applied. As this is a quadratic form, the same highly efficient numerical methods can be applied as for the optimization of SSD-based measures. Usually CC is not suited for multi-modality registration since a global linear transformation function of the grey values cannot be presumed. However, in a number of small neighborhoods the assumption of a linear relationship is valid and the cross-correlation coefficient can be used as an indicator of image similarity.

If we square and accumulate the local CC values (allowing for positive as well as negative correlated transitions) then also multi-modality images can be registered. The measure is denoted as local correlation

$$LC = \sqrt{\frac{1}{N} \sum_{S_j \in M} CC^2(S_j)},$$

where CC^2 is the square cross correlation coefficient for the j-th subregion S_j, and N is the number of subregions contained in N. LC has been successfully used for various medical rigid and deformable registration tasks.[6]

Image registration can also be considered within an information theoretic framework. The basic idea is to exploit a statistically significant relationship between the grey values of the input images. This relationship does not have to be explicitly known. The only fact used is that proper registration means proper alignment of significant grey value structures that — via their statistical relationship — lead to pronounced peaks in the joint grey value distribution detected as maxima of its mutual information or entropy. The mutual information

$$MI = - \sum_{j,k} \left(\frac{P_{j,k}^{2D}}{V} \log \frac{P_{j,k}^{2D}}{P_j^1 P_k^2} \right),$$

where V denotes the volume of overlap, P_j^1 and P_k^2 are the probabilities of grey values j and k in the two images respectively, and $P_{j,k}^{1,2}$ is the probability that grey values j and k occur in the fixed and at the corresponding position in the transforming image. MI has become the accepted standard for image registration, in particular for multi-modality applications. Over the last years, a large amount of publications demonstrate that MI can be used without need for pre-processing, user initialization and parameter tuning.[7]

The normalization of MI (NMI) with respect to the image overlap has proven as a useful extension of the measure. A drawback is that MI is not a least-squares criterion and the calculation of derivative information is not straightforward.[8] Steepest decent or simplex optimization schemes are frequently applied which may result in prohibitive computational costs for elastic transformations with a larger number of parameters. A dedicated Levenberg–Marquardt method for MI optimization can be found in.[9] This approach has recently been extended to higher order MI.[10]

MI is usually applied on image intensities directly. Recent work explores MI for measuring the similarity of voxel labels or image features by allowing different sized bins leading to probabilistic MI.[11] The registration is separated from the image space by integrating a pre-processing step that interprets grey values according to an underlying tissue class model.

2.1.2. *Contour-based measures*

Contour matching has been used to define boundary conditions for point-, surface or finite element model-based deformable registration algorithms. Basically, deformation is prescribed on the surfaces of ROI, which are then interpolated to the remaining voxels in the image by means of various deformation models.

Contour matching relies on previously delineated ROI in the image pairs. Several techniques to derive point-correspondences from corresponding contours have been developed, including manual identification and automated optimization to align the surface while minimizing distortion or energy.

Contour matching, through the manual identification of point correspondences on contours of the ROI on two images is limited to the accuracy with which one can identify corresponding points and is often used as a starting point for iterations that involve energy minimization.[12,13]

Energy minimization calculates the energy required to deform the contour by the displacement vector. By minimizing the energy that is required to deform the contoured representation of the ROI from one instance to another, the algorithm strives to model the true physiological deformation, which is governed by the path of least resistance.[14] Guided surface projection projects points, defined on the surface of one ROI, to a surface, defined by the second representation of the ROI. The projection is primarily perpendicular to the surface but allows flexibility in the projection to preserve the relationship between the points on the ROI surface.[15,16]

2.2. Deformation models

2.2.1. *Parametric transformations*

A common method for describing parametric elastic transformations is to view the transformation as a deformation field defined by a linear combination of a class of basis functions. Common choices of basis functions are thin-plate spline (TPS) models using radial basis functions, elastic body splines (EBS), or B-splines. The latter have the advantage of local support (basis functions with local support have also recently been applied for registration using TPS and EBS.[17,18] Using basis functions with compact support, a change of a parameter only affects the transformation in a spatially limited neighborhood while other parts of the deformation remain unchanged. Hence, with respect to image reformation, only the relevant part of the image has to be resampled, which significantly improves the computational performance.

2.2.1.1. **B-splines**

The 1D basis function of a B-spline is a piecewise polynomial with a uniform spacing between the control points, which is extended to higher dimensions by a tensor product. For example, a B-spline deformation field in 3D is defined as

$$\vec{u}(x, y, z) = \sum_{l=0}^{3} \sum_{m=0}^{3} \sum_{n=0}^{3} B_l(u) B_m(v) B_n(w) \phi_{i+l, j+m, k+n},$$

where B_l represents the lth basis function of a B-spline, $\phi_{i+l,j+m,k+n}$ is a control point on a uniform grid $n_x \times n_y \times n_z$, and x, y, z are the spatial 3D image coordinates. B-splines, in particular in combination with MI similarity, have shown potential for medical applications such as breast MRI.[10]

Although B-splines can be used within a multi-scale framework by first using coarse meshes which are constantly refined, the individual mesh resolution cannot be adapted to the structure of the underlying image. The mesh resolution can only be improved on the whole image requiring a large number of control points also in areas where the image does not provide much structure. This must also be considered when using advanced optimization schemes, for example when using a Gauss–Newton method in case of *SSD* similarity, since the linear systems to be solved during registration may become singular. A solution to this problem is to allow for a set of irregularly spaced control points which can be better adapted to the underlying image structures (see below).

Since the displacement of the control points is not constrained during optimization, a folding of the points may occur resulting in an inconsistent topology of the deformation field. To overcome this difficulty, several techniques for regularization are proposed such as adding an energy term to the similarity measure or using multi-level B-spline approximation techniques.[10,19]

2.2.1.2. Radial basis functions

Landmark-based registration methods are based on the framework of topologically consistent parametric deformations based on a mapping between corresponding control points (landmarks) in the floating and reference images. The landmark positions are usually selected manually, or (semi-) automatically, e.g., based on differential operators or fitting of deformable models.[20] Image intensity information is not explicitly used by these methods.

An interpolation transformation function or displacement field $\vec{u}(\vec{x}_i)$ based on point-landmarks must fulfill the constraint

$$\vec{u}(\vec{p}_i) = \vec{q}_i,$$

where $\vec{p}_i$ constitute a given set of point-landmarks (or control points) in the reference image, and $\vec{q}_i$ are the corresponding point-landmarks in the floating image. The displacement field is generally given by

$$\vec{u}(\vec{x}) = \sum_{i=1}^{N} \vec{c}_i U(r) + A\vec{x} + \vec{b},$$

where $A\vec{x} + \vec{b}$ is an affine transformation, N is the number of control points, and $U(r)$ is the basis function depending on the Euclidian distance $r = |\vec{x} - \vec{p}_i|$. Combining above equations results in a system of linear equations, which can be efficiently solved to calculate the coefficients $\vec{c}_i$ and the components of the affine transformation.

Intuitively, the coefficients have a meaning similar to force strengths, which are applied at the location of the control points $\vec{p}_i$ in order to move them on top of the corresponding points $\vec{q}_i$. To estimate the displacement that all forces yield at a particular location $\vec{x}$ in the image, the effect of each force in control point $\vec{p}_i$ at location $\vec{x}$ is accumulated.

The choice of the basis function $U(r)$ determines the characteristics of the displacement field away from the control points. Many basis functions have been proposed, but it is hard to give rules of thumb on how to select the best basis function, as the best choice is highly data-dependent.

2.2.1.3. Thin-plate splines (TPS)

The 3D TPS function is

$$U_{TPS}(r) = r,$$

which is analogous to the one used by Bookstein and has been used to analyze the variation of biological shapes.[21] The name "thin plate" refers to a physical analogy involving the bending of a thin sheet of metal orthogonal to the plate, such that it passes through given data points in elevation "z" of the plane, while taking a shape in which it is least bent. The TPS model produces radially symmetric transformations, which are globally distributed owing to the affine part.

2.2.1.4. Wendland functions

With the TPS, a landmark pair can influence the whole image. It has been argued that TPS has difficulties describing local deformations, if the control points are not well distributed over the image to prevent deformations in regions where no changes are desired. Fornefett *et al.* proposed Wendland basis functions for image registration, with

$$U_W(r) = \left(1 - \frac{r}{a}\right)^4_+ \left(4\frac{r}{a} + 1\right),$$

which produces radially symmetric local transformations that are zero for $r > a$.[17] The support radius a determines the spatial range of influence induced by a particular control point pair. The deformation induced by mapping $\vec{p}_i$ to $\vec{q}_i$ is zero outside of a spherical image region around $\vec{p}_i$ with radius a. Because this model is not invariant to affine transformations, the affine transformation parameters are estimated and applied prior to the deformable registration with Wendland functions.

2.2.1.5. Elastic body splines (EBS)

The EBS is a physically motivated model, which may be advantageous over the application of purely geometric transformations for registering follow-up data of the same subject. The EBS is an analytical solution to the Navier equation, describing the deformation of elastic bodies under the influence of externally applied forces.[3] A parametric representation with an analytical solution of the Navier equation can be derived if Gaussian-shaped forces are centered at the positions of the control points to elastically deform the image in a way that the prescribed corresponding control points (prescribed displacements) are preserved. This leads to the EBS function

$$U_{EBS}(r) = \frac{1+v}{8\Pi Y[1-v]}\{\Phi_1(\xi)I + \Phi_2(\xi)\vec{e}_r\vec{e}_r^T\},$$

with

$$\Phi_1(\xi) = \frac{1}{\sqrt{2}\sigma}\left\{\frac{(3-4v)erf(\xi)}{\xi} - \frac{\exp(-\xi^2)}{\xi^2\sqrt{\Pi}} + \frac{erf(\xi)}{2\xi^3}\right\},$$

and

$$\Phi_2(\xi) = \frac{1}{\sqrt{2}\sigma}\left\{\frac{erf(\xi)}{\xi} - \frac{3\exp(-\xi^2)}{\xi^2\sqrt{\Pi}} + \frac{3erf(\xi)}{2\xi^3}\right\},$$

where $\xi = r/\sqrt{2}\sigma$, $\vec{e}_r = (\vec{p} - \vec{q})/r$ is a unit vector pointing in the direction of r, and v and Y are the Poisson's ratio and Young's modulus controlling the compressibility and stiffness of the material.[18] Similar to the Wendland functions, the affine transformation is calculated prior to the registration with EBS, and the parameter σ can be used to define the locality of the transformation in order to cope with both small deformations of fine-detail and large (relatively to the image size) deformations. As opposed to TPS and Wendland functions, the model based on the Gaussian EBS results in local transformations that are not radially symmetric.

2.2.1.6. Irregular grids

Parametric registration using irregular grids can be considered as a generalization of landmark-based registration. The placement of landmarks is optimized jointly with the transformation parameters based on minimization of an objective function, which can potentially include the similarity measure between the images. This can be considered as a task of finding an optimal irregular grid of control points defining the transformation.

In Fornefett *et al.* the optimal landmark distribution was obtained through minimization of an energy function defined as a sum of the distance between the landmark positions in the reference and the transformed floating image and the TPS bending energy.[22] In this approach, however, the similarity measure was not included into the optimization procedure. In contrast, a registration method was proposed in Davis *et al.* where the optimal landmark distribution is selected, which maximizes the correlation coefficient between the images. A similar strategy has been pursued in Pekar *et al.* where optimal positions for Gaussian-shaped forces are determined by minimization of the squared difference between the images.[23,24]

An advantage of irregular grids is the potentially smaller number of parameters required compared to the regularly sampled grids. On the other hand, these methods may be computationally expensive, since the evaluation of the objective function to be minimized requires reformatting of the whole image, and global optimization requiring many evaluations may be needed to avoid local minima.

2.2.2. *Non-parametric transformations*

Non-parametric transformations rely on physical properties and functions to guide the registration process. Solving the transformation may be less efficient, but offer increased flexibility.

2.2.2.1. Linear elastic

Hooke's law of elasticity describes the strain, the deformation a body undergoes, when subjected to a stress, the force per unit area. Under Hooke's law this is a linear relationship described by

$$F = -kx,$$

where x is the change in length of the object, F is the restoring force exerted by the body, and k is the spring or force constant. Hooke's law can be rewritten, in terms of stress and strain, as

$$\sigma = E\varepsilon,$$

or as

$$\Delta L = \frac{1}{E} \times F \times \frac{L}{A} = \frac{1}{E} \times L \times \sigma.$$

2.2.2.2. Viscoelastic

In some materials, the relationship between stress and strain is not linear. A viscoelastic material exhibits hysteresis in the stress–strain curve and stress relaxation and creep occurs. As the linear elastic model is represented as a spring, a viscoelastic material is presented using springs and dashpots, connected in a series, a Maxwell material, or in parallel and series, a Kelvin material. In a viscoelastic model the stress and strain are a function of time.

2.2.2.3. Hyperelastic

The hyperelastic model, the most general type of nonlinear elastic behavior, assumes a strain energy density potential, U, which defines the stresses. The strain equation becomes:

$$\sigma = \frac{\partial U}{\partial \varepsilon},$$

where σ and ε are the work conjugate strain and stress measures.

2.2.2.4. Navier-Stokes equation

The standard partial differential equation (PDE) describing the deformation of a linear elastic object under equilibrium conditions is given by

$$\mu \nabla^2 \vec{u} + (\mu + \lambda)\nabla(\nabla^T \vec{u}) + \vec{F}(\vec{x}, \vec{u}) = 0,$$

where u is the displacement vector, F is the force on the object at x that depends on the deformation u, and μ and λ are Lames coefficients, determined from Young's Modulus (E) and Poisson's ratio (ν), through the equations

$$E = \frac{\mu(3\lambda + 2\mu)}{\lambda + \mu},$$

and

$$\nu = \frac{\lambda}{2(\lambda + \mu)}.$$

2.2.2.5. Viscous fluid

For an incompressible fluid, the conservation of energy, momentum, and mass lead to the Navier-Stokes equations to describe the motion of a fluid substance. In the viscous fluid model, μ is set to 1 and λ to 0, resulting in the simplified equation

$$\nabla^2 \vec{u} + \nabla(\nabla^T \vec{u}) + \vec{F}(\vec{x}, \vec{u}) = 0.$$

The force field $\vec{F}(\vec{x}, \vec{u})$ can be modified to maximize the intensity similarity between two images, i.e., using mutual information described above. Given two images $\mathcal{G}(\vec{x})$

and $\mathcal{F}(\vec{x} - \vec{u})$ F can be written as

$$\vec{F}(\vec{x}, \vec{u}) = \nabla_{\vec{u}} I = \frac{1}{V} \left[\frac{\partial \psi_h}{\partial i_l} L_{\vec{u}} \right] (\mathcal{F}(\vec{x} - \vec{u}), \mathcal{G}(\vec{x})) \nabla \mathcal{F}(\vec{x} - \vec{u}),$$

where $L_{\vec{u}}$ is a function of the mutual information in the images.

2.2.2.6. Diffusion or Demon's algorithm

The Demon's algorithm defines the deformation field as

$$\vec{u} = \frac{(m - s)\vec{\nabla} s}{|\vec{\nabla} s|^2 + (m - s)^2} = \frac{\vec{F}\vec{\nabla} s}{|\vec{\nabla} s|^2 + \vec{F}^2},$$

where $(m - s)$ is the external fore, or the differential force between the static and moving images

$$\vec{u}(|\vec{\nabla} s|^2 + \vec{F}^2) - \vec{F}\vec{\nabla} s = 0,$$

and

$$|\vec{\nabla} s|^2 \vec{u} + \vec{F}^2 \vec{u} - \vec{F}\vec{\nabla} s = 0,$$

where u is the displacement, s is the gradient of the static image.

2.2.2.7. Solving

There are two primary methods to solving the PDEs described above, the finite element method and the finite difference method. The finite element method approximates the solution using a mesh to describe the volume and solving the PDEs at the nodes in the mesh. The finite difference method approximates the differential equation, solving them using finite quantities instead of infinitesimal ones.

2.2.2.8. Finite element

The finite element method solves the above partial differential equations using finite elements, which approximates the solution of the equations using a mesh, which is a set of discrete sub-domains from a continuous domain. PDEs can be solved by eliminating the differential equation, using a stead state approach, or by converting the PDE into an equivalent ordinary differential equation. The finite element method numerically stable and allows the precision of the model to vary over the model domain, thereby increasing accuracy in areas where it is needed without increasing computational time for accuracy in areas where it is not needed. Finite element analysis is a computer simulation technique for the finite element method. The accuracy of the approximation can be improved by refining the mesh used to describe the problem, at the expense of increased computational times.

2.2.2.9. Finite difference

In the finite difference method, the PDEs are converted into a set of finite difference equations. These equations can be solved given the appropriate boundary conditions and imposing a regular grid over the domain. The approach can be implemented using the implicit method or explicit method. The implicit method solves a system of simultaneous linear equations using the backward difference. The method is always numerically stable and will converge, however, at the expense of being numerically intensive. The explicit method, proceeding backwards in small intervals using the appropriate boundary conditions, is numerically stable and convergent under specified certain step and grid sizes.

The errors of both the explicit and implicit methods are linear over the step and quadratic of the grid size. Several other formulas and methods exist, including the Crank-Nicolson method, which is numerically stable and convergent, numerically intensive, and accurate for small step sizes, the Du Fort-Frankel method, and the Laasonen method.

There are benefits to both the finite element and finite difference methods. The finite element method is better able to handle complex geometries, i.e., complex surfaces of structures, because the mesh is flexible. Finite difference relies on a rectangular grid, resulting in a less accurate approximation of surfaces that have a curved shape. Finite difference tends to be easier to implement than finite element. Although not always the case, the finite element approach tends to be more accurate than the finite difference method, largely due to the improved quality of the approximations between the grid points.

3. Applications

This section reviews RT applications where geometric changes are most prominent. The applications are organized according to location in the body — cancer of the head and neck, the lung, the liver, and the prostate. Each subsection provides a basic account of important issues specific to EBRT published evidence of geometric change, and potential and published applications of mono- and multi-modal image registration.

3.1. *Head and Neck*

The importance of deformable registration in radiotherapy treatment planning, delivery, and response assessment for the head and neck has been recently identified. Investigational studies show that the tumor and surrounding normal tissue change in shape and volume over the course of a standard fractionated treatment. In addition, the integration of MR and PET into the CT-based treatment planning process requires careful registration, including deformable registration when changes in neck flexion are present between scans, due to differences in patient position.

Treatment of the carcinoma in the head and neck requires highly conformal fields, in order to spare the many surrounding critical structures, such as the spinal cord and parotid glands, and image guidance to accurately deliver the treatment to the tumor.

Conformal treatment plans, i.e., plans that deliver a high dose to the tumor and have a rapid dose falloff outside of the tumor boundary, require 3D treatment planning. Although CT is the primary image dataset for radiotherapy, providing electron density information and a geometrically robust image, multi-modality imaging can improve the identification, and therefore delineation, of the tumor. When including multi-modality imaging, such as MRI and PET, registration and fusion must be performed to allow a correspondence between the secondary image and the primary image, used for dose calculation. Changes in patient position, due to neck flexion, and differences in internal anatomy, require deformable registration for integration of multi-modality imaging for treatment planning.

Characterization and validation of registration algorithms has been identified as an important area of research, whether using a rigid or deformable registration algorithm.[25,26] Phantom studies provide a robust method of quantifying the registration accuracy of rigid registration, however, are a simplification of the images obtained under clinical conditions, which include artifacts and deformations. Qualitative validation of deformable registration has been performed by applying the deformation map to the contours generated on the reference image to map them to the secondary image. These auto-contours are then compared to manual contours on the secondary image. Contour variation is also a factor in this method of evaluation and it does not ensure the accuracy of the deformation of the internal structure of the contoured structure.

The benefit of multi-modality imaging to improve variability of target definition by different observers (inter-observer variability) has also been investigated. Results have been mixed, with some indicating improved consistency, while others show no improvement, depending on anatomical site and type of multi-modality imaging. It is important, however, to ensure that the images are properly registered before comparing volumes, which may often require deformable registration.

Changes in tumor and normal tissue shape and volume have been observed over the multi-fraction course of treatment for cancers in the head and neck.[27] The gross tumor volume had a median relative loss of 69.5% over the course of treatment and a median center of mass displacement of 3.3 mm. The parotid glands, a radiosensitive normal tissue, saw a median decrease in volume of 0.19 cc/day and a median medial shift of 3.1 mm. These anatomical changes can result in a deviation of the delivered dose from the planned dose, resulting in a potential increase in dose to normal tissue and a decrease in dose to the tumor. These deviations may result in an unacceptable plan, either exceeding the normal tissue dose limitations or delivering a dose that it lower than the dose expected to lead to local tumor control for the tumor. Adapting the treatment plan during the course of treatment to account for these changes has been the subject of recent research, which relies on accurate deformable registration. Deformable registration allows the anatomical structures, as defined on the mid-treatment images, to be mapped back to the planning image. This allows an accurate accumulation of delivered dose to be generated. Once the accurate accumulated dose is generated, a new optimized plan can be created to maintain the initial planning goals for the tumor and the normal tissue.

The advancement of volumetric imagining in the treatment room, using in-room CT, kV cone-beam CT (kVCBCT), MV cone-beam CT (MVCBCT) and MV CT imaging (MVCT), has provided the imaging data needed to perform ART. Lu *et al.* investigated the application of deformable registration using a fast intensity-based free-form deformable registration technique to correlate MVCT images acquired at the time of treatment with a kVCT image obtained for treatment planning for five head and neck patients.[28] Prior to deformable registration, the MVCT images were smoothed using an edge-preserving smoothing function. The free-form deformable registration produced a deformation map between the reference and test (MVCT) images. This same deformation map was used to accumulate the dose by calculating the dose on the MVCT and then using the deformation map to relate this dose back to the kVCT, which is used as the reference frame. This dose accumulation was performed for each fraction, as an MVCT was obtained at each fraction to provide the deformation map. The accuracy was assessed by using the deformation map to automatically recontour the MVCT using the contours generated on the kVCBCT. The correlation between the automatic contours and the physician generated contours, on the MVCT, provided a metric for qualitative evaluation of the deformable registration accuracy. The dose accumulation indicated that without replanning to account for anatomical changes, the dose to both parotid glands increased due to weight loss.

Wang *et al.* also investigated the role of deformable registration to facilitate adaptive planning for the head and neck using an accelerated "demons" algorithm and an in-room CT scanner.[29] The accelerated demons algorithm includes an active force based on the gradient information of the moving image. Qualitative evaluation of the registration was performed by using the deformation map to automatically segment the anatomical structures in the in-room CT images, similar to the study previously described. The ability to automatically contour subsequent images of th e same patient is a substantial time savings in the radiotherapy environment and makes adaptive planning clinically feasible. CT to MR.

Sharpe *et al.* investigated the benefit of ART for head and neck cancer using linear elastic body deformable registration, based on surface mesh propagation and weekly MR images registered to a planning kVCT image.[30] The study investigated the benefits of an offline adaptive planning technique, which generated a new treatment plan each week over the course of radiotherapy, in the limit of reducing PTV margins. The study showed that setup uncertainties and anatomic changes produced significant dose variation over the course of treatment when the original treatment plan was delivered over the entire course of radiotherapy. Although the tumor dose was maintained with an adequate PTV margin, the dose to the normal tissues increased, including a dose increase to the parotid glands of up to 30% more than the initial treatment plan and spinal cord dose of up to 10% higher. Performing weekly adaptive planning, tumor coverage could be achieved with no PTV margin, which permitted reduced cord and mean parotid gland dose of 5% and 12%, respectively.

3.2. *Thorax and upper abdomen*

The need for deformable registration in the thorax and upper abdomen is widely accepted and the subject of much research. Breathing motion, stomach filling, and patient positioning demand careful registration between repeat images of the same modality and the integration of multi-modality imaging. Respiration correlated imaging has also improved the ability to quantify and understand the respiration process and deformable registration between these images can improve the quantification and accuracy of these assessments.

Conformal radiotherapy, tightly shaping the high dose region around the target, has improved the application of radiation therapy in the treatment of tumors in the thorax and upper abdomen, by allowing sparing of normal tissue, which in turn can facilitate increased dose to the tumor. Precise definition of the tumor and the critical normal tissues is critical to this process and can be improved through the integration of multi-modality imaging, e.g., MRI, which provides improved soft tissue contrast, and PET, which provides functional information. Precise reproducibility of the patient between imaging sessions is extremely challenging due to changes in the breath hold position, which is necessary for an artifact free image, stomach filling, and patient alignment. Deformable registration is often required to reduce the geometric discrepancies between the images to allow accurate correlation of the unique imaging information available from each modality.

Mattes *et al.* have integrated PET with CT images of the thorax using free-form deformations and mutual information.[31] The accuracy of the algorithm was studied on image sets from 27 patients imaged for lung cancer staging (Fig. 3). Two expert observers visually assessed the accuracy using a split window. The errors ranged 0–6 mm.

Slomka *et al.* investigated an automated 3D registration of stand alone FDG whole body PET with CT, which compensates the non-linear deformation due to the breath hold at which the CT image is obtained, whereas the PET image is obtained while the patient is free breathing.[32] The algorithm uses a mutual information based cost function of the PET emission and transmission scans to provide registration to the CT scan. The first step was a linear registration, allowing for translation, rotation, and an isotropic scaling. A nonlinear step followed, to account for any remaining differences. The nonlinear registration significantly

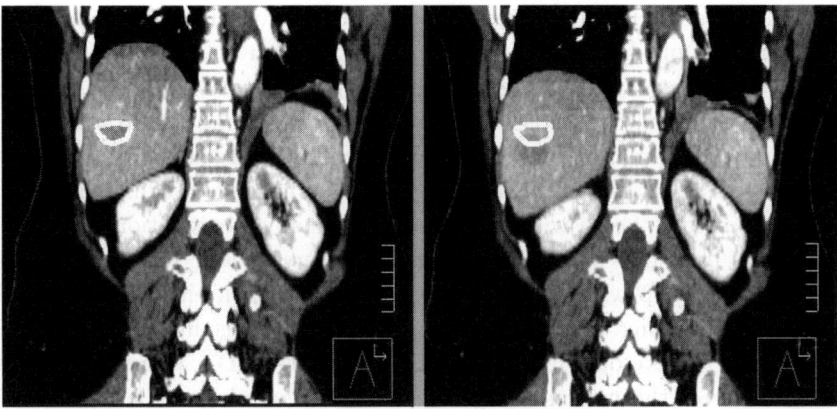

Fig. 3. Illustration of the motion observed in a patient with liver cancer in the exhale (left) and inhale (right) breathing phase. The overlaid contour delineates the primary liver tumor at exhale. Images courtesy Radiation Medicine Program, Princess Margaret Hospital.

improved the registration in 10 of the 18 patients. Lung volumes measured on the transmission PET image after deformable registration closely matched the lung volume defined on the CT image.

Brock *et al.* have investigated the use of a finite element model-based deformable registration algorithm that is driven by the alignment of the surface contours of selected organs to integrate MR imaging with CT for radiotherapy of the liver.[33] The MR and CT images were obtained at exhale breath hold and a radiation oncologist contoured the liver and tumor on each image. Quantitative accuracy was calculated using vessel bifurcations identified on the CT and MR images. The mean residual error following deformable registration was 0.42 cm, vector magnitude, which is approximately half of the MR voxel size, 0.73–0.82 cm. The tumor concordance increased with deformable registration for all cases, the average increase was 28%, although discrepancies still remained between the contours indicating an inconsistency in the definition of tumor on across the modalities.

In addition to precise definition of the tumor, the expected motion of the tumor and surrounding normal tissue due to breathing is important in the definition of the PTV margin. Deformable registration between inhale and exhale breath hold images, or inhale and exhale images obtained from a respiration correlated, or "4D" CT can provide this information. 4D CT images are obtained by repeated imaging the same region of anatomy over a breathing cycle prior to advancing the table, while obtaining information on the breathing phase at each time of treatment[34−38] The images are then retrospectively sorted into breathing phases, typically eight, including end inhale and end exhale, as well as intermediate breathing states.

The use of deformable registration to provide a detailed deformation map of the breathing motion from 4D CT scans of the thorax has been the subject of recent investigation. Keall *et al.* used a viscous-fluid flow and mean square error based deformable registration algorithm to generate a deformation map between all eight phases of a 4D CT image of the thorax.[39] Bifurcations identified on each phases indicated an accuracy of less than 4 mm, which was within one CT slice thickness. Reitzel et al. used a B-spline free-form deformation model and the sum of the squared differences between 4D CT images of the lung and liver.[40]

Both methods can also be used to map the contours of one phase of the 4D CT scan to all subsequent phases, which can save valuable time in clinical integration. Zhang et al. used a fast variational-based deformable registration algorithm to map contours from one phase of the 4D CT image to each subsequent phase.[41] The deformation map was also used to generate a motion envelope for the PTV for treatment planning. Pevsner et al. applied a viscous fluid model of tissue deformation to achieve deformable registration between 4D CT images.[23] Contour differences between the automatically mapped contours, using the deformation field, and the manually drawn contours for the GTV had a mean of 2.6 mm, the inter-observer variations in contouring the GTV had a mean of 2.1 mm. The mean discrepancy between predicted and actual bifurcations in the lung was 2.9 mm, inter-observer discrepancies were 2.8 mm.

Inhale and exhale breath hold images have also been used to define a deformation map for the thorax and upper abdomen. Brock et al. used a TPS and MI algorithm to register the inhale breath hold image of the liver to the exhale breath hold image.[42] The accuracy, 1.0–1.4 mm in each direction, was determined via identified bifurcations in the liver. Coselmon et al. also used a TPS and MI registration algorithm for application in the lung.[43] The accuracy, determined from identified bifurcations in the lung, ranged from 1.7 mm in the left-right direction, to greater than 3 mm in the anterior-posterior and superior-inferior directions. Lu et al. implemented a energy minimization function for breath hold images of the lung to generate a deformation map due to breathing motion.[44] The algorithm substantially improved the cross correlation of the images. Brock et al. implemented a finite element model-based deformable registration algorithm for breath hold image registration for both the lung and liver[16] The accuracy ranged from 1.4–2.0 mm in each direction for the liver to 2.2 mm in each direction for the lung. Zhang et al. applied a finite element model based registration algorithm using contact elements to breath hold images of the lung.[14] Qualitative registration showed good agreement between the predicted (i.e., the deformed inhale image into the exhale position) and actual exhale images. Rohlfing et al. applied a cubic B-spline and MI based algorithm to MR images of the liver at various breathing states.[45] Quantitative accuracy was determined by comparing the distance to agreement of the mapped liver surface to the contoured liver surface, mean difference range of 2.5–4.6 mm, and the position of the inferior vena cava and hepatic artery, range of 1.7–4.3 mm.

Once the deformation map is determined, methods of integration into the radiotherapy process can be investigated. There are three primary options: (1) account for the motion in the PTV margin and in the accumulated dose by performing deformable dose accumulation, (2) suspending the patients breathing during the delivery of each beam or only turning the beam on during the correct phase of breathing and (3) tracking the breathing motion of the patient with the beam. Option 2, which suspends the patients' breathing, known as active breath hold.[46,47], or suspends the treatment beam, known as gating.[48-51], does not require a deformation map, and therefore will not be discussed further here.

The application of the deformation field to calculated the true dose delivered in the presence of motion has been investigated for the liver and the lung. Brock *et al.* demonstrated that using an individualized prescription dose for each liver patient based on the irradiation of the normal liver, the change in prescribed dose when including deformation compared to the standard method of calculated dose on the static image only ranged from −4.1 to 1.7 Gy.[52] This exceeded the treatment fraction size of 1.5 Gy. Rosu *et al.* investigated the effect of deformation in dose accumulation in the lung, during free breathing treatment. Dose calculations were performed using dose planning method (DPM) Monte Carlo code on six patients using the inhale and exhale breath hold images. The mean lung dose was found to not change significantly when including deformation, as the hot and cold regions are averaged out in the large volume of lung.[53] The inclusion of deformation, however, was found to have a larger impact for neighboring organs, such as the esophagus. Rietzel *et al.* showed the necessity of patient specific PTV margins over standardized PTV margins by comparing the overlap and under-coverage of standard margins.[54] An under-overage of up to 19% was calculated, depending on standard margin used. This indicates the possibility of tumor under dosing. Flampouri *et al.* investigated the true delivered dose using a B-spline and mean square difference-based deformable registration and 4D CT on six lung cancer patients.[55] Investigations into the minimum number of breathing phases required recreating the dose computed using all 10 phases of the 4D CT indicated that using three phases had a 3% or greater error in up to 2.5% of the CTV volume, which decreases to 0.5% of the volume when five phases are used.

Tumor tracking, or 4D RT, involves calculating the deformation field and then applying this information to the treatment delivery process. As the tumor is moving and deforming, the multi-leaf collimator, which shapes the beam to the position and shape of the tumor, is continuously moving to account for this motion and deformation. This method relies on an updated position of the tumor, either through an external surrogate or imaging information. Research has investigated the potential benefits of this technique. Keall *et al.* have investigated the feasibility of this approach.[39] Initial testing has shown reductions in the dose delivered to normal tissues, including the cord, heart, and normal lung.

In addition, novel applications of deformable registration are being investigated. Thorndyke *et al.* have applied deformable registration to reduce the artifacts in PET images using a method coined retrospective stacking.[56] Respiration sorted images are combined using a B-spline approach to increase the contrast to noise (CNR) in the final image. Phantom results showed a three-fold CNR improvement over gated images and a five-fold increase over un-gated data. Schreibmann *et al.* and Sarrut *et al.* have applied deformable registration algorithms to generate the intermediate phases of 4D CT data from inhale and exhale CT data.[57,58] This has the potential to reduce the radiation dose required to collect breathing motion data and reduce artifacts in the intermediate phases of traditional 4D CT. Xu *et al.* investigated the potential for deformable registration to eliminate the need for an external surrogate in 4D CT acquisition by deforming each 2D image slice to a reference CT image.[59] The method also reduces imaging dose and has the potential to increase image quality through reduction in artifacts.

3.3. *Pelvis*

The scenarios of relevance for deformable registration in prostate cancer RT include motion management, dose accumulation, and image fusion of CT, MRI and MRI using endo-rectal coils (ERC) for improved target definition.

The treatment of prostate cancer with EBRT includes the definition of a target volume of the prostate and periprostatic tissues. The dose to the anterior rectal wall and urinary bladder are limited to reduce complications.

The main goal of motion management is to improve treatment by improving target coverage, reducing treatment toxicity, enabling potential dose escalation. There are several strategies and aspects of motion management in EBRT, including patient positioning and immobilization, PTV treatment margin design, quantification and minimization of target organ motion, visualization of target organ position during treatment.

More recently, deformable registration is investigated for the simulation and quantification of dose in deforming geometry, and the design of treatment schemes that adapt to the deforming geometry during the course of therapy. In order to estimate the dose that each volume element actually received over the course of therapy, it is necessary to track the trajectory of each volume element from one image to the next. This is again a classical correspondence problem approached by image registration techniques.

3.3.1. *Measurement of organ motion*

Prostate motion has been differentiated into inter-fraction (day-to-day), intra-fraction (observed during daily treatment), and respiratory (as a special case of intra-fraction) motion. The range of reported prostate motion varies highly among studies, depending on population size, method of measurement (prostate surface, prostate center-of-gravity, implanted fiducial markers; CT, US, MRI), and time between measurements. The type of patient positioning (prone vs. supine) and immobilization (full vs. empty bladder and rectum) also has a substantial impact on motion.

Prostate motion has been characterized using various surrogates and definitions: Estimating mean or center-of-gravity (COG) displacement of seed markers physically implanted in the prostate, imaged using MV projection, kV CBCT volumetric images, CT or MRI; COG displacement of the contoured prostate gland in MRI or CT; and contour least-square alignment of contoured prostates. Markers are more reproducible, but may degrade image quality, are invasive and do not provide information about normal tissue volume, while purely image-based techniques do not require seed placement but are affected by the reproducibility of the (manual) contouring process.

The optimal method and the clinical significance of the difference between the various measurement techniques are still being debated. Current practice is to reposition the couch based on manual rigid alignment of planning CT and on-line measurement, using fiducials or bony anatomy imaged with MV projections, kV CBCT or US imaging.

A vast amount of studies on prostate motion (i.e., translation and rotation) have been reported.[60,61] The main origins of organ motion are pressure from bowel, gas, feces, and urine in the urinary bladder.

Generally, the largest shifts were found from day-to-day, and found to be greatest at the gland base. Largest inter-fraction motion was observed in the AP and SI directions (3-7 mm mean, 1.5–4.1 mm SD for AP, 1.7–4.5 mm for SI), and least in lateral direction (0.7–1.9 mm). Maximum displacements of prostate centre-of-mass have been reported between 7 and 12 mm (data reviewed in Byrne et al.).[61] Ghilezan et al. reported rectal filling to be the most significant predictor of prostate displacement; a prostate displacement of <3 mm (90%) can be expected for the 20 min after the moment of initial imaging for patients with an empty rectum.[62]

Measurements of intra-fraction motion vary substantially across studies, ranging from 5–10 mm for 80% of prostate movement measurements using cine MRI,.[63] to 0.01 ± 0.4 mm (LR), 0.2 ± 1.3 mm (AP), and 0.1 ± 1.0 mm using prostate surface alignment in US.[64]

Respiratory induced prostate motion in prone position was reported with 0.9–5.1 mm (cranial-caudal) and maximum of 3.5 mm (AP) in the prone position,[65] and 1 mm maximum in all directions in supine positioning.[66]

Recently, Jaffray et al. evaluated the geometric surface discrepancy remaining after marker-based alignment due to prostate deformation.[67] They concluded that markers must be recognized as surrogates of prostate motion, and 48% of the patients had more than 10% of the surface with a discrepancy >3 mm after marker-based alignment.

3.3.2. *Application of deformable registration*

The main applications of deformable image registration in prostate EBRT include quantification of prostate and OAR motion, dose accumulation in deforming geometry, and multi-modality image fusion. The approaches are discussed along with their accuracy performance.

3.3.2.1. Quantification of organ motion and dose tracking

Yan *et al.* investigated the use of a biomechanical model of an elastic body to quantify patient organ motion.[15] They applied a finite element method with boundary conditions obtained from multiple daily CT measurements to track volume elements and accumulate dose. The same group reported deformations as much as 3–5 cm for the bladder.[68]

Wang *et al.* applied a fast grey-value based "demons" algorithm to CT of a physically deformable pelvic phantom, and to CT acquired on several days.[69] They reported 0.5 ± 1.5 mm (mean $\pm$ SD) based on phantom experiments.

Schaly *et al.* report a clinical prostate case exhibiting significant localized dose differences due to systematic inter-fraction motion of 23%, 32% and 18% in rectum, bladder and seminal vesicles.[70] They use a TPS method where the corresponding points are selected by a combination of closest-point search between corresponding manually drawn contours and a heuristic set of rules.

Lu *et al.* present a free-form variational method that minimizes SSD between two images.[44] They use calculus of variations to represent the optimization problem as a set of nonlinear elliptic partial differential equations, which results in an efficiently solvable linear system of equations.

Foskey *et al.* use an SSD-based large-deformation diffeomorphism PDE approach to register daily CT imagery of prostate RT patients.[71] They address the problem of missing grey-value correspondence due to daily variations in bowel filling by automatically identifying and "painting" gas regions to coincide with the grey value levels of the remaining rectal filling. In addition to dose tracking, they propose the application of automatic segmentation of secondary images by means of deformable registration and contour propagation from the primary CT.

3.3.2.2. Image fusion

A prominent application of multi-modality integration is the fusion of MRI to CT. MRI provides improved soft tissue contrast, enabling improved appreciation of the true extent of the tumor. The goal is to transfer geometrical information from the MRI to the CT, which requires compensation of motion occurring between imaging sessions, and compensation of reduced geometrical accuracy observed in MRI.

Recently, there have been a number of approaches publish to align high-resolution MRI (and in some cases MRI/MRSI) using endo-rectal coils (ERC) with US or CT imagery.[72] ERCs introduce anatomical shifts, tilts and deformations, which need to be compensated when fusing with CT. Kim *et al.* measured prostate translation, rotation and deformation using rigid and expandable ERCs. The degree of geometric change could be reduced using rigid coil to some extent. However, remaining distortions were measured in both the rigid and the expandable coil (AP 4.1 ± 3.0 mm vs. 1.2 ± 2.2 mm; LR 3.8 ± 3.7 mm vs. 1.5 ± 3.1 mm).

4. Conclusions and Outlook

Several applications of deformable registration exist in the radiotherapy environment. It has been shown that deformable registration has the potential to improve current treatment strategies, and with the integration of additional imaging beyond planning CT, enables the exploration of current existing treatment shortcomings and the extension of the application range of RT.

Currently, the application of deformable registration exists mainly in retrospective research studies. The introduction of deformable registration for target delineation, treatment planning, and treatment delivery will require a paradigm shift for radiation oncologists, which in turn requires careful clinical implementation in addition to ensuring quality assurance.

A large variety of registration techniques have been developed and applied to clinical applications specific to radiation therapy. The extent of quantitative validation varies substantially between studies, which makes it currently difficult to judge as to which approach performs optimally. Registration accuracy of the liver and prostate tends to be on the order of 1.5 mm, where accuracy of the lung tends to be larger, likely due to the increased complexity in motion and deformation. Initiatives towards benchmarking of approaches based on the same image data sets using the same metrics are under way.

Another important aspect of clinical implementation is computation time. While some approaches already compute results within a minute, several deformable registration techniques require efficiency improvements without substantially compromising accuracy.

Advances in imaging for radiotherapy, prior to, during, and following the completion of treatment will create a further demand for deformable registration as information on anatomical changes are revealed, e.g., in treatment of the cervix and sarcoma. This will require that deformable registration algorithms are expandable and able to adapt to changes in the information presented and the requirements for accuracy.

Acknowledgments

MRK wishes to thank the Scientists of Philips Research, Germany, as a ceaseless source of expertise. KKB wishes to thank the team of physicists, physicians, and therapists at Princess Margaret Hospital for their discussions on the role of deformable registration in radiotherapy.

References

1. G. T. Chen, J. H. Kung and K. P. Beaudette. Artifacts in computed tomography scanning of moving objects, *Semin. Radiat. Oncol.* **14**(1) (2004) 19–26.
2. G. S. Mageras. Introduction: management of target localization uncertainties in external-beam therapy, *Semin. Radiat. Oncol.* **15**(3) (2005) 133–135.
3. R Bajcsy and S Kovacic, Multiresolution elastic matching, *Comput. Vis. Graph.* **46** (1989) 1–21.
4. J. V. Hajnal, D. L. G. Hill and D. J. Hawkes. *Medical Image Registration* (CRC Press, 2001).
5. T. Netsch, P. Roesch, A. van Muiswinkel and J. Weese. Towards real-time multimodality 3d medical image registration, in *Proc. 8th Int. Conf. Comput. Vision* (Vancouver, Canada, 2001, 2006).
6. J. Weese, P. Roesch, T. Netsch, T. Blaffert and M. Quist. Gray-value based registration of CT and MR images by maximation of local correlation. In: C. Taylor, A. Colchester (Eds): MICCAI'99, Lecture Notes in Computer Science **1679** (1999) 656–663.
7. J. P. Pluim, J. B. Maintz and M. A. Viergever. Mutual-information-based registration of medical images: a survey, *IEEE Trans. Med. Imaging* **22**(8) (2003) 986–1004.
8. F. Maes, D. Vandermeulen and P. Suetens. Comparative evaluation of multiresolution optimization strategies for multimodality image registration by maximization of mutual information, *Med. Image Anal.* **3**(4) (1999) 373–386.
9. P. Thevenaz and M. Unser. Optimization of mutual information for multiresolution image registration, *IEEE Trans. Image Process.* **9**(12) (2000) 2083–2099.
10. D. Rueckert, L. I. Sonoda, C. Hayes, D. L. Hill, M. O. Leach and D. J. Hawkes. Nonrigid registration using free-form deformations: application to breast MR images, *IEEE Trans. Med. Imaging* **18**(8) (1999) 712–721.
11. T. Rohlfing, D. B. Russakoff, M. J. Murphy and C. R. Maurer Jr. An intensity-based registration algorithm for probabilistic images and its application for 2-D and 3-D image registration, *Proc. SPIE Med. Imaging* **4684** (2002) 581–591.
12. K. K. Brock, S. J. Hollister, L. A. Dawson and J. M. Balter. Technical note: creating a four-dimensional model of the liver using finite element analysis, *Med. Phys.* **29**(7) (2002) 1403–1405.
13. M. Kaus, K. Brock, V. Pekar, L. Dawson, A. Nichol and D. Jaffray. Assessment of a model-based deformable image registration approach for radiation therapy planning, *IJROBP* **68**(2) (2007) 572–580.
14. T. Zhang, N. P. Orton, T. R. Mackie and B. R. Paliwal. Technical note: A novel boundary condition using contact elements for finite element based deformable image registration, *Med. Phys.* **31**(9) (2004) 2412–2415.
15. D. Yan, D. A. Jaffray and J. W. Wong. A model to accumulate fractionated dose in a deforming organ, *Int. J. Radiat. Oncol. Biol. Phys.* **44**(3) (1999) 665–675.
16. K. K. Brock, M. B. Sharpe, L. A. Dawson, S. M. Kim and D. A. Jaffray. Accuracy of finite element model (FEM)-based multi-organ deformable image registration, *Med. Phys.* **32**(6) (2005) 1647–1659.
17. M. Fornefett, K. Rohr and H. S. Stiehl. Radial basis functions with compact support for elastic registration of medical images, *Image Vision Comput.* **19** (2001) 87–96.
18. J. Kohlrausch, K. Rohr and S. Stiehl. A new class of elastic body splines for nonrigid registration of medical images, *J. Math. imaging vision* **23**(3) (2005) 253–280.
19. J. A. Schnabel, C. Tanner, A. D. Castellano-Smith, A. Degenhard, M. O. Leach, D. R. Hose, D. L. Hill and D. J. Hawkes. Validation of nonrigid image registration using finite-element methods: application to breast MR images, *IEEE Trans. Med. Imaging* **22**(2) (2003) 238–247.

20. S. Frantz, K. Rohr and H. S. Stiehl. Localization of 3D anatomical point landmarks in 3D tomographic images using deformable models, *Proc. MICCAI* (2000) 492–501.
21. F. L. Bookstein. Principal warps: thin-plate splines and the decomposition of deformations, *IEEE Trans. Pattern Analy. Machine Intelli.* **11**(6) (1989) 567–585.
22. M. Fornefett, K. Stiehl and H. S. Stiehl. Elastic medical image registration using surface landmarks with automatic finding of correspondences, *Proc. Bildverarbeitung in der Medizin* (2000) 8–52.
23. A. Pevsner, B. Davis, S. Joshi, A. Hertanto, J. Mechalakos, E. Yorke, K. Rosenzweig, S. Nehmeh, Y. E. Erdi, J. L. Humm, S. Larson, C. C. Ling and G. S. Mageras. Evaluation of an automated deformable image matching method for quantifying lung motion in respiration-correlated CT images, *Med. Phys.* **33**(2) (2006) 369–376.
24. V. Pekar, E. Gladilin and K. Rohr. An adaptive irregular grid approach for 3D deformable image registration, *Phys. Med. Biol.* **51**(2) (2006) 361–377.
25. C. S. Moore, G. P. Liney and A. W. Beavis. Quality assurance of registration of CT and MRI data sets for treatment planning of radiotherapy for head and neck cancers, *J. Appl. Clin. Med. Phys.* **5**(1) (2004) 25–35.
26. J. F. Daisne, M. Sibomana, A. Bol, G. Cosnard, M. Lonneux and V. Gregoire. Evaluation of a multimodality image (CT, MRI and PET) coregistration procedure on phantom and head and neck cancer patients: accuracy, reproducibility and consistency, *Radiother. Oncol.* **69**(3) (2003) 237–245.
27. J. Barker, A. Garden, L. Dong, J. O'Daniel, H. Wang, L. Court, W. Morrison, D. Rosenthal, C. Chao, R. Mohan and K. Ang. Radiation-induced anatomic changes during fractionated head and neck radiotherapy: a pilot study using an integrated CT-LINAC system, *Int. J. Radiat. Oncol. Biol. Phys.* **57**(2 Suppl) (2003) S304.
28. W. Lu, G. H. Olivera, Q. Chen, K. J. Ruchala, J. Haimerl, S. L. Meeks, K. M. Langen and P. A. Kupelian. Deformable registration of the planning image (kVCT) and the daily images (MVCT) for adaptive radiation therapy, *Phys. Med. Biol.* **51**(17) (2006) 4357–4374.
29. H. Wang, L. Dong, J. O'Daniel, R. Mohan, A. S. Garden, K. K. Ang, D. A. Kuban, M. Bonnen, J. Y. Chang and R. Cheung. Validation of an accelerated 'demons' algorithm for deformable image registration in radiation therapy, *Phys. Med. Biol.* **50**(12) (2005) 2887–2905.
30. M. B. Sharpe, K. K. Brock, H. Rehbinder, C. Forsgren, A. Lundin, L. A. Dawson, G. Studer, B. O'Sullivan, T. R. McNutt, M. R. Kaus, J. Lof and D. A. Jaffray. Adaptive planning and delivery to account for anatomical changes induced by radiation therapy of head and neck cancer, *Int. J. Radiat. Oncol. Biol. Phys.* **63**(Suppl 1) (2006) S3.
31. D. Mattes, D. R. Haynor, H. Vesselle, T. K. Lewellen and W. Eubank. PET-CT image registration in the chest using free-form deformations, *IEEE Trans. Med. Imaging* **22**(1) (2003) 120–128.
32. P. J. Slomka, D. Dey, C. Przetak, U. E. Aladl and R. P. Baum. Automated 3-dimensional registration of stand-alone (18)F-FDG whole-body PET with CT, *J. Nucl. Med.* **44**(7) (2003) 1156–1167.
33. K. K. Brock, L. A. Dawson, M. B. Sharpe, D. J. Moseley and D. A. Jaffray. Feasibility of a novel deformable image registration technique to facilitate classification, targeting and monitoring of tumor and normal tissue, *Int. J. Radiat. Oncol. Biol. Phys.* **64**(4) (2006) 1245–1254.
34. M. Endo, T. Tsunoo, S. Kandatsu, S. Tanada, H. Aradate and Y. Saito. Four-dimensional computed tomography (4D CT) — concepts and preliminary development, *Radiat. Med.* **21**(1) (2003) 17–22.

35. T. Ichikawa and T. Kumazaki. 4D-CT: a new development in three-dimensional hepatic computed tomography, *J. Nippon Med. Sch* **67**(1) (2000) 24–27.
36. P. J. Keall, G. Starkschall, H. Shukla, K. M. Forster, V. Ortiz, C. W. Stevens, S. S. Vedam, R. George, T. Guerrero and R. Mohan. Acquiring 4D thoracic CT scans using a multislice helical method, *Phys. Med. Biol.* **49**(10) (2004) 2053–2067.
37. S. A. Nehmeh, Y. E. Erdi, T. Pan, A. Pevsner, K. E. Rosenzweig, E. Yorke, G. S. Mageras, H. Schoder, P. Vernon, O. Squire, H. Mostafavi, S. M. Larson and J. L. Humm. Four-dimensional (4D) PET/CT imaging of the thorax, *Med. Phys.* **31**(12) (2004) 3179–3186.
38. T. Pan, T. Y. Lee, E. Rietzel and G. T. Chen. 4D-CT imaging of a volume influenced by respiratory motion on multi-slice CT, *Med. Phys.* **31**(2) (2004) 333–340.
39. P. J. Keall, S. Joshi, S. S. Vedam, J. V. Siebers, V. R. Kini and R. Mohan. Four-dimensional radiotherapy planning for DMLC-based respiratory motion tracking, *Med. Phys.* **32**(4) (2005) 942–951.
40. E. Rietzel, G. T. Chen, N. C. Choi, C. G. Will *et al.* Four-dimensional image-based treatment planning: Target volume segmentation and dose calculation in the presence of respiratory motion, *Int. J. Radiat. Oncol. Biol. Phys.* **61**(5) (2005) 1535–1550.
41. T. Zhang, N. P. Orton and W. A. Tome. On the automated definition of mobile target volumes from 4D-CT images for stereotactic body radiotherapy, *Med. Phys.* **32**(11) (2005) 3493–3502.
42. K. M. Brock, J. M. Balter, L. A. Dawson, M. L. Kessler and C. R. Meyer. Automated generation of a four-dimensional model of the liver using warping and mutual information, *Med. Phys.* **30**(6) (2003) 1128–1133.
43. M. M. Coselmon, J. M. Balter, D. L. McShan and M. L. Kessler. Mutual information based CT registration of the lung at exhale and inhale breathing states using thin-plate splines, *Med. Phys.* **31**(11) (2004) 2942–2948.
44. W. Lu, M. L. Chen, G. H. Olivera, K. J. Ruchala and T. R. Mackie. Fast free-form deformable registration via calculus of variations, *Phys. Med. Biol.* **49**(14) (2004) 3067–3087.
45. T. Rohlfing, C. R. Maurer, Jr., W. G. O'Dell and J. Zhong. Modeling liver motion and deformation during the respiratory cycle using intensity-based nonrigid registration of gated MR images, *Med. Phys.* **31**(3) (2004) 427–432.
46. L. A. Dawson, K. K. Brock, S. Kazanjian, D. Fitch, C. J. McGinn, T. S. Lawrence, R. K. Ten Haken and J. Balter. The reproducibility of organ position using active breathing control (ABC) during liver radiotherapy, *Int. J. Radiat. Oncol. Biol. Phys.* **51**(5) (2001) 1410–1421.
47. J. W. Wong, M. B. Sharpe, D. A. Jaffray, V. R. Kini, J. M. Robertson, J. S. Stromberg and A. A. Martinez. The use of active breathing control (ABC) to reduce margin for breathing motion, *Int. J. Radiat. Oncol. Biol. Phys.* **44**(4) (1999) 911–919.
48. C. R. Ramsey, D. Scaperoth, D. Arwood and A. L. Oliver. Clinical efficacy of respiratory gated conformal radiation therapy, *Med. Dosim.* **24**(2) (1999) 115–119.
49. S. S. Vedam, P. J. Keall, V. R. Kini and R. Mohan. Determining parameters for respiration-gated radiotherapy, *Med. Phys.* **28**(10) (2001) 2139–2146.
50. G. D. Hugo, N. Agazaryan and T. D. Solberg. The effects of tumor motion on planning and delivery of respiratory-gated IMRT, *Med. Phys.* **30**(6) (2003) 1052–1066.
51. P. Keall, S. Vedam, R. George, C. Bartee, J. Siebers, F. Lerma, E. Weiss and T. Chung. The clinical implementation of respiratory-gated intensity-modulated radiotherapy, *Med. Dosim.* **31**(2) (2006) 152–162.
52. K. K. Brock, D. L. McShan, R. K. Ten Haken, S. J. Hollister, L. A. Dawson and J. M. Balter. Inclusion of organ deformation in dose calculations, *Med. Phys.* **30**(3) (2003) 290–295.

53. M. Rosu, I. J. Chetty, J. M. Balter, M. L. Kessler, D. L. McShan and R. K. Ten Haken. Dose reconstruction in deforming lung anatomy: dose grid size effects and clinical implications, *Med. Phys.* **32**(8) (2005) 2487–2495.

54. E. Rietzel, A. K. Liu, K. P. Doppke, J. A. Wolfgang, A. B. Chen, G. T. Chen and N. C. Choi. Design of 4D treatment planning target volumes, *Int. J. Radiat. Oncol. Biol. Phys.* **66**(1) (2006) 287–295.

55. S. Flampouri, S. B. Jiang, G. C. Sharp, J. Wolfgang, A. A. Patel and N. C. Choi. Estimation of the delivered patient dose in lung IMRT treatment based on deformable registration of 4D-CT data and Monte Carlo simulations, *Phys. Med. Biol.* **51**(11) (2006) 2763–2779.

56. B. Thorndyke, E. Schreibmann, A. Koong and L. Xing. Reducing respiratory motion artifacts in positron emission tomography through retrospective stacking, *Med. Phys.* **33**(7) (2006) 2632–2641.

57. E. Schreibmann, G. T. Chen and L. Xing. Image interpolation in 4D CT using a BSpline deformable registration model, *Int. J. Radiat. Oncol. Biol. Phys.* **64**(5) (2006) 1537–1550.

58. D. Sarrut, V. Boldea, S. Miguet and C. Ginest. Simulation of four-dimensional CT images from deformable registration between inhale and exhale breath-hold CT scans, *Med. Phys.* **33**(3) (2006) 605–617.

59. S. Xu, R. H. Taylor, G. Fichtinger and K. Cleary. Lung deformation estimation and four-dimensional CT lung reconstruction, *Acad. Radiol.* **13**(9) (2006) 1082–1092.

60. K. M. Langen and D. T. Jones. Organ motion and its management, *Int. J. Radiat. Oncol. Biol. Phys.* **50**(1) (2001) 265–278.

61. T. E. Byrne. A review of prostate motion with considerations for the treatment of prostate cancer, *Med. Dosim.* **30**(3) (2005) 155–161.

62. M. J. Ghilezan, D. A. Jaffray, J. H. Siewerdsen, M. van Herk, A. Shetty, M. B. Sharpe, Jafri S. Zafar, F. A. Vicini, R. C. Matter, D. S. Brabbins and A. A. Martinez. Prostate gland motion assessed with cine-magnetic resonance imaging (cine-MRI), *Int. J. Radiat. Oncol. Biol. Phys.* **62**(2) (2005) 406–417.

63. A. R. Padhani, V. S. Khoo, J. Suckling, J. E. Husband, M. O. Leach and D. P. Dearnaley. Evaluating the effect of rectal distension and rectal movement on prostate gland position using cine MRI, *Int. J. Radiat. Oncol. Biol. Phys.* **44**(3) (1999) 525–533.

64. L. A. Dawson, D. W. Litzenberg, K. K. Brock, M. Sanda, M. Sullivan, H. M. Sandler and J. M. Balter. A comparison of ventilatory prostate movement in four treatment positions, *Int. J. Radiat. Oncol. Biol. Phys.* **48**(2) (2000) 319–323.

65. S. Malone, J. M. Crook, W. S. Kendal and J. Szanto. Respiratory-induced prostate motion: quantification and characterization, *Int. J. Radiat. Oncol. Biol. Phys.* **48**(1) (2000) 105–109.

66. J. Liang and D. Yana. Reducing uncertainties in volumetric image based deformable organ registration, *Med. Phys.* **30**(8) (2003) 2116–2122.

67. H. Wang, L. Dong, M. F. Lii, A. L. Lee, R. de Crevoisier, R. Mohan, J. D. Cox, D. A. Kuban and R. Cheung. Implementation and validation of a three-dimensional deformable registration algorithm for targeted prostate cancer radiotherapy, *Int. J. Radiat. Oncol. Biol. Phys.* **61**(3) (2005) 725–735.

68. B. Schaly, J. A. Kempe, G. S. Bauman, J. J. Battista and J. Van Dyk. Tracking the dose distribution in radiation therapy by accounting for variable anatomy, *Phys. Med. Biol.* **49**(5) (2004) 791–805.

69. M. Foskey, B. Davis, L. Goyal, S. Chang, E. Chaney, N. Strehl, S. Tomei, J. Rosenman and S. Joshi. Large deformation three-dimensional image registration in image-guided radiation therapy, *Phys. Med. Biol.* **50**(24) (2005) 5869–5892.

70. Y. Kim, I. C. Hsu, J. Pouliot, S. M. Noworolski, D. B. Vigneron and J. Kurhanewicz. Expandable and rigid endorectal coils for prostate MRI: impact on prostate distortion and rigid image registration, *Med. Phys.* **32**(12) (2005) 3569–3578.
71. E. Huang, L. Dong, A. Chandra, D. A. Kuban, I. I. Rosen, A. Evans and A. Pollack. Intrafaction prostate motion during IMRT for prostate cancer, *Int. J. Radiat. Oncol. Biol. Phys.* **53**(2) (2002) 261–268.
72. D. A. Jaffray, K. K. Brock, A. Nichol, D. Moseley, C. Catton, P. Warde. An analysis of inter-fraction prostate deformation relative to implanted fiducial markers using finite element modelling, *Proc. AAPM* (2004) S229.

CHAPTER 2

IMAGE-BASED COMPUTATIONAL HEMODYNAMICS METHODS AND THEIR APPLICATION FOR THE ANALYSIS OF BLOOD FLOW PAST ENDOVASCULAR DEVICES

J. R. CEBRAL*, R. LÖHNER and S. APPANABOYINA

Center for Computational Fluid Dynamics
George Mason University, Fairfax, Virginia
*jcebral@gmu.edu

C. M. PUTMAN

Interventional Neuroradiology
Inova Fairfax Hospital, Falls Church, Virginia

Knowledge of the hemodynamic conditions in intracranial aneurysms before and after endovascular treatment is important to better understand the mechanisms responsible for aneurysm growth and rupture, and to optimize and personalize the therapies. Unfortunately, there are no reliable imaging techniques for *in vivo* quantification of blood flow patterns in cerebral aneurysms. Patient-specific, image-based computational models provide an attractive alternative since they can handle any vascular geometry and physiologic flow condition. However, computational modeling of the hemodynamics in cerebral aneurysms after their endovascular treatment is a challenging problem because of the high degree of geometric complexity required to represent and mesh the vascular anatomy and the endovascular devices simultaneously. This paper describes an image-based methodology for constructing patient-specific vascular computational fluid dynamics models and an adaptive grid embedding technique to simulate blood flows around endovascular devices. The methodology is illustrated with several examples ranging from idealized vascular models to patient-specific models of cerebral aneurysms after deployment of stents and coils. These techniques have the potential to be used to select the best therapeutic option for a particular individual and to optimize the design of endovascular devices on a patient-specific basis.

Keywords: Hemodynamics; cerebral aneurysms; stents; computational fluid dynamics; embedded grids.

1. Introduction

1.1. *Cerebral aneurysms and their treatment*

Cerebral aneurysms are pathological dilatations of the arterial wall frequently located near arterial bifurcations in the circle of Willis.[1-3] The most serious consequence is their rupture and intracranial hemorrhage into the subarachnoid space, with an associated high mortality and morbidity rate.[4-7] Intracranial aneurysms are particularly difficult to treat, and often do not produce symptoms before they rupture.[8] Greater availability and improvement of neuroradiological

29

techniques have resulted in more frequent detection of unruptured aneurysms. Because prognosis of subarachnoid hemorrhage is still poor, preventive surgery is increasingly considered as a therapeutic option. Planning elective surgery requires a better understanding of the process of aneurysm formation, progression, and rupture so that a sound judgment between the risks and benefits of possible therapies can be made. The genesis, progression and rupture of cerebral aneurysms are not well understood. However, their pathogenesis is believed to be due to the dynamic forces of the blood on a weakened vascular wall. Previous studies.[1,9] have identified the major factors involved in these processes: (a) arterial hemodynamics, (b) wall biomechanics and mechanobiology, and (c) peri-aneurysmal environment.

Traditional surgical treatments for vascular disease attempted to normalize of lumen of the blood vessel. For ischemic disease, this meant physically re-opening the vessel back to its nominal caliber. For cerebral aneurysms, it meant excluding it from the circulation. This paradigm was based upon the correlation between clinical symptoms and a visible blood vessel abnormality. We now consider the physiology of vascular lesions as a more important component of the disease process. Previously, simple detection of an anatomical abnormality was the end of the diagnostic process, but contemporary treatment attempts to further characterize the lesion with physiologic measures. Despite accumulating extensive experience with cerebral aneurysms, we cannot currently predict which aneurysm will grow, rupture or remain stable. Two similar aneurysms in different patients may show dramatically different responses to treatment, so simply detecting the aneurysm is insufficient to help the patient and the treating physician determine the appropriate course of therapy.

A cerebral aneurysm that ruptures has an associated rate of fatality of 50%, with another 20% suffering significant morbidity. This terrible burden can be reduced by the appropriate aneurysm treatment, but every treatment carries a risk, which sometimes matches or exceeds the yearly risk of aneurysm rupture. Therefore, the best patient care would be to treat only those patients who are likely to rupture.[10–12] Treatment by either traditional surgical clipping or endovascular intra-aneurysmal occlusion has been proven to dramatically reduced re-rupture rates from the natural history rate.[13]

Surgical and endovascular procedures are two of the most common methods used to treat cerebral aneurysms.[14] Surgical clipping consists in placing a metal clip across the neck of the aneurysm to isolate the aneurysm from the flow of blood, whereas endovascular procedures such as coiling and stenting consist in implanting intravascular devices to limit the flow of blood into aneurysm and promote thrombus formation in the sac. The most used method to treat aneurysms is coiling, which consist in packing platinum coils in the aneurysm sac to stop the blood flow. The main limitation of this type of treatment is the potential for aneurysm recurrence due to coil compaction and aneurysm refilling. Presumably, coil compaction is the result of the interaction between the aneurysm wall, the reparative tissue, the coils and the hemodynamic forces exerted on the coil mass. In the setting of incomplete reparative response, the coils can be moved by the chronic, repetitive hemodynamic forces of the flow stream impaction. Some aneurysm such as those with wide necks or fusiform aneurysms are difficult or impossible to coil because the aneurysm geometry will not allow a stable coil position without adversely affecting the parent artery flow. In these cases, placement of stents in the parent artery, across the neck of the aneurysm, can be performed in order to limit the flow into the aneurysm or to hold coils inside the aneurysm sac. Recently, there has been increasing interest in using stents as flow diverters that deviate the inflow jet away from the aneurysm, and thus reduce the risk of rupture.

The current challenges of aneurysm treatment are many. First and foremost is the selection of aneurysms for treatment. Numerous studies to determine the factors that are associated with rupture have been performed, but these studies have relied on anatomic or clinical factors only. For example, increasing size seems to correlate well with rupture, and smoking and hypertension seem to have a minor influence. Certain locations seem to have a higher risk than others for similarly sized aneurysms. The highest associated risk is a previous rupture of the same aneurysm. Other factors are also believed to be associated, such as irregularity (daughter saccules) of the aneurysm. Most investigators believe that wall characteristics and flow forces are responsible for the growth and change in aneurysms. This concept is fundamental to fluid dynamics in all areas. In vascular medicine, there is no validated method to characterize, model, confirm measurements of these parameters, and test their utility on patient datasets.[15-23] Even with the generally accepted belief that flow is a major determinant of aneurysm formation and growth, this has not been systematically studied.

In vitro and numerical models have shown that the most important factors to determine the flow into an aneurysm are the geometry of the aneurysm neck, and flow characteristics and geometry of the parent artery. Clinically, a physician can alter the flow into an aneurysm by changing the flow in the parent artery (flow diversion or reversal) using parent artery occlusion devices, or alter the neck geometry using coils packed into an aneurysm or stents in the parent artery. Studies have shown that the size and amount of coils and the porosity of the stent have the most important effect on intra-aneurysmal flow.[22,24-26] Adapting these studies to clinical situations is problematic because idealized models were used for these studies that do not represent the conditions found in clinical situations. Ideally, personalized models could be used for patient evaluation and planning of endovascular procedures. Patient-specific computational fluid dynamics (CFD) models of cerebral aneurysms constructed from medical images are an attractive method to study flow alterations induced by different endovascular treatment options.[27-31]

1.2. *Patient-specific hemodynamics*

Knowledge of patient-specific *in vivo* blood flow patterns is important for understanding the role of hemodynamics in a variety of vascular diseases. In particular, wall shear stress is known to regulate mechanobiological processes associated with cell apoptosis.[32-34] and arterial wall remodeling and degeneration.[35-38] These processes play an important role in vascular diseases such as atherosclerosis and aneurysms. However, to date there are no reliable techniques for non-invasive *in vivo* imaging of blood flow patterns and wall shear stress distribution.

Phase-contrast magnetic resonance (PC-MR) can provide reliable estimations of bulk flow rates in the major cerebral arteries and reasonable measurements of velocity profiles in the largest vessels. The major drawback is limited time and spatial resolution and signal losses in regions of slowly moving fluid. Doppler ultrasound (DUS) can be used to obtain point-wise measurements of blood velocity with great temporal resolution. However, this technique is strongly operator dependent, it can only measure velocity components aligned with the detector, and the signal is obstructed by bone. Transcranial Doppler ultrasound (TCD) can be used to measure velocity in intracranial vessels, but the exact location of the measurement is unknown. Animal models have been used to study the *in vivo* hemodynamic patterns. In particular, blood flow patterns have been quantified in surgically created or flow induced aneurysms in animal models.[17,39-46]

Patient-specific *in vitro* models of vascular structures can be constructed using rapid prototyping techniques from anatomical images.[44,47,48] The male casts produced by the rapid prototyping machines are used as molds to construct hollow models that can be placed in a flow through circuit. Pulsatile pumps are used to obtain flow rate curves that mimic the physiologic flow conditions encountered *in vivo*. The working fluid is typically a mixture of water and glycerol in order to achieve the viscosity of blood without altering significantly the refractive index of water. More refined models use blood mimicking fluids with non-Newtonian viscosity properties similar to blood. Time-dependent velocity distributions are commonly measured with particle image velocimetry (PIV) techniques.[24,49] For this purpose, small particles are added to the fluid and are illuminated with a laser. Usually one plane is measured at a time and the in-plane velocity components are quantified. The 3D velocity components are obtained by either imaging in a set of perpendicular planes or by using stereo-PIV techniques.[49] Wall shear stress measurements can be obtained by measuring the velocity at a point close to the vessel wall with laser Doppler velocimetry (LDV) techniques.[47] The wall shear stress is then obtained from $\tau = \mu dv/dx$, where μ is the viscosity, v is the velocity, and dx is the distance to the wall and assuming that the velocity at the wall is zero (no-slip condition). Producing maps of wall shear stress distribution would require measuring at many points along the vessel wall, which is very labor intensive. Differential pressure or pressure drops can be measured directly with pressure transducers placed at different locations of the model.[50] Blood flow patterns *in vitro* models have also been measured with PC-MR techniques.[51,52] These experimental techniques allow very detailed measurement of several hemodynamic variables, however they are quite expensive and time consuming. Therefore, using patient-specific *in vitro* models is impractical for individual treatment planning.

Idealized CFD models have been used to understand the influence of hemodynamics in the initiation and progression of vascular diseases. These models have been helpful to understand the hemodynamic characteristics in "general" or "average" anatomical configurations.

The use of animal, *in vitro*, and idealized computational models has characterized the complexity of blood flow patterns in many vascular structures. Because these approaches do not use patient specific anatomies, they do not allow connection of the observed hemodynamic variables to clinical events.

Although current imaging techniques are limited for *in vivo* quantification of blood flow patterns, they can provide accurate measurements of the geometrical shape of blood vessels. Therefore, realistic image-based computational models can be constructed from anatomical images. This is an attractive alternative because of the ability of computational models to handle any vessel geometry. Image-based CFD has been applied to the study of a variety of vascular diseases.[27,28,30,53–55] In addition, computational models can be used not only to study the current hemodynamic conditions of a given patient (as any imaging modality would do), but also they provide the possibility of asking what-if questions. For instance, it is possible to study the alterations of the blood flow patterns of a particular patient induced by surgical procedures such as bypass surgery[56] or endovascular interventions such as stenting and aneurysm coiling.[57] This opens the possibility of choosing the best therapeutic alternative for a given patient, and also of personalizing and optimizing the treatment for the particular anatomical and hemodynamic structures of each individual. This predictive character of patient-specific image-based computational models cannot be reproduced with any imaging modality.

2. Image-based Computational Hemodynamics Models

The process of simulation of patient-specific hemodynamics from medical images can be divided into two major stages: (a) anatomical modeling and (b) blood flow modeling. Each of these stages can be further subdivided into more basic steps: (a1) image processing, (a2) geometric modeling, (a3) grid generation, (b1) flow simulation, (b2) post processing and (b3) visualization. The set of sequential modeling stages is called a computational modeling pipeline or chain. Several alternative approaches exist for each of the stages of the modeling chain, and different investigators have used different combinations of computational tools to assemble their pipelines. In what follows a description of the pipeline used by the authors is provided.[58]

2.1. *Anatomical modeling: image processing*

Patient-specific anatomical models can be constructed from a variety of imaging modalities such as 3D rotational angiography (3DRA), computed tomography angiography (CTA) and magnetic resonance angiography (MRA). Rotational angiography is an invasive technique that requires an intra-arterial injection of contrast material and exposition to a low dose of X-rays, but provides the highest resolution and contrast between vascular structures and the surrounding tissue. This imaging modality is limited to visualizing only one vascular tree (e.g. from the left or right internal carotid artery (ICA)) at a time. Visualization of the entire circulation requires multiple injections. However, it is still the preferred imaging modality for numerical modeling because of its superior quality depicting the vascular structures and simplicity for constructing anatomical models. CTA is a less invasive technique that requires an intra-venous injection of contrast material and exposition to X-rays. The resolution is less than that of rotational angiography and other non-vascular structures such as bone appear bright in these images, complicating the anatomical modeling process. However, these images can be very helpful to characterize the peri-aneurysmal environment, i.e. contact between the vessels and bone or dura matter. MRA does not use any ionizing radiation but suffers from signal loss in regions of decreased or disturbed flow patterns. This signal loss can be reduced with the use of contrast enhancement via endovenous injection of paramagnetic material. As in the case of CTA, in MRA images tissues other than blood vessels are also visualized, complicating the segmentation process. However, MRI can also provide flow information in the parent vessel using PC-MR techniques.

After obtaining the clinical data set, the first step in the construction of a patient-specific anatomical model is to filter the anatomical image in order to reduce the noise and increase the contrast between the blood vessels and surrounding tissue. The sharpness of an image is increased using a sigmoid function to map the pixel intensities.[59] Defining

$$I^* = I_0 + \frac{1}{2}\left[\frac{1}{2}\left(\sin\left(I_0 - 1/2\right)\pi + 1\right) - I_0\right] \tag{1}$$

where I_0 is the original image intensity, the sharpened image is:

$$I = \begin{cases} 1 & \text{if } I^* > 1 \\ 0 & \text{if } I^* < 0 \\ I^* & \text{otherwise} \end{cases} \tag{2}$$

Several techniques can be used to smooth anatomical images. The simplest method is the convolution with a Gaussian kernel or blurring operation:[60]

$$I^{\text{smooth}} = G \otimes I, \quad G = \frac{1}{\sqrt{2\pi}\sigma}e^{-r^2/\sigma^2} \tag{3}$$

where I is the image intensity, G is the Gaussian kernel, r is the distance, and σ is the kernel size constant. Typically, a $3 \times 3 \times 3$ window is employed for blurring operations.

The main drawback of this approach is that it diffuses the vascular structures, i.e. it is not edge-preserving. More sophisticated techniques include inhomogeneous and anisotropic diffusion methods.[61] These edge-preserving smoothing techniques are based on the solution of partial differential equations (PDEs), typically non-linear advection-diffusion equations, using finite difference methods. The general form of the equation is

$$I_{,t} = \nabla \cdot (\mathbf{D} \nabla I) \tag{4}$$

where $\mathbf{D}$ is the diffusion tensor that depends on the image intensity I. Different methods define different forms of the diffusion tensor, and inhomogeneous diffusion methods use a scalar edge detection function for D. In particular, the Gaussian smoothing method is the solution of the linear diffusion equation with a constant scalar diffusivity coefficient. Vessel enhancement filters based on the local structure of the image intensity distribution have also been designed.[62] These techniques aim at smoothing our non-vascular structures and at the same time increase the contrast of tubular structures in the images.

The second step in the model construction process is the segmentation of vascular structures. The result of this process is the classification of the image voxels into blood vessels and other tissues. Several techniques can be used for this process. The selection of the appropriate technique for a particular image is done on a trial and error basis, and usually depends on the complexity of the vascular structure being segmented, the quality of the anatomical image and the contrast between the blood vessels and surrounding tissues. The simplest method is thresholding[60] in which an iso-surface is directly extracted from the image intensity level. However, this can fail because in many cases the image intensity distribution is not homogeneous within the blood vessels and there may be other tissues with similar intensities. A seeded region growing approach can be used to segment simple vascular structures.[59,60] This approach consists in manually selecting a seed voxel within the desired vascular tree and marking all voxels connected to it within a specified intensity range. The main drawback of this technique is that the growth process can leak into non-vascular structures adjacent to blood vessels that have similar image intensity (e.g. bone in CTA images).

Level set techniques are based on the solution of a partial differential equation describing the evolution of a function whose zero level set represents the boundary of the blood vessels.[63] Again non-linear advection-diffusion equations are used, and different expressions for the advection velocity are used in different methods.

$$\phi_{,t} + \alpha F|\nabla\phi| - \beta(g|\nabla\phi| + \nabla g \nabla\phi) = 0, \tag{5}$$

where ϕ is the level set function, F is a speed function that controls the normal velocity of the propagating front, α and β are user defined parameters, and g is a classical edge detector function defined as:

$$g = \frac{1}{1 + |\nabla I|^2} \tag{6}$$

with I the image intensity level. The simplest methods define a propagation velocity F based on the local image intensity distribution and other more sophisticated methods use a velocity function based on estimations of the local probability that each voxel belongs to different tissue classes.[64,65] These techniques have been applied with success to 3DRA and CTA images.[29,30,55]

Another class of vessel reconstruction techniques is the so called deformable models. The basic idea behind this approach is to construct an initial surface representing the blood vessels that has the correct vascular topology. Then, the surface is allowed to deform under internal elastic forces between neighboring nodes and external forces derived from the local image intensity gradient.[66] The image force applied to node i of the surface model is given by:

$$\mathbf{F}_i^{\text{image}} = \alpha(\mathbf{n}_i \cdot \nabla G \otimes |\nabla G \otimes I|)\, \mathbf{n}_i, \tag{7}$$

where α is a constant, G is the Gaussian kernel, I is the image intensity and $\mathbf{n}_i$ is the unit normal to grid point i. The elastic force applied to node i of the model is given by:

$$\mathbf{F}_i^{\text{elastic}} = \beta \sum_j (\mathbf{x}_j - \mathbf{x}_i) - [(\mathbf{x}_j - \mathbf{x}_i) \cdot \mathbf{n}_i]\, \mathbf{n}_i, \tag{8}$$

where β is a constant and the summation is taken over the points j adjacent to node point i. In addition, a torsional force or moment is applied to the triangles:

$$\mathbf{M}_i = \mathbf{n}_i \times \mathbf{n}_i^{\text{neighbors}}, \tag{9}$$

where $\mathbf{n}_i^{\text{neighbors}}$ is the unit vector whose direction is determined by taking the resultant of the normal vectors of the adjacent triangles. The deformation due to the moment is then:

$$\Delta \mathbf{x}_i^{\text{rotational}} = \gamma\, (\mathbf{l}_{ji} \times \mathbf{M}_i) \tag{10}$$

where γ is a constant and $\mathbf{l}_{ji}$ the vector moment arm from the jth vertex to the center of mass of the ith triangle.

In tubular deformable models,[67] the initial surface is a cylinder constructed along the vessel skeleton or centerline. With this approach, one vessel is segmented at a time minimizing leaks into surrounding anatomical structures. In iso-surface deformable models,[66,68] the initial surface model is constructed via iso-surface extraction from the original image or from a segmented image using any of the previously described methods. Deformable models are quite useful as the last step in the vessel segmentation process for correcting the geometry of the vascular model since they tend to place the surface nodes at the boundaries of vascular structures. They have been applied with success to 3DRA and MRA images.[50,54,69-71] In some difficult cases, a combination of the segmentation techniques described above is used to produce the final segmentation.

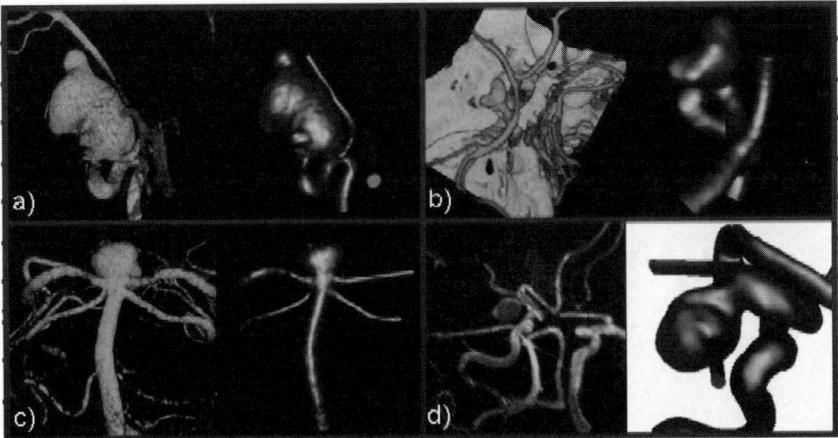

Fig. 1.   Examples of aneurysm models constructed from anatomical images of different modalities: (a,c) 3D rotational angiography, (b) computed tomography angiography, (d) time-of-flight magnetic resonance angiography.

Once the image has been segmented, a geometrical model (surface triangulation) is constructed via iso-surface extraction using either marching cubes[60] or marching tetrahedra[59] methods. Examples of anatomical models constructed from different imaging modalities (3DRA, CTA and MRA) are presented in Fig. 1. The figure shows volume renderings of the anatomical images and the reconstructed vascular models for four intracranial aneurysms.

2.2. *Anatomical modeling: geometric modeling*

The generation of computational grids for the numerical solution of the fluid flow equations requires a proper description of the computational domain, i.e. a watertight anatomical model. In many situations, it is advantageous to reconstruct different portions of the vascular tree independently, i.e. using a component-based approach. For instance when a single segmentation technique fails to reconstruct the entire vascular tree because of large variations of the image intensity inside blood vessels, or when vessels touch each other, or when multiple injection 3DRA images are used to construct models of complex vascular networks. In these cases, a complete anatomical model is obtained by fusing the different surface components using an adaptive voxelization technique.[72] This method is based on the construction of a background grid composed of tetrahedral elements that covers the entire computational domain. Then, the distance vector from each grid point to the closest surface is computed. The background grid is adaptively refined close to the anatomical surface in order to increase the resolution of the method. Typically two to four levels of mesh refinement are used. A watertight surface model is then obtained by extracting the zero-level iso-surface of the signed distance map computed on the background grid. An example is presented in Fig. 2.[73] In this case,

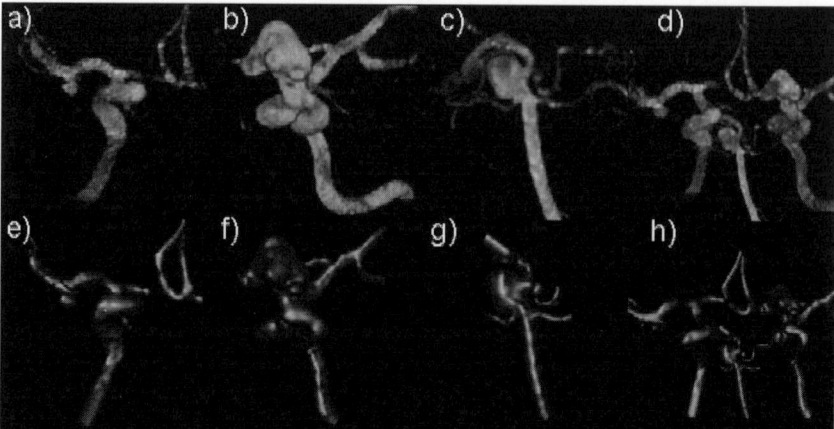

Fig. 2.   Example of component-based approach for constructing a model of the entire circle of
Willis of a patient with five cerebral aneurysms: (a) right ICA 3DRA, (b) left ICA 3DRA, (c) basilar
3DRA, (d) co-registered 3DRA images, (e) model from right ICA image, (f) model from left ICA
image, (g) model from basilar image, (h) complete model after fusing surface components.

a model of the circle of Willis of a patient with five intracranial aneurysms was
constructed from three rotational angiography images (a,b,c) which were manually
co-registered (d). From each 3DRA image, a piece of the arterial network was
reconstructed (e,f,g) and merged into a single vascular model (h).

Before proceeding to unstructured grid generation the vascular model is further
processed. It is smoothed using a non-shrinking smoothing algorithm[74] in order to
filter out high frequency noise from the coordinates of the surface triangulation.
The quality of the surface triangulation is improved using edge-collapsing and
diagonal swapping algorithms[59] that remove highly stretched or very small elements,
and minimize the maximum angle of the triangular elements. The vascular model
is then manually cut perpendicularly to the vessel axis at desired locations in
order to apply boundary conditions for the flow simulations. If desired, the vessel
boundaries are extruded along the vessel direction in order to minimize the effect of
boundary conditions on the computed flow patterns. In some difficult cases where
the segmentation algorithms fail to separate blood vessels that are in close proximity,
the surface triangulation is interactively edited, opening and closing holes in order
to correct the topology of the vascular model.

2.3. Anatomical modeling: grid generation

The process of grid generation for CFD simulations can be divided into two parts:
(a) surface meshing, (b) volume meshing. Surface grids can be generated from
a representation of the computational domain via analytical surface patches or
directly from a surface triangulation. In the former case, an extra step is required
in order to create a set of non-overlapping analytical surface patches such as Coon's

patches or NURBS from the reconstructed vascular model. In the latter approach, the reconstructed model is directly used as the description of the computational domain. Our methodology is based on this latter approach. The surface grid can be constructed by improving and refining the original surface grid, or by generating an entirely new mesh on top of the original triangulation. We use this latter strategy. The new surface grid is generated using an advancing front method that places newly created points on the original surface triangulation by linear or quadratic interpolation.[75]

Once the surface mesh has been generated, the space within the anatomical model is filled with tetrahedral elements. Several approaches can be used for this purpose including Delaunay triangulations, quad-tree meshing, or advancing front methods.[76–78] We use the advancing front method. The idea of the advancing front method is to place all the triangles into a list or front. Then, the smallest triangle is extracted from this front and a new tetrahedral element is formed by adding one point and checking that the new element does not intersect with any other element already generated. The triangular faces of the newly created element are inserted into the front. The process is repeated until no triangles are left in the front.

The distribution of element sizes is prescribed using background grids and source functions.[79] Adaptive background grids are used to increase the mesh resolution in regions where the anatomical model has a large surface curvature. Source points, lines and triangles are interactively placed in the anatomical model in order to specify the element size as a linear function of the distance from the source element. These sources are used to prescribe the desired element sizes for example along small vessels.

2.4. *Flow modeling: computational fluid dynamics*

Blood may be considered an incompressible flow, described at the continuum level by the Navier-Stokes equations:[78,80]

$$\rho \mathbf{v}_{,t} + \rho \mathbf{v} \cdot \nabla \mathbf{v} + \nabla p = \nabla \mu \nabla \mathbf{v} \tag{11}$$

$$\nabla \cdot \mathbf{v} = 0, \tag{12}$$

where ρ denotes the (constant) density, p the pressure, $\mathbf{v}$ the velocity vector and μ the viscosity. By taking the divergence of Eq. (11) and using Eq. (2) we can immediately derive the so-called pressure-Poisson equation:

$$\nabla^2 p = -\nabla \cdot \mathbf{v} \nabla \mathbf{v} \tag{13}$$

What sets incompressible flow solvers apart from compressible flow solvers is the fact that the pressure is not obtained from an equation of state $p = p(\rho, T)$, but from the divergence constraint. This implies that the pressure field establishes itself instantaneously (reflecting the infinite speed of sound assumption of incompressible fluids) and must therefore be integrated implicitly in time.

2.4.1. *Spatial discretization*

The spatial discretization of the computational domain is carried out using unstructured grids in order to: (a) approximate arbitrary domains, (b) generate highly stretched grids in near-wall boundary layer regions, (c) use advanced automatic grid generators for arbitrary domains and (d) perform adaptive refinement in a straightforward manner, i.e. without changes to the solver.

We briefly recall how, for any operator (e.g. the Navier-Stokes operator given by Eqs. (11) and (12) one can derive a discrete set of ordinary differential equations or algebraic equations for unstructured grids using the Finite Element method, so that the final system can be solved on a computer. Assume an operator of the form:

$$L(u) = 0 \qquad (14)$$

The unknowns u are approximated by a set of shape functions N^i that have local spatial support and that can easily be defined on the element level.[78] Then the approximate value of u, given by u^h, may be obtained from:

$$u \approx u^h = N^i \hat{u}_i \qquad (15)$$

where the Einstein summation convention has been adopted. The Galerkin weighted residuals method is obtained by setting:

$$\int_\Omega N^j L(u^h) d\Omega = 0 \quad \forall j \qquad (16)$$

i.e. by orthogonalizing $L(u^h)$ against all shape functions. If we assume, for the moment, a linear operator of the form $L(u) = Ku + s$, this results in

$$\int_\Omega \left(N^j K N^i \hat{u}_i + N^j s \right) d\Omega = 0 \qquad (17)$$

which may be written as

$$\mathbf{K}\,\mathbf{u} = \mathbf{s} \qquad (18)$$

In order to simplify the coding logic, the integrals are evaluated at the element level, i.e. the global domain integral is written as a sum of sub-domain integrals:

$$\sum_{el} \int_{\Omega_{el}} N^j L(u^h) d\Omega_{el} = 0 \qquad (19)$$

For low-order elements, and in particular for linear tetrahedra, it is convenient to rewrite the loops over elements as loops over edges, as this results in a much lower operation count, as well as much lower indirect addressing requirements.[78]

2.4.2. *The advection operator*

As with the compressible Euler/Navier-Stokes equations, there are three ways of modifying the unstable Galerkin discretization of the advection terms: (a) integration along characteristics, (b) Taylor-Galerkin (or streamline diffusion) and (c) edge-based upwinding. In what follows we consider the last option, based on the derivation of consistent numerical fluxes for edge-based solvers. The Galerkin approximation for the advection terms yields a residual (or right-hand side) of the form:

$$r^i = D^{ij} F_{ij} = D^{ij} (\mathbf{f}_i + \mathbf{f}_j), \tag{20}$$

where the $\mathbf{f}_i$ are the "fluxes along edges"

$$\mathbf{f}_i = S_k^{ij} \mathbf{F}_i^k, \quad S_k^{ij} = \frac{d_k^{ij}}{D^{ij}}, \quad D^{ij} = \sqrt{d_k^{ij} d_k^{ij}} \tag{21}$$

$$\mathbf{f}_i = \left(S_k^{ij} \mathbf{v}_i^k \right) \mathbf{v}_i, \quad \mathbf{f}_j = \left(S_k^{ij} \mathbf{v}_j^k \right) \mathbf{v}_j. \tag{22}$$

A consistent numerical flux is given by

$$F_{ij} = \mathbf{f}_i + \mathbf{f}_j - |\mathbf{v}^{ij}|(\mathbf{v}_i - \mathbf{v}_j), \tag{23}$$

where

$$\mathbf{v}^{ij} = \frac{1}{2} S_k^{ij} (\mathbf{v}_i^k + \mathbf{v}_j^k) \tag{24}$$

As before, this first-order scheme can be improved by reducing the difference $\mathbf{v}_i - \mathbf{v}_j$ through (limited) extrapolation to the edge center.[81]

2.4.3. *The divergence operator*

A persistent difficulty with incompressible flow solvers has been the derivation of a stable scheme for the divergence constraint (12). The stability criterion for the divergence constraint is also known as the Ladyzenskaya–Babuska–Brezzi or LBB condition.[82] The classic way to satisfy the LBB condition has been to use different functional spaces for the velocity and pressure discretization.[83] Typically, the velocity space has to be richer, containing more degrees of freedom than the pressure space. Elements belonging to this class are the $p1/p1+$ bubble mini-element,[84] the $p1/iso$-$p1$ element,[85] and the $p1/p2$ element.[86] An alternative way to satisfy the LBB condition is through the use of artificial viscosities,[87] "stabilization",[88–90] or the use of consistent numerical fluxes. We consider this last option. The resulting fluxes are given by

$$F_{ij} = \mathbf{f}_i + \mathbf{f}_j, \quad \mathbf{f}_i = S_k^{ij} v_i^k, \quad \mathbf{f}_j = S_k^{ij} v_j^k. \tag{25}$$

A consistent numerical flux may be constructed by adding pressure terms of the form:

$$F_{ij} = \mathbf{f}_i + \mathbf{f}_j - |\lambda^{ij}|(p_i - p_j), \tag{26}$$

where the eigenvalue λ^{ij} is given by the ratio of the characteristic advective timestep of the edge Δt and the characteristic advective length of the edge l:

$$\lambda^{ij} = \frac{\Delta t^{ij}}{l^{ij}}. \tag{27}$$

Higher order schemes can be derived by reconstruction and limiting, or by substituting the first-order differences of the pressure with third-order differences:

$$F_{ij} = \mathbf{f}_i + \mathbf{f}_j - |\lambda^{ij}| \left(p_i - p_j + \frac{l^{ij}}{2}(\nabla p_i + \nabla p_j) \right). \tag{28}$$

This results in a stable, low-diffusion, fourth-order damping for the divergence constraint.

2.4.4. *Temporal discretization: projection schemes*

The hyperbolic character of the advection operator and the elliptic character of the pressure-Poisson equation have led to a number of so-called projection schemes. The key idea is to predict first a velocity field from the current flow variables without taking the divergence constraint into account. In a second step, the divergence constraint is enforced by solving a pressure-Poisson equation. The velocity increment can therefore be separated into an advective and pressure increment:

$$\mathbf{v}^{n+1} = \mathbf{v}^n + \Delta\mathbf{v}^a + \Delta\mathbf{v}^p = \mathbf{v}^{**} + \Delta\mathbf{v}^p. \tag{29}$$

For an explicit integration of the advective terms, one complete timestep is given by:

(a) Advective/diffusive prediction: $\mathbf{v}^n \to \mathbf{v}^{**}$

$$\left[\frac{1}{\Delta t} - \nabla\mu\nabla \right] \cdot (\mathbf{v}^{**} - \mathbf{v}^n) + \mathbf{v}^n \cdot \nabla\mathbf{v}^n = \nabla\mu\nabla\mathbf{v}^n \tag{30}$$

(b) Pressure correction: $p^n \to p^{n+1}$

$$\nabla \cdot \mathbf{v}^{n+1} = 0, \quad \mathbf{v}^{n+1} + \Delta t\nabla p^{n+1} = \mathbf{v}^{**} \quad \Rightarrow \quad \nabla^2 p^{n+1} = \frac{\nabla \cdot \mathbf{v}^{**}}{\Delta t} \tag{31}$$

(c) Velocity correction: $\mathbf{v}^{**} \to \mathbf{v}^{n+1}$

$$\mathbf{v}^{n+1} = \mathbf{v}^{**} - \Delta t\nabla p^{n+1}. \tag{32}$$

This scheme was originally proposed by,[91] and has since been used repeatedly within finite difference,[92] finite volume,[93] finite element,[94–97] and spectral element[98] solvers. The main drawback of this scheme is that the residuals of the pressure correction do not vanish at steady state, implying that the results depend on the timestep Δt. This situation can be remedied by considering the pressure for the advective/diffusive predictor. The resulting scheme is given by:

(a) Advective-diffusive prediction: $\mathbf{v}^n \to \mathbf{v}^*$

$$\left[\frac{1}{\Delta t} - \nabla \mu \nabla\right] \cdot (\mathbf{v}^* - \mathbf{v}^n) + \mathbf{v}^n \cdot \nabla \mathbf{v}^n + \nabla p^n = \nabla \mu \nabla \mathbf{v}^n \qquad (33)$$

(b) Pressure correction: $p^n \to p^{n+1}$

$$\nabla \cdot \mathbf{v}^{n+1} = 0, \quad \frac{\mathbf{v}^{n+1} - \mathbf{v}^*}{\Delta t} + \nabla(p^{n+1} - p^n) = 0 \ \Rightarrow \ \nabla^2(p^{n+1} - p^n) = \cdot \quad (34)$$

(c) Velocity correction: $\mathbf{v}^* \to \mathbf{v}^{n+1}$

$$\mathbf{v}^{n+1} = \mathbf{v}^* - \Delta t \nabla(p^{n+1} - p^n). \qquad (35)$$

At steady state, the residuals of the pressure correction vanish, implying that the result does not depend on the timestep Δt. Another advantage of this scheme as compared to the one given by Eqs. (30)–(32) is that the "pressure-Poisson" equation (34) computes increments of pressures, implying that the Dirichlet and Neumann boundary conditions simplify.

The forward Euler integration of the advection terms imposes rather severe restrictions on the allowable timestep. For this reason, alternative explicit integration schemes have been used repeatedly.[99] Many authors have used multilevel schemes, such as the second-order Adams-Bashforth scheme. The problem with schemes of this kind is that they use the values at the current and previous timestep, which makes them awkward in the context of adaptive refinement, moving meshes, and local or global remeshing. Single step schemes are therefore preferable. Lax-Wendroff or Taylor-Galerkin schemes offer such a possibility, but in this case the result of steady-state calculations depends (albeit weakly) on the timestep (or equivalently the Courant-number) chosen. This leads us to single step schemes whose steady-state result does not depend on the timestep. Schemes of this kind (explicit advection with a variety of schemes, implicit diffusion, pressure-Poisson equation for the pressure increments) have been widely used.[81,87,100–102]

The resulting large, but symmetric systems of equations given by Eqs. (30)–(32) and Eqs. (33)–(35) are of the form:

$$\mathbf{K}\,\mathbf{u} = \mathbf{r}. \tag{36}$$

For large 3-D grids, iterative solvers are well suited for such systems. Preconditioned conjugate gradient (PCG) solvers[103] are most often used to solve Eq. (36). For isotropic grids, simple diagonal preconditioning has proven very effective. For highly stretched RANS grids, linelet preconditioning has proven superior.[100,104] We remark in passing that we have attempted repeatedly to use multigrid as a solver,[105] but that for most cases to date the simpler, highly optimized PCG solvers have proven superior.

2.4.5. *Temporal discretization: implicit schemes*

Using the notation

$$u^{\theta} = (1-\theta)\,u^n + \theta\,u^{n+1} \quad \text{or} \quad u^{n+1} - u^n = \frac{u^{\theta} - u^n}{\theta} \tag{37}$$

an implicit time-stepping scheme may be written as follows:

$$\frac{\mathbf{v}^{\theta} - \mathbf{v}^n}{\theta\,\Delta t} + \mathbf{v}^{\theta}\nabla\mathbf{v}^{\theta} + \nabla p^{\theta} = \nabla\mu\nabla\mathbf{v}^{\theta} \tag{38}$$

$$\nabla \cdot \mathbf{v}^{\theta} = 0. \tag{39}$$

Following similar approaches for compressible flow solvers,[106] this system can be interpreted as the steady-state solution of the pseudo-time system:

$$\mathbf{v}^{\theta}_{,\tau} + \mathbf{v}^{\theta}\nabla\mathbf{v}^{\theta} + \nabla p^{\theta} = \nabla\mu\nabla\mathbf{v}^{\theta} - \frac{\mathbf{v}^{\theta} - \mathbf{v}^n}{\theta\,\Delta t} \tag{40}$$

$$\nabla \cdot \mathbf{v}^{\theta} = 0 \tag{41}$$

Observe that the only difference between these equations and the original incompressible Navier-Stokes equations is the appearance of new source-terms. These source terms are point-wise dependent on the variables being integrated ($\mathbf{v}$), and can therefore be folded into the left hand side for explicit time-stepping without any difficulty. The idea is then to march Eqs. (40)–(41) to steady state in the pseudo-time τ using either an explicit-advection projection scheme or an explicit artificial compressibility scheme using local timesteps. For steady flows, the use of a time-accurate scheme with uniform timestep Δt in the domain will invariably lead to slow convergence. In order to obtain steady results faster, a number of possibilities can be explored. Among that have been reported in the literature, the following have proven the most successful: (a) local timesteps, (b) reduced iteration for the pressure, (c) sub-stepping for the advection terms, (d) implicit treatment of the advection terms and (e) fully implicit treatment of advection, diffusion and pressure.

2.4.6. *Implicit treatment of the advection terms*

Any explicit integration of the advective terms implies that information can only travel at most one element per timestep. In order to allow for a faster transfer of information and larger timesteps, the advective terms have to be integrated implicitly:[107]

$$\left[\frac{1}{\Delta t} - \mathbf{v}^* \cdot \nabla - \nabla \mu \nabla\right] \cdot (\mathbf{v}^* - \mathbf{v}^n) + \mathbf{v}^n \cdot \nabla \mathbf{v}^n + \nabla p^n = \nabla \mu \nabla \mathbf{v}^n \qquad (42)$$

leading to a non-symmetric system of equations of the form:

$$\mathbf{A} \cdot \Delta \mathbf{v} = \mathbf{r}. \qquad (43)$$

This may be rewritten as

$$\mathbf{A} \cdot \Delta \mathbf{v} = (\mathbf{L} + \mathbf{D} + \mathbf{U}) \cdot \Delta \mathbf{v} = \mathbf{r}, \qquad (44)$$

where $\mathbf{L}, \mathbf{D}, \mathbf{U}$ denote the lower, diagonal and upper diagonal entries of $\mathbf{A}$. Classic relaxation schemes to solve this system of equations include:

(a) Gauss-Seidel, given by:

$$\begin{aligned} (\mathbf{L} + \mathbf{D}) \cdot \Delta \mathbf{v}^1 &= \mathbf{r} - \mathbf{U} \cdot \Delta \mathbf{v}^0 \\ (\mathbf{D} + \mathbf{U}) \cdot \Delta \mathbf{v} &= \mathbf{r} - \mathbf{L} \cdot \Delta \mathbf{v}^1 \end{aligned} \qquad (45)$$

(b) Lower-Upper Symmetric Gauss-Seidel (LU-SGS), given by:

$$(\mathbf{L} + \mathbf{D}) \cdot \mathbf{D}^{-1} \cdot (\mathbf{D} + \mathbf{U}) \cdot \Delta \mathbf{v} = \mathbf{r} \qquad (46)$$

These relaxation schemes have been optimized over the years, resulting in very efficient edge-based compressible flow solvers.[108,109] Key ideas include:

(i) Using the spectral radius ρ_A of $\mathbf{A}$ for the diagonal entries $\mathbf{D}$; for the advection case, $\rho_A = |\mathbf{v}|$, resulting in:

$$\mathbf{D} = \left[\frac{1}{\Delta t} \mathbf{M}_l^i - \frac{1}{2} \sum \mathbf{C}^{ij} |\mathbf{v}|_{ij} + \sum \mathbf{k}^{ij}\right], \qquad (47)$$

where $\mathbf{C}, \mathbf{k}$ denote the edge coefficients for the advective and viscous fluxes and $\mathbf{M}_l^i$ the lumped mass matrix at node i;

(ii) Replacing:

$$\mathbf{A} \cdot \Delta \mathbf{v} \approx \Delta \mathbf{F} \Rightarrow \Delta \mathbf{F} = \mathbf{F}(\mathbf{v} + \Delta \mathbf{v}) - \mathbf{F}(\mathbf{v}). \qquad (48)$$

The combined effect of these simplifications is a family of schemes that are matrix free, require no extra storage as compared to explicit schemes, and (due to lack of

limiting) per relaxation sweep are faster than conventional explicit schemes. For the
LU-SGS scheme, each pass over the mesh proceeds as follows:

Forward Sweep:

$$\Delta \hat{\mathbf{v}}^i = \mathbf{D}^{-1} \left[\mathbf{r}^i - \frac{1}{2} \sum \mathbf{C}^{ij} \cdot \left(\Delta \hat{\mathbf{F}}_{ij} - |\mathbf{v}|_{ij} \Delta \hat{\mathbf{v}}_j + \sum_{j<i} \mathbf{k}^{ij} \Delta \hat{v}_j \right) \right]. \quad (49)$$

Backward Sweep:

$$\mathbf{r} = \mathbf{D} \cdot \Delta \hat{\mathbf{v}} \quad (50)$$

$$\Delta \mathbf{v}^i = \mathbf{D}^{-1} \left[\mathbf{r}^i - \frac{1}{2} \sum \mathbf{C}^{ij} \cdot \left(\Delta \mathbf{F}_{ij} - |\mathbf{v}|_{ij} \Delta \mathbf{v}_j + \sum_{j>i} \mathbf{k}^{ij} \Delta \hat{v}_j \right) \right]. \quad (51)$$

Luo et al.[108] have shown that no discernable difference could be observed when
taking central or upwind discretizations for $\Delta \mathbf{F}$. As the CPU requirements of
upwind discretizations are much higher, all relaxation passes are carried out using
central schemes. Given that the same loop structure ($\mathbf{L}$, $\mathbf{D}$, $\mathbf{U}$) is required for
both the Gauss-Seidel, the LU-SGS and the GMRES matrix-vector products, it is
possible to write a single "sweep" subroutine that encompasses all of these cases.
The initialization of the Gauss-Seidel loop is accomplished with an LU-SGS pass.

2.4.7. *Blood viscosity*

Modeling the rheological behavior of blood is important not only for computing
arterial blood flow patterns but also for modeling blood clotting and thrombus
formation. Rheological models can be divided into two main groups: (a) microscopic
models and (b) macroscopic models. Microscopic models attempt to model explicitly
the interaction between the different cells embedded in the blood stream. These
cells interact with other cells, with the endothelium, and with endovascular devices
deployed into the vessels. Macroscopic models aim at describing the blood as a
continuous fluid accounting for these interactions implicitly. In what follows we
only consider macroscopic models that do not include clot formation mechanisms.
This latter topic is an important one, especially for endovascular device modeling
and should be further investigated.

The simplest rheological model for blood is a Newtonian fluid, which assumes
a constant viscosity: $\mu = \mu_0$. This implies a linear relationship between the stress
and strain rate:

$$\tau = \mu \, \gamma \quad (52)$$

where τ is the stress, γ is the strain rate. Typical values used for blood are
$\rho = 1.105 \, \text{g/cm}^3$ and $\mu = 0.04 \, \text{dyne s/cm}$. However, blood can be thought of as a
suspension of particles (red blood cells) in an aqueous medium (plasma). Thus, it is

neither homogeneous nor Newtonian. The rheological properties of blood are mainly dependent on the hematocrit, or the volume fraction of red blood cells in the blood. One of the most commonly used non-Newtonian fluid models for blood is the model of Casson,[80] which assumes a stress–strain-rate relation of the form:

$$\sqrt{\tau} = \sqrt{\tau_0} + \sqrt{\mu_0 \gamma}, \tag{53}$$

where τ_0 is the yield stress and μ_0 the Newtonian viscosity. The existence of a yield stress implies that blood requires a finite stress before it begins to flow, a fact that has been observed experimentally. Assuming a stress–strain rate relationship of the form of Eq. (52), the apparent viscosity of the Casson model can be written as:

$$\mu = \left(\sqrt{\tau_0/\gamma} + \sqrt{\mu_0} \right)^2. \tag{54}$$

Since this expression diverges as the strain-rate becomes zero, it is typically modified in the following way:[110]

$$\mu = \left[\sqrt{\tau_0(1 - e^{-m\gamma})/\gamma} + \sqrt{\mu_0} \right]^2, \tag{55}$$

where the parameter m controls the maximum viscosity obtained when γ tends to zero. In the numerical calculations, the strain rate γ is computed as the second invariant of the strain rate tensor, which for incompressible fluids can be written as:[111]

$$\gamma = 2\sqrt{\varepsilon_{ij}\varepsilon_{ij}}, \quad \varepsilon_{ij} = \frac{1}{2} \left(\frac{\partial \mathbf{v}_i}{\partial x_j} + \frac{\partial \mathbf{v}_j}{\partial x_i} \right). \tag{56}$$

Typical values used for the model constants for blood are: $\tau_0 = 0.04 \, \text{dyne/cm}^2$, $\mu_0 = 0.04 \, \text{dyne s/cm}$ and $m = 100$.

2.4.8. Boundary conditions

Physiologic inflow conditions can be derived from PC-MR measurements of blood flow rates obtained in the major cerebral vessels.[54,70] Time-dependent flow rates are obtained by integration of the measured velocity profile over the vessel cross-section. The region of integration is either manually drawn on cross-sectional views or via threshold segmentation of the magnitude images. The curve is decomposed into Fourier modes:

$$Q(t) = \sum_{n=0}^{N} Q_n e^{in\omega t}, \tag{57}$$

where N is the number of modes and ω is the angular frequency obtained from the period of the cardiac cycle. The velocity profile corresponding to this flow rate curve can be computed from the Womersley solution.[112] The Womersley profile is the analytic solution for a fully developed sinusoidally varying flow of an incompressible

Newtonian fluid in a rigid circular pipe. The velocity profile is then obtained as a superposition of Womersley solutions corresponding to each Fourier mode:[113]

$$v(r,t) = \frac{2Q_0}{\pi a^2}\left[1 - \left(\frac{r}{a}\right)^2\right] + \sum_{n=1}^{N}\frac{2Q_n}{\pi a^2}\left[\frac{1 - \dfrac{J_0(\beta_n r/a)}{J_0(\beta_n)}}{1 - \dfrac{2J_1(\beta_n)}{\beta_n J_0(\beta_n)}}\right]e^{in\omega t}, \qquad (58)$$

where

$$\beta_n = i^{3/2}\alpha_n = i^{3/2}\sqrt{\frac{n\omega}{\nu}} \qquad (59)$$

with α_n the Womersley number (a dimensionless parameter characterizing the frequency of the pulsatile flow) and ν the kinematic viscosity. In order to impose pulsatile flow boundary conditions, this velocity profile is mapped to the inflow boundary.

The flow division among different arterial branches is determined by the impedance of the distal arterial tree. Different authors have used different approaches for prescribing outflow boundary conditions, depending on the availability of flow measurements in the different branches of the models. The different options are: (a) impose traction free boundary conditions in all the model outlets with the implicit assumption that all vascular trees have the same impedance,[28,30] (b) impose flow divisions determined by the area ratio of the outflow vessels which implies that the distal impedance is proportional to the area,[44,48] (c) prescribe flow impedances computed from arterial tree models generated for each outflow boundary,[54,114,115] (d) couple the 3D simulations to 1D models of the systemic circulation,[116] and (e) impose flow rates measured in all the model outlets.[117,118]

At the vessel wall, the no-slip boundary condition implies that the fluid velocity must be equal to the velocity of the arterial wall. If the vessel walls are assumed rigid, this implies a zero velocity at the wall. Vessel wall compliance is an important effect that may alter the local hemodynamics. Vessel wall compliance can be incorporated into the models in two basic ways: (a) directly impose the motion of the vessel wall measured using dynamic imaging techniques such as 4D-CTA or high frame-rate biplane angiography,[119,120] and (b) perform coupled fluid-solid interaction simulations.[117,118,121–123] The former option is very attractive as recent advances in dynamic imaging modalities are making this possibility a reality. The latter option has several difficulties, such as a proper model for the solid or biomechanical modeling of the vessel wall, estimations of the distribution of the wall elasticity and thickness, estimation of the intra-arterial pressure waveform required for proper boundary condition specification, larger CPU requirements, etc. However, this approach can yield detailed biomechanical information useful for studying the interplay of hemodynamics and wall mechanobiology. Although the vessel walls are known to pulsate during the cardiac cycle, the effects on the hemodynamic are not well understood. Preliminary studies have shown differences between compliant and rigid models of cerebral aneurysms were found, but the overall intraaneurysmal flow pattern and wall shear stress distributions had similar characteristics.[119] It is not clear whether incorporating wall compliance into the numerical models is important for clinical purposes. This is an important question that needs further study.

2.5. *Flow modeling: post processing*

The results of CFD simulations are the velocity and pressure field at all the mesh nodes and the wall shear stress at all the nodes on the surface of the model, and for all time steps. This information is usually post-processed in order to compute clinically relevant quantities and to produce visualizations and animations that help us understand the complex unsteady flow patterns.

Since blood flows are periodic in time, in addition to the instantaneous values of hemodynamic variables, it is important to compute the time average and the variability during the cardiac cycle of the hemodynamic quantities. Typically the time average or mean wall shear stress is computed as:

$$\bar{\tau} = \int \tau \, dt = \int \sigma \cdot \mathbf{n} \, dt, \tag{60}$$

where σ is the strain rate tensor and $\mathbf{n}$ is the surface normal. The oscillatory shear index (OST) defined as:[124]

$$\text{OSI} = \frac{1}{2} \left(1 - \frac{|\bar{\tau}|}{|\overline{\tau}|} \right) \tag{61}$$

is a measure of the degree of angular deviation of the shear stress force with respect to the mean shear stress during the cardiac cycle.

A very useful technique to visualize the unsteady 3D flow fields in aneurysms is to produce particle animations. For this purpose, massless particles that move with the local flow velocity are used. The equation of motion for each particle is simply

$$\frac{d\mathbf{x}_i}{dt} = \mathbf{v}(\mathbf{x}_i, t), \tag{62}$$

where t is the time, $\mathbf{x}_i$ is the position of particle i and $\mathbf{v}$ is the fluid velocity field. These equations are integrated explicitly in time using a four stage Runge-Kutta scheme. Each particle is advected independently, therefore this scheme is very easy to parallelize. Assuming that the velocity field is periodic in time, only one cardiac cycle is stored. As the particles move, the velocity field is spatially interpolated to the position of the particles. Spatial interpolation on unstructured grids is efficiently performed using a neighbor-to-neighbor search algorithm to find the element that contains the particle.[125] Once this host element has been found, the velocity field is linearly interpolated to the particle position using the element shape functions evaluated at the particle position. If the host element is saved,

in the next time step the neighbor-to-neighbor search starts with the previous
host element and the new host element is typically found in one or two steps,
making this algorithm very efficient. Since the time intervals at which the flow
field was stored may be different from the timestep used to advect the particles,
it is also necessary to interpolate the velocity field to the current time of each
particle. This could be a linear interpolation between two fluid timesteps or a
higher order spline interpolation using more timesteps. The timestep used to move
a particle is computed from the condition that the particle does not move more
than a fraction of the current host element size. The element size is computed for
example as the minimum of the lengths of the edges of the host element. This
condition ensures that particles do not jump over mesh elements. In addition to
the hemodynamic variables (velocity, pressure, shear stress, etc.) interpolated from
the flow field to the particle positions, extra variables are computed as the particles
move through the flow field. These include the particle residence time (the time
elapsed from the particle injection to the current time), the length of the particle
path, etc. Variables such as the particle residence time are important for example
to identify regions of the flow field where thrombus formation or particle-wall
adhesion may take place. Examples of flow visualizations using particles are shown
in Fig. 3. The first example (top row) corresponds to an anterior communicating
artery aneurysm. In this case the particles were colored according to the injection
site in order to visualize the mixing of the two inflow jets from the left and right
ICA inside the aneurysm. The second example (bottom row) corresponds to a
giant aneurysm of the ICA. In this case the particles were colored according to
the residence time.

Another technique that is useful for visualizing intraaneurysmal flow structures
is the so called "virtual angiography".[126,127] The basic idea is to simulate the passage
of a bolus of contrast material or dye and visualize the filling and washout of the
vascular model. For this purpose, the flow velocity field is assumed periodic and
the solution for one cardiac cycle is stored. Using this unsteady velocity field $\mathbf{v}$, the
transport or advection-diffusion equation is solved in order to compute the evolution

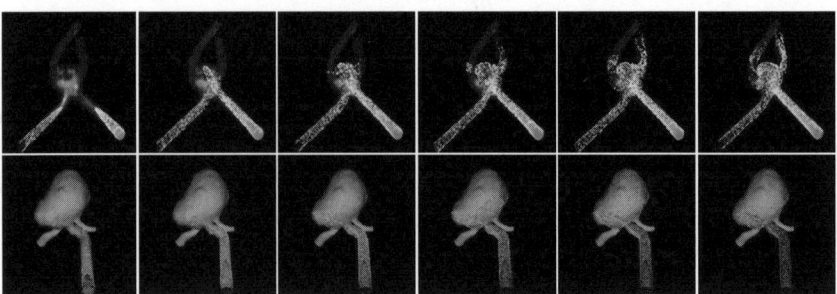

Fig. 3.   Example of particle animations in two aneurysm models. Top row: anterior communicating
artery aneurysm. Bottom row: internal carotid artery aneurysm.

of the dye concentration field C for several cardiac cycles:

$$\frac{\partial C}{\partial t} + \mathbf{v} \cdot \nabla C = k \nabla^2 C, \tag{63}$$

where k is a user defined diffusivity constant. At the inlet, a uniform concentration field is imposed as boundary condition. The time-dependence of this boundary condition simulates the injection of contrast material. At the model outlets, natural boundary conditions are prescribed. The solution of the transport equation is obtained using an implicit finite element formulation.[126] Once the dye concentration field is computed, volume rendering techniques are used to visualize the distribution of contrast material within the vascular model. In addition to providing flow information in a familiar way for Neuroradiologists, virtual angiograms can be used to compare numerical simulations to conventional angiograms.[127] These comparisons are useful to demonstrate that patient-specific CFD simulations can realistically reproduce flow structures observed *in vivo*. An example is presented in Fig. 4 for an ICA aneurysm model constructed from rotational angiography images. The 3DRA image and the vascular model are shown in the top panel from three different viewpoints. The bottom panel shows the concentration of the virtual dye at different instants of time during a simulated injection of approximately eight cardiac cycles. This sequence of images depicts the filling pattern of the aneurysm, the location and size of the inflow jet and flow impaction zone, and the primary intraaneurysmal flow structures.

2.6. *Flow modeling: visualization*

Anatomical images and models are usually visualized using volume rendering and surface rendering techniques. Volume renderings can be obtained via ray-casting or 3D texture mapping. Ray casting consists in computing the opacification of a light ray as it travels from a pixel in the screen through the volumetric image. Texture mapping techniques consist in rendering a series of polygonal surfaces (usually rectangles) from back to front with transparencies mapped from the volumetric

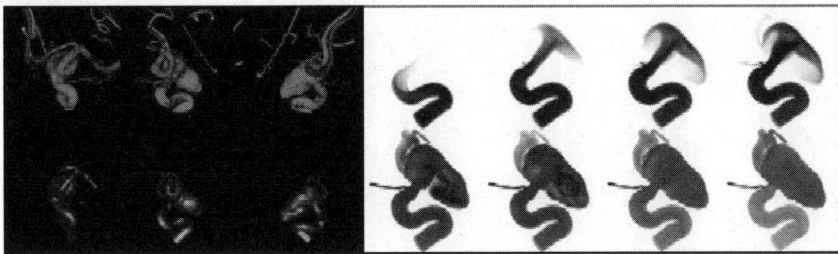

Fig. 4. Example of virtual angiography. Left panel: 3D rotational angiography image (top row) and anatomical model (bottom row) from three viewing points. Right panel: sequence of virtual angiography images showing the filling of the aneurysm with a simulated contrast agent.

image. Both techniques are view dependent and can become slow for large images. Anatomical surface models are directly rendered as shaded triangulations. Examples of volume renderings and surface renderings of anatomical images of cerebral aneurysms are shown in Figs. 1 and 2.

A variety of techniques can be used to visualize the blood flow patterns and distributions of hemodynamic forces. The distribution of wall shear stress (mean or instantaneous) and OSI are easily visualized as color mapped surfaces. Figures 5(b) and (c) show the mean WSS in a cerebral aneurysm from two viewpoints. Figures 5(e) and (f) show the distribution of OSI in the same model and from the same two viewpoints.

Understanding the intra-aneurysmal flow structure is usually more complicated. Streamlines rendered as illuminated ribbons are a powerful tool for understanding the aneurysmal flow patterns. Streamlines are computed by integrating $d\mathbf{x}/dt = \mathbf{v}$ starting from a set of initial positions interactively placed. The twist of the ribbons is computed from the rotation of the fluid elements (vorticity) along the streamlines. Propagating the streamlines from the initial positions forward and backwards in time simplifies the specification of the origins as they can be placed in the locations where one wants to see the flow structure and therefore it is not necessary to guess where these streamlines came from. An example is presented in Fig. 5(a). While streamlines give a good representation of the 3D flow field, they may fail to visualize flow features if the streamline origins are not placed at the correct location. The velocity distribution can also be visualized by cutting the computational domain

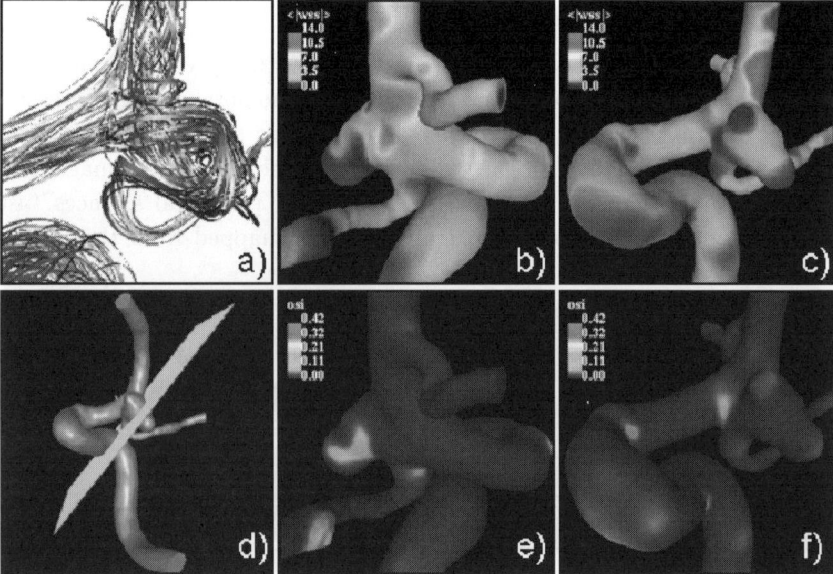

Fig. 5. Visualization examples: (a) streamlines at peak systole, (b,c) mean wall shear stress magnitude, (e,f) oscillatory shear index, (d) definition of a cut-plane for velocity visualization.

with a plane and interpolating the velocities to that plane. Then, the plane is rendered as a velocity color mapped shaded surface. Figure 5(d) shows the definition of a cut plane used to visualize the intra-aneurysmal velocity distribution, and Fig. 6 (top row) shows the velocity distribution on this plane at four instants of time during the cardiac cycle. These visualizations show in 2D the inflow jet and flow impaction zone. The time-dependent inflow jet is visualized in Fig. 6 (middle row) as a velocity iso-surface, at the same four instants during the cardiac cycle. These visualizations show a relatively flat inflow jet that enters the aneurysm through the distal part of the neck and spreads over a relatively large portion of the distal part of the aneurysm body. This region of flow impaction coincides with the region of highest wall shear stress in the aneurysm (Figs. 5(b) and (c)). The velocity pattern in the vicinity of the aneurysm wall can be visualized by first calculating an iso-surface of constant distance to the wall. This iso-surface is parallel to the aneurysm wall but at a constant distance towards the interior of the computational domain, where the velocity is non-zero. An example is shown in Fig. 6 (bottom row), for the same aneurysm and instants of time.

Another technique that can be used to visualize the flow structure in more detail is line integral convolution (LIC).[128–130] This technique was originally designed visualization of vector fields in 2D or on 3D surfaces. Extensions to 3D flow fields have also been developed. An example is presented in Fig. 7 for a bifurcation

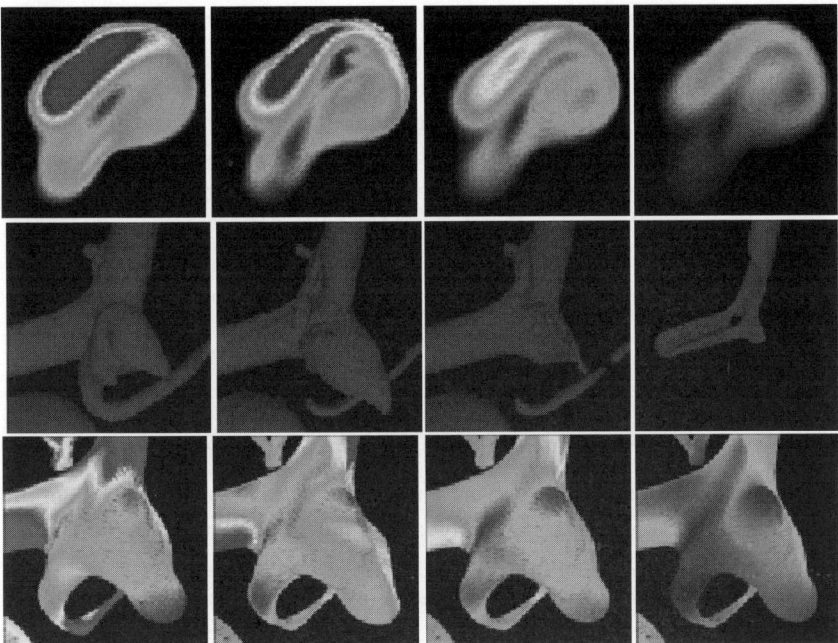

Fig. 6.   Unsteady visualization examples. Top row: velocity magnitudes on cut-plane shown in Figure 5 at four instants during the cardiac cycle. Middle row: iso-velocity surfaces at the same instants of time. Bottom row: velocity vectors on a surface near the vessel wall at the same times.

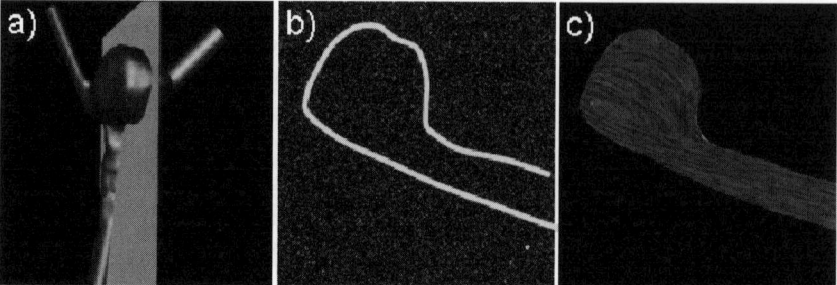

Fig. 7. Flow visualization using line integral convolution (LIC): (a) cut plane considered for 2D visualization of flow structure in a bifurcation aneurysm, (b) white noise image used as input for the LIC visualization – the yellow line indicates the region of the vascular model, (c) visualization of flow structure on the plane using LIC.

aneurysm. The basic idea of the method is as follows. A plane-cut is first computed for the 2D visualization of the flow field on this plane (Fig. 7(a)). Second, an image that covers the 2D domain is created and initialized with white noise, i.e. a uniform distribution of random gray values between 0 and 1 (Fig. 7(b)). Then, the image is locally smoothed along the streamlines. This is done by convolving the image with a Gaussian kernel that is locally displaced from the current pixel in the positive and negative velocity directions (along the local streamline). The new image is then texture mapped to the 2D geometry and rendered as a shaded surface. The result is a visualization of the local direction of the vector field (Fig. 7(c)). The advantage of this technique is that it yields a more dense visualization of the vector fields than streamlines since in a sense is similar to computing streamlines from each pixel in the image. Therefore, depending on the image resolution selected, small scale details of the vector fields can be effectively visualized. Animated LIC visualization techniques have also been developed in order to visualize not only the direction of flow but also its sense. Color mapped LIC methods can be used to visualize together with the direction and sense of the vector field some extra variable such as its magnitude.

3. Hemodynamics Simulations and Endovascular Devices

Computer models of blood flow past endovascular devices are useful for understanding the alterations in the hemodynamics patterns induced by deployment of such devices. This information is important for two main purposes: (a) designing better endovascular devices and (b) choosing the best treatment option for a particular patient, i.e. personalizing the treatment. In the former case, it may be enough to work with geometrically idealized models since one is interested in the general characteristics of the endovascular devices and the flow alterations they produce. However, in the latter case, it is necessary to model the patient-specific anatomy in order to understand the effects of different devices on the hemodynamic patterns of each individual patient.

Creating patient-specific models with endovascular devices is a challenging problem due to the high degree of geometric complexity. The main difficulty is that one needs to generate a volumetric grid filling the space inside the blood vessels and around the endovascular devices. In turn this requires a proper representation of the geometry (surface) of the computational domain. In addition to the difficulties associated with the construction of realistic vascular models from medical images, these two tasks are extremely difficult for a number of reasons: (a) it is necessary to construct a geometrical model that properly represents the intersection between the endovascular devices such as stents and the vessel walls, (b) devices such as coils can have extremely complex shapes that are in self contact thus creating topologically complex domains, (c) the contact between the devices and the vessel can create small gaps that are difficult to mesh and (d) creating a surface model of the device alone can be a challenging task in itself, etc.

The meshing problem is complicated if one is restricted to body fitted grids. These are grids that conform to the geometry of the computational domain. In other words, the surface of the computational grid coincides exactly with the surface of the computational domain (the vessel and the endovascular device). However, there are other possible computational approaches, namely grid embedding or immersed boundary methods. These methods are based on the idea of generating a mesh that *covers* the surface model, and then approximating the geometry by the external faces of the elements that are cut by the domain surface. These techniques are commonly used with finite difference solvers that require structured grids, by masking off grid points that fall outside the computational domain. These techniques have been combined with adaptive unstructured grids into hybrid approaches that are very flexible and can deal with the geometric complexity required for modeling blood flows past endovascular devices in realistic arterial modes.[57] A description of this approach is given below and example applications in the next section.

3.1. *Embedded grid techniques*

As seen before, the numerical solution of PDEs is usually accomplished by performing a spatial and temporal discretization with subsequent solution of a large algebraic system of equations. The transition from an arbitrary surface description to a proper mesh still represents a difficult task. This is particularly so when the surface description is based on data that does not originate from CAD-systems, such as data from medical imaging or fluid-structure interaction problems.

So far, the discussion has centered on grids that are body-conforming, i.e. grids where the external mesh faces match up with the surface (body surfaces, external surfaces, etc.) of the domain. The subsequent section will consider the case then elements and points do not match up perfectly with the body. Solvers or methods that employ these non body-conforming grids are known by a variety of names: embedded mesh, fictitious domain, immersed boundary, Cartesian method etc. The key idea is to place the bodies in the flow field (e.g. a medical device) inside the body-conforming mesh (or a large mesh surrounding all bodies), and treat the elements close to the immersed body surfaces so that the proper flow boundary conditions are enforced. At every timestep, the elements/edges/points close to the embedded/immersed surface are identified and proper boundary conditions are applied in their vicinity. While used extensively[131–135] this solution strategy also exhibits some shortcomings: (a) the boundary, which, in the absence of field sources has the most profound influence on the ensuing physics, is also the place where the worst elements/approximations are found, (b) near the boundary, the embedding boundary conditions need to be applied, reducing the local order of approximation for the PDE, (c) no stretched elements can be introduced to resolve boundary layers, (d) adaptivity is essential for most cases and (e) for problems with moving boundaries the information required to build the proper boundary conditions for elements close to the surface can take a considerable amount of time.

In nearly all cases reported to date, embedded or immersed boundary techniques were developed as a response to the treatment of problems with: (a) "dirty geometries",[132,133] (b) moving/sliding bodies with thin/vanishing gaps,[136,137] and (c) physics that can be handled with isotropic grids (potential flow, Euler, RANS/LES with law of the wall).

Two basic approaches have been proposed to modify field solvers in order to accommodate embedded surfaces. They are based on either kinetic or kinematics boundary conditions near the surface or inside the bodies in the fluid. The first type applies an equivalent balancing force to the flow field in order to achieve the kinematic boundary required at the embedded surface or within the embedded domain.[135,137] The second approach is to apply kinematic boundary conditions at the nodes close to the embedded surface.[132,133]

It may appear somewhat contradictory to even consider a general unstructured grid solver in conjunction with surface embedding. Most of the work carried out to date was in conjunction with Cartesian solvers,[131–134] the argument being that flux evaluations could be optimized due to coordinate alignment. However, the achievable gains of such coordinate alignment may be limited due to the following mitigating factors: (a) for most of the high resolution schemes the cost of limiting and the approximate Riemann solver far outweigh the cost of the few scalar products required for arbitrary edge orientation, (b) the fact that any of these schemes (Cartesian, unstructured) requires mesh adaptation in order to be successful immediately implies the use of indirect addressing; given current trends in microchip design, indirect addressing, present in both types of solvers, may outweigh all other factors and (c) three specialized (x, y, z) edge-loops versus one general edge-loop, and the associated data reorganization implies an increase in software maintenance costs.

For a general unstructured grid solver, surface embedding represents just another addition in a toolbox of mesh handling techniques (mesh movement, overlapping grids, remeshing, h-refinement, deactivation, etc.), and one that allows to treat "dirty geometry" problems with surprising ease. It also allows for a combination of different surface treatment options. A good example where this was used very effectively is the modeling of endovascular devices such as coils and stents.[57] The arterial vessels were gridded using a body-fitted unstructured grid while the endovascular devices were treated via an embedded technique.

In what follows, we denote by CSD faces the surface of the computational domain that is embedded. We implicitly assume that this information is given by a triangulation, which typically is obtained from a CAD package via STL files, remote sensing data, medical images or from a CSD code (hence the name) in coupled fluid-structure applications. For immersed methods we assume that the embedded object is given by a tetrahedral mesh.

3.1.1. *Kinetic treatment of embedded objects*

As stated before, one way of treating embedded objects is via the addition of suitable force-functions that let the fluid "feel" the presence of the surface, and push away any fluid trying to penetrate the same. If we consider a rigid, closed body, as sketched in Fig. 8, an obvious aim is to enforce, within the body, the condition $\mathbf{v} = \mathbf{v}_b$. This may be accomplished by applying a force term of the form:

$$\mathbf{f} = -c_0(\mathbf{v}_b - \mathbf{v}) \tag{64}$$

for points that are inside of the body. This particular type of force function is known as the penalty force technique.[138]

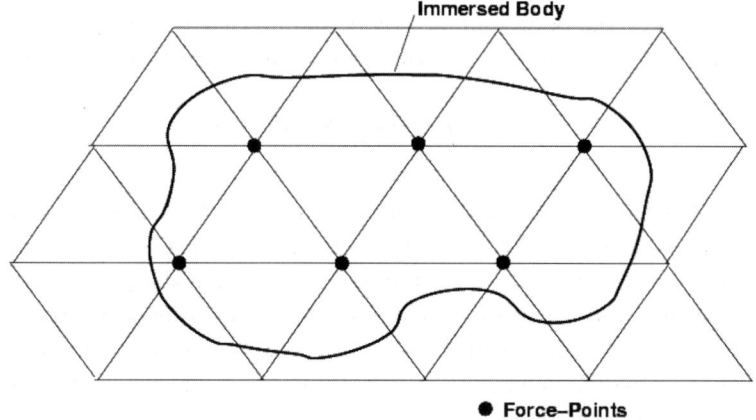

Fig. 8.   Kinetic treatment of embedded surfaces.

Of course, other functional forms of $\mathbf{v}_b - \mathbf{v}$ are possible, e.g. the quadratic form:

$$\mathbf{f} = -c_0|\mathbf{v}_b - \mathbf{v}|(\mathbf{v}_b - \mathbf{v}) \tag{65}$$

exponential forms, etc. The damping characteristics in time for the relaxation of a current velocity to the final state will vary, but the basic idea is the same. The advantage of the simple linear form given by Eq. (64) is that a point-implicit integration of the velocities is possible, i.e. the stiffness of the large coefficient c_0 can be removed with no discernable increase in operations.[137] The main problem with force fields given by Eqs. (64) and (65) is the choice of the constants c_0. Values that are too low do not allow the flow to adjust rapidly enough to the body, values that are too high may produce artificial stiffness. Moreover, for body motions that are not completely divergence-free a large pressure buildup is observed (see Ref. 137 for a case of lobe-pumps). A major improvement was put forward by Ref. 138, who proposed to evaluate first the usual right-hand side for the flow equations at immersed points (or cells), and then add a force such that the velocity at the next timestep would satisfy the kinematic boundary conditions. Writing the spatially discretized form of the momentum equations at each point (or cell) i as:

$$\mathbf{M}\frac{\Delta \mathbf{v}_i}{\Delta t} = \mathbf{r}_i + \mathbf{f}_i, \quad \mathbf{f}_i = \mathbf{M}\frac{\mathbf{w}_i^{n+1} - \mathbf{v}_i^n}{\Delta t} - \mathbf{r}_i. \tag{66}$$

Here $\mathbf{w}_i$ denotes the velocity of the immersed body at the location of point (or cell) i, and n the timestep. For explicit time-stepping schemes, this force function in effect imposes the (required) velocity of the immersed body at the new timestep. Schemes of this kind have been used repeatedly in conjunction with fractional step/projection methods for incompressible flow. In this case, while the kinematic boundary condition $\mathbf{v}^{n+1} = \mathbf{w}^{n+1}$ is enforced strictly by Eq. (66) in the advective-diffusive prediction step, during the pressure correction step the condition is relaxed, offering the possibility of imposing the kinematic boundary conditions in a "soft" way.

For cases where the bodies are not rigid, and all that is given is the embedded surface triangulation and movement, the force-terms added take the general form:

$$\mathbf{f} = \int_\Gamma \mathbf{F}\,\delta(\mathbf{x} - \mathbf{X}_\Gamma)\,d\Gamma, \tag{67}$$

where Γ denotes the location of the embedded surface, $\mathbf{X}_\Gamma$ the nearest embedded surface point to point $\mathbf{x}$ and $\mathbf{F}$ is the force. In theory, the $\mathbf{F}$ should be applied to the fluid using a Dirac delta function δ in order to obtain a sharp interface. In most cases the influence of this delta-function is smeared over several grid points, giving rise to different methods. If instead of a surface we are given the volume of the immersed body, then the penalization force may be applied at each point of the flow mesh that falls into the body.

While simple to program and employ, the force-based enforcement is particularly useful if the "body thickness" covers several CFD mesh elements.

This is because the pressures obtained are continuous across the embedded surface/immersed body. This implies that for thin embedded surfaces such as shells, where the pressure is different on both sides, this method will not yield satisfactory results.

The search operations required for the imposition of kinetic boundary conditions can be performed as follows:

- Initialization:
  - Store all CFD mesh points in a bin, octree, or any other similar data structure;
- Loop over the immersed body elements:
  - Determine the bounding box of the element;
  - Find all points in the bounding box;
  - Detailed analysis to determine the shape function values.

If the immersed body only covers a small portion of the CFD domain, one can reduce the list of points stored or points checked via the bounding box of all immersed body points. This approach is easily parallelized on shared memory machines.

3.1.2. *Kinematic treatment of embedded surfaces*

Embedded surfaces may be alternatively be treated by applying kinematic boundary conditions at the nodes close to the embedded surface. Depending on the required order of accuracy and simplicity, a first or second-order (higher-order) scheme may be chosen to apply the kinematic boundary conditions. Figure 9 illustrates the basic difference between these approaches. Note that in both cases the treatment of infinitely thin surfaces with fluid on both sides (e.g. fluid-structure interaction simulations) is straightforward.

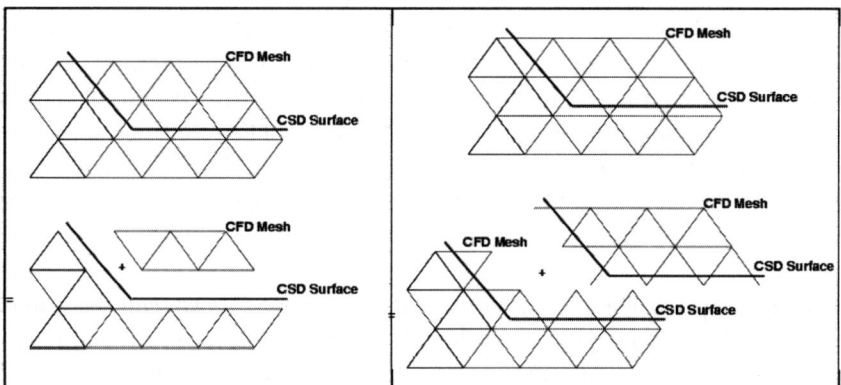

Fig. 9. Treatment of embedded surfaces. Left panel: first order treatment. Right panel: second order treatment.

A first-order scheme can be achieved by:

- Eliminating the edges crossing the embedded surface;
- Forming boundary coefficients to achieve flux balance;
- Applying boundary conditions for the end-points of the crossed edges based on the normals of the embedded surface.

A second-order scheme can be achieved by:

- Duplicating the edges crossing the embedded surface;
- Duplicating the end-points of crossed edges;
- Applying boundary conditions for the end-points of the crossed edges based on the normals of the embedded surface.

Note that in either case CFD edges crossed by CSD faces are modified/ duplicated. Given that an edge/face crossing is essentially the same in 2D and 3D, these schemes are rather general.

The following sections describe in more detail each one of the steps required, as well as near-optimal techniques to realize them.

3.1.3. *Determination of crossed edges*

Given the CSD triangulation and the CFD mesh, the first step is to find the CFD edges cut by CSD faces. This is performed by building a fast spatial search data structure, such as an octree or a bin for the CSD faces. Without loss of generality, let us assume an octree for the CSD faces. Then, a (parallel) loop is performed over the edges. For each edge, the bounding box of the edge is built. From the octree, all the faces in the region of the bounding box are found. This is followed by an in-depth test to determine which faces cross the given edge. The crossing face closest to each of the edge end-nodes is stored. This allows resolving cases of thin gaps or cusps. Once the faces crossing edges are found, the closest face to the end-points of crossed edges is also stored. This information is required to apply boundary conditions for the points close to the embedded surface. For cases where the embedded surfaces only cut a small portion the CFD edges, a considerable speedup may be realized by removing from the list of edges tested all those that fall outside the global bounding box of the CSD faces. The resulting list of edges to be tested in depth may be reduced further by removing all edges whose bounding boxes do not fall into an octree or bin covering that spatial region. One typically finds that the list of edges to be tested in detail has been reduced by an order of magnitude.

For transient problems, the procedure described above can be improved considerably. The key assumption is that the CSD triangulation will not move over more than 1–2 elements during a timestep. If the topology of the CSD triangulation has not changed, the crossed-edge information from the previous timestep can be re-checked. The points of edges no longer crossed by a face crossing them in the previous timestep are marked, and the neighboring edges are checked for crossing. If the topology of the CSD triangulation has changed, the crossed-edge information from the previous timestep is no longer valid. However, the points close to cut edges in the previous timestep can be used to mark 1–2 layers of edges. Only these edges are then re-checked for crossing.

3.1.4. *First order treatment*

The first order scheme is the simplest to implement. Given the CSD triangulation and the CFD mesh, the CFD edges cut by CSD faces are found and deactivated. Considering an arbitrary field point i, the time-advancement of the unknowns $\mathbf{u}^i$ for an explicit edge-based time integration scheme is given by:

$$M^i \Delta \mathbf{u}^i = \Delta t \sum_j C^{ij} (F_i + F_j). \tag{68}$$

Here C, F, M denote, respectively, the edge-coefficients, fluxes and mass-matrix. For any edge ij crossed by a CSD face, the coefficients C^{ij} are set to zero. This implies that for a uniform state $\mathbf{u} = \text{const.}$ the balance of fluxes for interior points with cut edges will not vanish. This is remedied by defining a new boundary point to impose total/normal velocities, as well as adding a "boundary contribution", resulting in:

$$M^i \Delta \mathbf{u}^i = \Delta t \left[\sum_j C^{ij} (F_i + F_j) + C_\Gamma^i F_i \right]. \tag{69}$$

The point-coefficients C_Γ^i are obtained from the condition that $\Delta \mathbf{u} = 0$ for $\mathbf{u} = \text{const.}$ Given that gradients (e.g. for limiting) are constructed using a loop of the form:

$$M^i \mathbf{g}^i = \sum_j C^{ij} (\mathbf{u}_i + \mathbf{u}_j) \tag{70}$$

it would be desirable to build the C_Γ^i coefficients in such a way that the constant gradient of a linear function $\mathbf{u}$ can be obtained exactly. However, this is not possible, as the number of coefficients is too small. Therefore, the gradients at the boundary are either set to zero or extrapolated from the interior of the domain.

The mass-matrix M^i of points surrounded by cut edges must be modified to reflect the reduced volume due to cut elements. The simplest possible modification of M^i is given by the so-called "cut edge fraction" method (see Fig. 10).

In a pass over the edges, the smallest "cut edge fraction" ξ for all the edges surrounding a point is found. The modified mass-matrix is then given by:

$$M_*^i = \frac{1 + \xi_{\min}}{2} M^i \tag{71}$$

Note that the value of the modified mass-matrix can never fall below half its original value, implying that timestep sizes will always be acceptable.

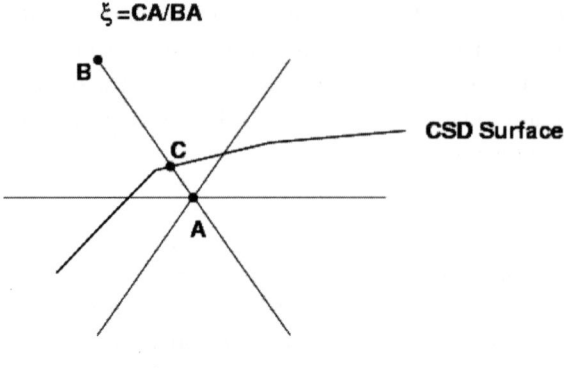

Fig. 10.   Cut edge fraction method.

For the new boundary points belonging to cut edges the proper PDE boundary conditions are required. In the case of flow solvers, these are either an imposed velocity or an imposed normal velocity. For limiting and higher-order schemes, one may also have to impose boundary conditions on the gradients. The required surface normal and boundary velocity are obtained directly from the closest CSD face to each of the new boundary points.

These low-order boundary conditions may be improved by extrapolating the velocity from the surface with field information. The location where the flow velocity is equal to the surface velocity is the surface itself, and not the closest boundary point. As shown in Fig. 11 (top panel), for each boundary point the closest point on the CSD face is found. Then, two (three) neighboring field

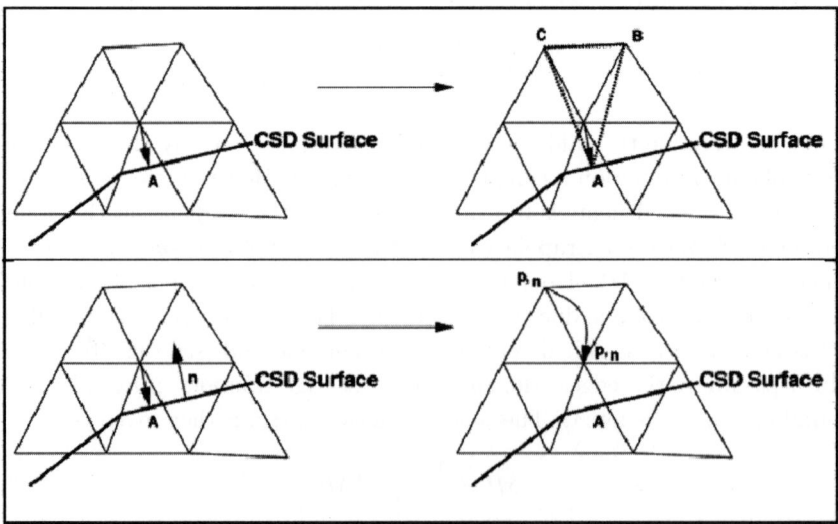

Fig. 11.   Top panel: extrapolation of velocity. Bottom panel: extrapolation of normal pressure gradient.

(i.e. non-boundary) points are found and a triangular (tetrahedral) element that contains the boundary point is formed. The velocity imposed at the field point is then found by interpolation. In this way, the boundary velocity "lags" the field velocities by one timestep.

The normal gradients at the boundary points can be improved by considering the "most aligned" field (i.e. non-boundary) point to the line formed by the boundary point and the closest point on the CSD face (see Fig. 11 – bottom panel).

3.1.5. *Higher order treatment*

As stated before, a higher-order treatment of embedded surfaces may be achieved by using ghost points or mirrored points to compute the contribution of the crossed edges to the overall solution. This approach presents the advantage of not requiring the modification of the mass matrix as all edges (even the crossed ones) are taken into consideration. It also does not require an extensive modification of the various solvers. On the other hand, it requires more memory due to duplication of crossed edges and points, as well as (scalar) CPU time for renumbering/reordering arrays. Particularly for moving body problems, this may represent a considerable CPU burden.

By duplicating the edges, the points are treated in the same way as in the original (non-embedded) case. The boundary conditions are imposed indirectly by mirroring and interpolating the unknowns as required. Figure 12 depicts the contribution due to the edges surrounding point i. A CSD boundary crosses the CFD domain. In this particular situation point j, which lies on the opposite side of the CSD face, will have to use the flow values of its mirror image j' based on the crossed CSD face.

The flow values of the mirrored point are then interpolated from the element the point resides in using the following formulation for the Euler (gliding wall) case:

$$p_m = p_i, \quad \mathbf{v}_m = \mathbf{v}_i - 2[(\mathbf{v}_i - \mathbf{w}_{csd}) \cdot \mathbf{n}]\,\mathbf{n}, \tag{72}$$

where $\mathbf{w}_{csd}$ is the average velocity of the crossed CSD face, $\mathbf{v}$ the flow velocity, p the pressure and $\mathbf{n}$ the unit surface normal of the face. Proper handling of the

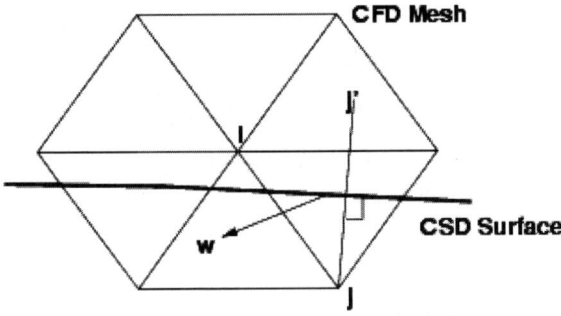

Fig. 12.   Higer order boundary conditions.

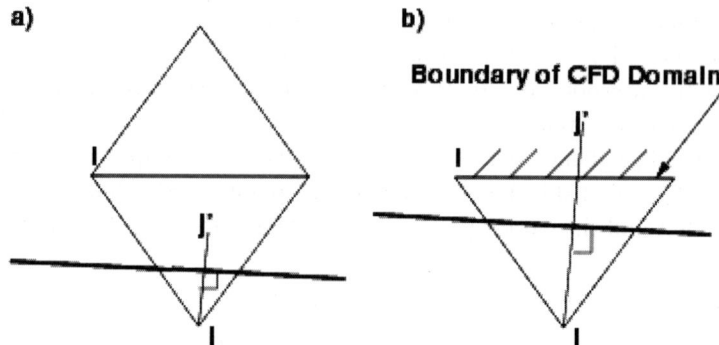

Fig. 13.   Problematic cases: (a) element used for interpolation crossed, (b) no available element for interpolation.

interpolation is also required as the element used for the interpolation might either be crossed (Fig. 13(a)) or not exist (Fig. 13(b)).

A more accurate formulation of the mirrored pressure and density can also be used taking into account the local radius of curvature of the CSD wetted surface:

$$p_m = p_i - \rho_i \frac{[\mathbf{v}_i - (\mathbf{v}_i - \mathbf{w}_{csd}) \cdot \mathbf{n}]^2}{R_i} \Delta \tag{73}$$

where R_i is the radius of curvature and Δ the distance between the point and its mirror image. This second formulation is more complex and requires the computation of the two radii (3D) of curvature at each CSD point. The radius of curvature plays an important role for large elements but this influence can be diminished by the use of automatic h-refinement.

For problematic cases such as the one shown in Fig. 14 the interpolation will be such that the point at which the information is interpolated may not be located at the same normal distance from the wall as the point where information is required.

With the notation of Fig. 14, and assuming a linear interpolation of the velocities, the velocity values for the viscous (i.e. no-slip) case are interpolated as:

$$\mathbf{w} = (1 - \xi_\omega)\mathbf{v}_c + \xi_\omega \mathbf{v}_i, \quad \xi_\omega = \frac{h_0}{h_0 + h_i}, \tag{74}$$

i.e.

$$\mathbf{v}_c = \frac{1}{1 - \xi_\omega}\mathbf{w} - \frac{\xi_\omega}{1 - \xi_\omega}\mathbf{v}_i. \tag{75}$$

Here $\mathbf{w}$ is the average velocity of the crossed CSD face, $\mathbf{v}_i$ the interpolated flow velocity and the distance factor $\xi_\omega < 0.5$.

3.1.6. *Deactivation of interior regions*

For highly distorted CSD surfaces, or for CSD surfaces with thin reentrant corners, all edges surrounding a given point may be crossed by CSD faces (see Fig. 15). The best way to treat such points is to simply deactivate them.

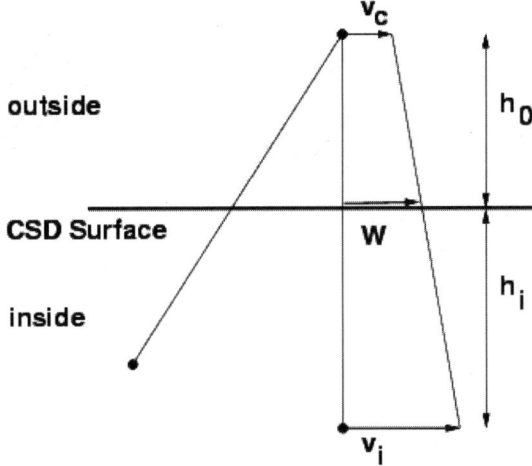

Fig. 14.   Navier-Stokes boundary conditions.

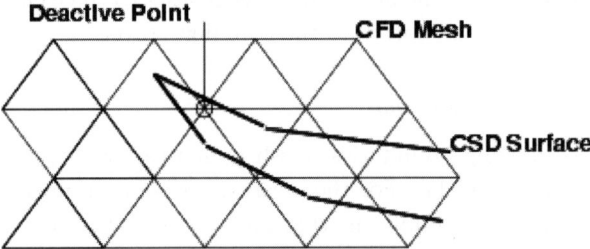

Fig. 15.   Deactivation of CFD interior points that are inside the embedded surfaces.

This deactivation concept can be extended further in order to avoid unnecessary work for regions inside solid objects. Two approaches were pursued in this direction: seed points and automatic deactivation.

(a) *Seed Points*: In this case, the user specifies a point inside an object. The closest CFD field point to this so-called seed point is then obtained. Starting from this point, additional points are added using an advancing front (nearest neighbor layer) algorithm, and flagged as inactive. The procedure stops once points that are attached to crossed edges have been reached.

(b) *Automatic Deactivation*: For complex geometries with moving surfaces, the manual specification of seed points becomes impractical. An automatic way of determining which regions correspond to the flow field one is trying to compute and which regions correspond to solid objects immersed in it is then required. The algorithm employed starts from the edges crossed by embedded surfaces. For the end-points of these edges an in/outside determination is attempted. This is non-trivial, particularly for thin or folded surfaces (Fig. 16). A more reliable way to determine whether a point is in/outside the flow field is obtained by storing, for the

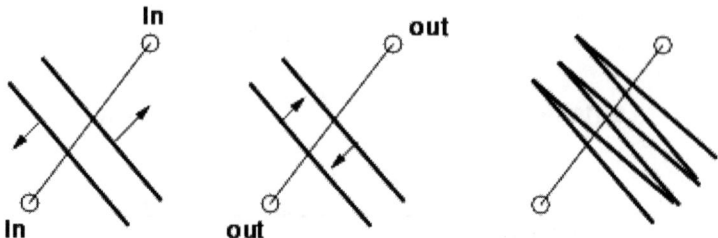

Fig. 16.   Edges with multiple crossing faces.

crossed edges, the faces closest to the end-points of the edge. Once this in/outside determination has been done for the end-points of crossed edges, the remaining points are marked using an advancing front algorithm. It is important to remark that in this case both the inside (active) and outside (deactive) points are marked at the same time. In the case of a conflict, preference is always given to mark the points as inside the flow domain (active). Once the points have been marked as active/inactive, the element and edge-groups required for vectorization are inspected in turn. The idea is to move the active/inactive if-tests to the element/edge-groups level in order to simplify and speed up the core flow solver.

3.1.7. Extrapolation of the solution

For problems with moving boundaries, mesh points can switch from one side of a surface to another (see Fig. 17). For these cases, the solution must be extrapolated from the proper state. The conditions that have to be met for extrapolation are as follows:

- The edge was crossed at the previous timestep and is no longer crossed;
- The edge has one field point (the point donating unknowns) and one boundary point (the point receiving unknowns); and
- The CSD face associated with the boundary point is aligned with the edge.

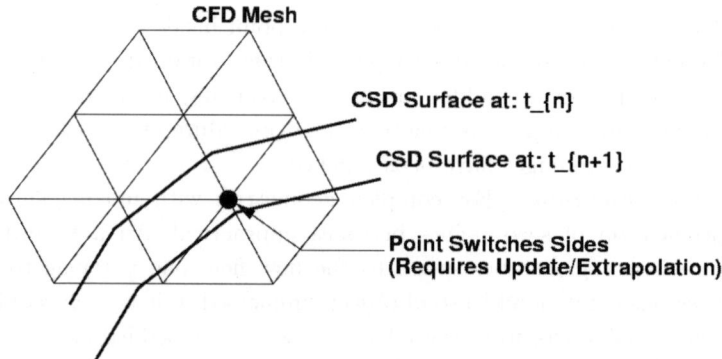

Fig. 17.   Extrapolation of solution.

3.1.8. *Adaptive mesh refinement*

Adaptive mesh refinement is very often used to reduce CPU and memory requirements without compromising the accuracy of the numerical solution. For transient problems with moving discontinuities, adaptive mesh refinement has been shown to be an essential ingredient of production codes. For embedded CSD triangulations, the mesh can be refined automatically close to the surfaces. This has been done in the present case by including two additional refinement indicators (on top of the usual ones based on the flow variables). The first one looks at the edges cut by CSD faces, and refines the mesh to a certain element size or refinement level. The second, more sophisticated indicator, looks at the surface curvature, and refines the mesh only in regions where the element size is deemed insufficient.

3.1.9. *Direct link to particles*

One of the most promising ways to treat discontinuous media is via so-called discrete element methods (DEMs) or discrete particle methods (DPMs). A considerable amount of work has been devoted to this area in the last two decades, and these techniques are being used for the prediction of soil, masonry, concrete and particulates.[139] The filling of space with objects of arbitrary shape has also reached the maturity of advanced unstructured grid generators[140] opening the way for widespread use with arbitrary geometries. Adaptive embedded grid techniques can be linked to DPMs in a very natural way. The discrete particle is represented as a sphere. Discrete elements, such as polyhedra, may be represented as an agglomeration of spheres. The host element for each one of the discrete particles is updated every timestep and is assumed as given. All points of host elements are marked for additional boundary conditions. The closest particle to each of these points is used as a marker. Starting from these points, all additional points covered by particles are marked (see Fig. 18).

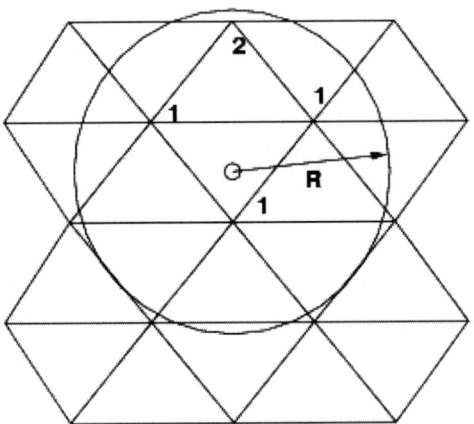

Fig. 18.   Link to discrete particle methods.

All edges touching any of the marked points are subsequently marked as crossed. From this point onwards, the procedure reverts back to the usual embedded mesh technique. The velocity of particles is imposed at the endpoints of crossed edges.

4. Numerical Examples

In this section a number of computer simulations of blood flows past endovascular devices are provided. The examples provided range from simple idealistic geometries to complex patient-specific geometries with endovascular devices. These examples show that grid embedding and immersed boundary methods yield results consistent with body fitted grids and that they can readily be used for device design and treatment personalization.

4.1. *Flow past a circular cylinder*

The first example consists in the flow past a circular cylinder. This example was chosen because of its simplicity and the availability of experimental results that can be used to estimate the accuracy of the numerical models.[141] The problem was solved with the three approaches: (a) a body conforming grid, (b) embedded grids and (c) immersed boundary methods. For the embedded and immersed approaches, different levels of mesh refinement were considered in order to assess the grid resolution needed to achieve an accurate solution. The diameter of the cylinder was 0.01 cm. This dimension was chosen to match those of typical endovascular devices. Blood was modeled as a Newtonian incompressible fluid, and the kinematic viscosity was set to $\nu = 0.04\,\mathrm{cm}^2/\mathrm{s}$. With a typical aneurysmal inflow velocity of 100 cm/s these parameters yield a Reynold's number of $\mathrm{Re} = 25$.

The geometry of the domain and the computational grids used for the numerical simulations are shown in Fig. 19(a), (b) and (c). Visualizations of the velocity distributions obtained with each method are also presented in Fig. 19(d), (e) and (f). Figure 19 also shows a superposition of velocity contours obtained with the body fitted grid and contours obtained with embedded grids after two (g) and four (h) levels of mesh refinement. It can be seen that the velocity field obtained with the embedded approach closely match the velocity field obtained with body fitted grids.

The value of the drag coefficient for a circular cylinder at $\mathrm{Re} = 25$ was measured experimentally.[141] A comparison of the drag coefficient obtained with the body fitted method and with the grid embedding technique with different levels of mesh refinement are is presented in Table 1. This table also lists the relative errors with respect to the experimental value. It can be seen that the relative error decreases as the number of mesh refinement levels is increased.

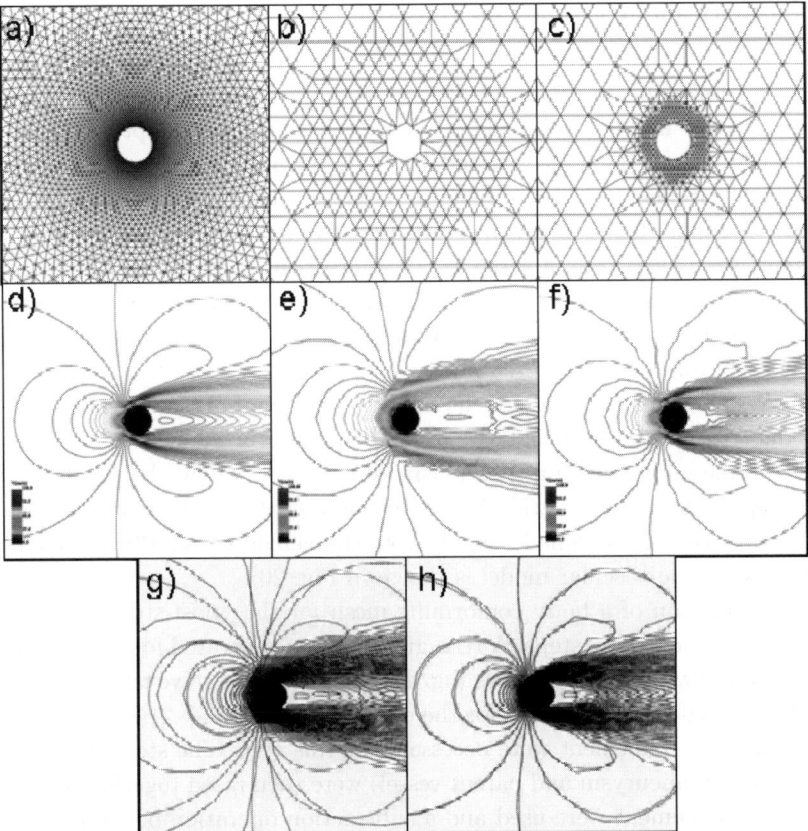

Fig. 19. (a) body fitted grid, (b) embedded grid after two levels of refinement, (c) embedded grid after four levels of refinement, (d) velocity contours obtained on the body conforming grid, (e) velocity contours computed on the embedded grid with two levels of refinement, (f) velocity contours computed on the embedded grid with four levels of refinement, (g) superposition of velocity contours of the body fitted grid and embedded after two refinement levels, (h) superposition of velocity contours of the body fitted grid and embedded after four refinement levels.

Table 1. Drag coefficient for a circular cylinder at $\mathrm{Re} = 25$ and relative errors with respect to experimental value obtained with the grid embedding technique for different levels of grid refinement.

Experiment	1.8597					
Body fitted	1.8437					
Error	0.85%					
Embedded						
Refinement level	2	3	4	5	6	7
Drag coefficient	2.1323	2.0699	1.9132	1.8727	1.8876	1.8536
Error	14.7%	11.3%	2.9%	0.7%	1.5%	0.3%

4.2. *Idealized aneurysm stenting model*

The second example corresponds to stenting of an idealized aneurysm that was constructed following the work of Stuhne *et al.*[142] In this case, flow calculations were carried out using a body conforming mesh as well as adaptive unstructured grid embedding and immersive boundary methods. The parent vessel was modeled as a straight circular cylinder of 0.35 cm diameter. The aneurysm was modeled as a sphere of radius 0.466 cm displaced 0.4 cm from the axis of the parent vessel. The stent was modeled as a series of 12 intersecting helices of 0.01 cm thickness (diameter of the wires) and 0.5 cm long. The helices were regularly distributed along the circumference of the parent vessel with alternating directions of rotation, and one turn from one end to the other.

The vascular model of the aneurysm and the parent vessel was constructed by fusing the triangulations of the cylinder and the sphere. This was carried out with the surface merging algorithm previously described using two levels of refinement of the adaptive background grid. A finite element grid was generated for this "pre-stent" configuration contained roughly 760,000 elements and 138,000 nodes. The construction of the vascular model is shown in Fig. 20.

The generation of a body conforming mesh for the "post-stent" configuration consisted in the following steps. A triangulation was generated for each of the wires of the stent following each helix (see Fig. 21(a)). Then, all twelve triangulations were fused into a single surface model for the entire stent (see Fig. 21(b)). Four levels of background grid refinement were necessary for this step. The stent model and the vascular model (aneurysm and parent vessel) were then fused together. In this case, six levels of refinement were used and a subtraction operation between the surface triangulations was used instead of the union operation used previously. The resulting surface triangulation, was smoothed and used as the final geometric model. A finite element grid was then generated using this geometric model. The element size distribution was specified by using line sources along the axis of each stent wire. For a line source, the element size at a given position in space is computed as an analytic function of the distance to the line segment. The final grid contained approximately 10.2 million tetrahedral elements and 1.8 million nodes (see Fig. 21(c–f). Although illustrated with an idealized case, this procedure for constructing finite element grids

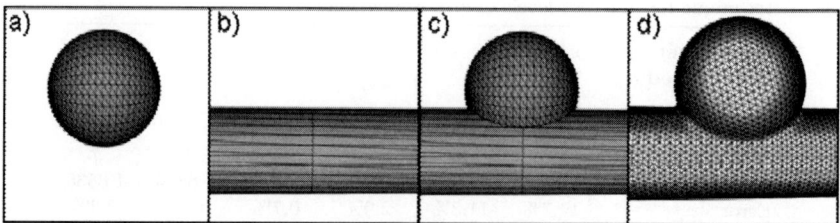

Fig. 20.   Idealized stent model: (a) aneurysm model, (b) vessel model, (c) superposed aneurysm and vessel models, (d) finite element grid.

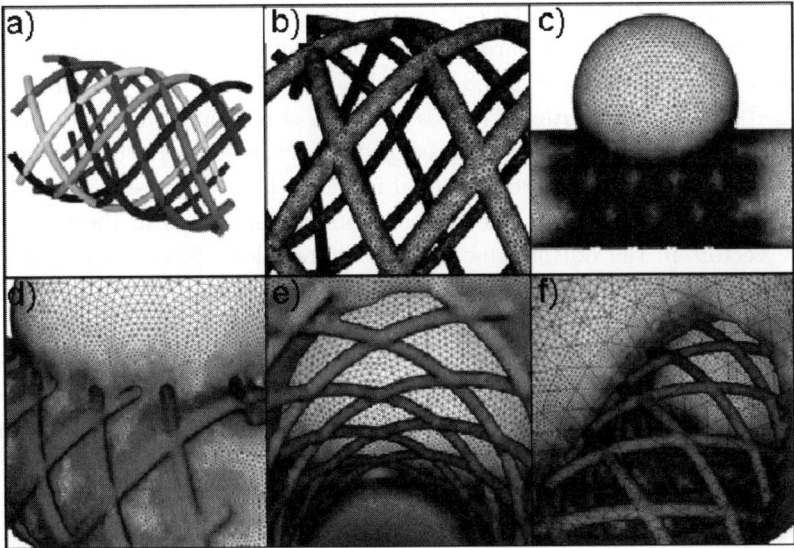

Fig. 21.   Construction of body conforming grid for idealized stented aneurysm: (a) stent components, (b) stent surface model, (c) finite element grid, (d,e,f) details of body fitted grid.

of stented aneurysms is general and can in principle be applied to patient-specific models.

A second representation of the stent geometry was constructed for flow calculations using embedded and immersed grid methods. In this case, the stent was simply modeled as a sequence of overlapping spheres or beads along each helix (Fig. 22(a–b)). The "pre-stent" grid was then adaptively refined around the stent. For this purpose, the edges of the grid cut by the spheres representing the stent were identified and the tetrahedral elements connected to these edges were marked for refinement. Groups of elements entirely surrounded by cut edges are removed from the grid for the embedded approach (see Fig. 22(c)). In contrast, in the immersed approach these elements are kept but represent physically disconnected domains (Fig. 22(d)). The embedded and grid contained approximately 2.8 million elements and 506,000 nodes.

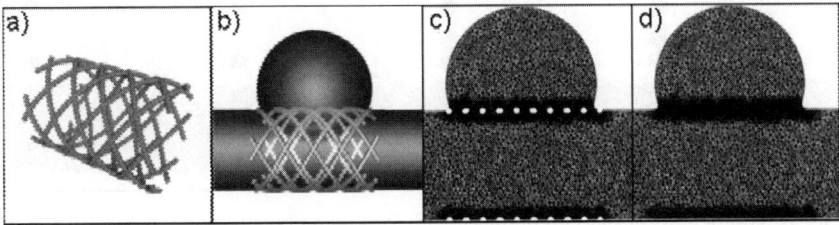

Fig. 22.   Embedded aneurysm model: (a) stent model constructed as beads of spheres, (b) stent in vascular model, (c) cut through mesh used for embedded simulation, (d) cut through mesh used for immersed simulation.

A total of four CFD calculations were performed under steady flow conditions before and after stenting. A parabolic velocity profile was prescribed at the inlet corresponding to a flow rate of 4.8 ml/s. Traction-free boundary conditions were prescribed at the model outlet. The post-stenting simulations were performed with the body fitted, embedded and immersed grid approaches. For the case of embedded and immersed grids, results are presented for three levels of mesh refinement. The results are shown in Fig. 23. Velocity contours are presented in the top row and velocity vectors in the bottom row. In this figure, blood flows from right to left. In the pre-stent configuration (Fig. 23(a,e)) the inflow zone is located at the distal end of the aneurysm neck and the intraaneurysmal flow pattern is dominated by a single vortex structure rotating in the clockwise direction. The post-stenting flow patterns obtained with the different approaches are in very good agreement (Fig. 23(b–d) and (f–h)). These results are in agreement with those obtained by Stuhne et al. using body fitted grids.[142] It is interesting to note that after the stent deployment, the inflow zone is located at the proximal end of the aneurysm neck and the intraaneurysmal flow circulates in the counter-clockwise direction. This observation is consistent with similar results obtained by Lieber *et al.*[24] with PIV techniques on idealized *in vitro* models.

4.3. *Idealized model of stented perforating artery*

This example illustrates the use the adaptive unstructured grid embedding technique for studying the flow reduction in a perforating artery after deployment of a micro-porous stent. The anatomical model was constructed by fusing a cylinder of 0.3 cm in diameter representing a cerebral artery with another cylinder of 0.03 cm

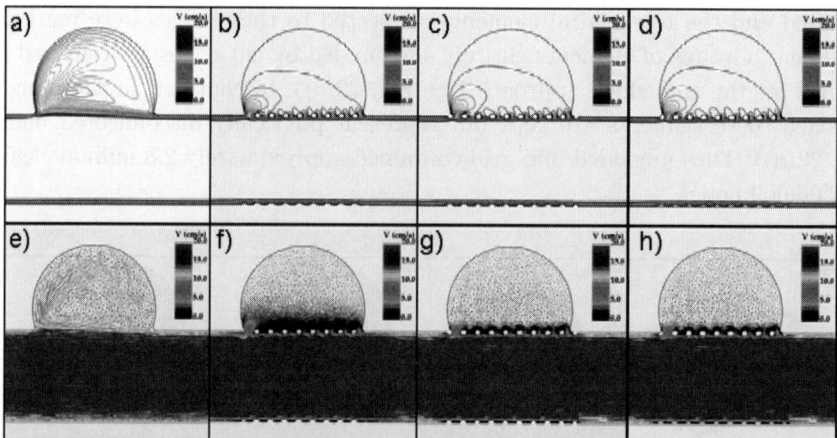

Fig. 23.   Results of flow calculations obtained with the different approaches: (a) velocity contours – body fitted (pre-stenting), (b) velocity contours – body fitted, (c) velocity contours – embedded, (d) velocity contours – immersed, (e) velocity vectors – body fitted (pre-stenting), (f) velocity vectors – body fitted, (g) velocity vectors – embedded, (h) velocity vectors – immersed.

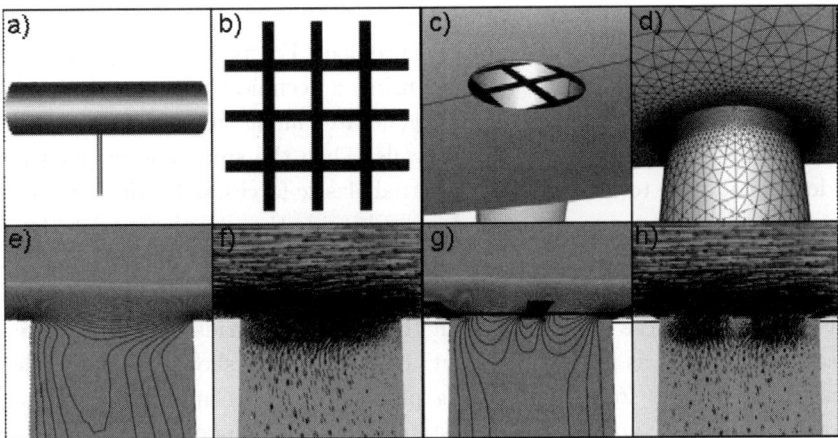

Fig. 24. Simulation of flow reduction in perforating artery by micro-porous stent: (a) vascular model, (b) stent design, (c) occlusion of perforating artery by stent, (d) detail of the finite element grid, (e) velocity contours before stent deployment, (f) velocity vectors before stent deployment, (g) velocity contours after stent deployment, (f) velocity vectors after stent deployment.

diameter branching off at a right angle representing the perforating artery. The stent consisted in squared holes of 0.01 cm and the strut thickness was 0.003 cm (see Fig. 24(b)). Only the portion of the stent near the origin of the perforator was considered. At the model entrance, a steady flow of 2.0 ml/s was prescribed and traction-free boundary conditions were specified at the model outflows. Blood flow simulations were performed with and without the stent, and the flow rate through the perforating vessel was recorded. Visualizations of the resulting flow fields are shown in Fig. 24. The results show that although the stents occludes approximately 69% of the inflow area at the origin of the perforator, the flow rate through the perforator is reduced by only approximately 18%. Whether this is a clinically significant reduction that could put the patient at risk of stroke is not known.

4.4. Patient specific aneurysm stenting model

This case exemplifies the use of patient-specific computational models to test the performance of different stent designs for a patient with a cerebral aneurysm in the ICA. In this case, the vascular model was constructed from a 3D RA image using the modeling pipeline described earlier. For the flow simulations, physiologic pulsatile flow rates were prescribed at the inlet of the ICA. The flow rate was derived from PC-MR measurements performed on a normal subject in the same artery. Traction-free boundary conditions were imposed at the model outlets.

The flow alterations produced by two different stent designs were simulated. The first stent (stent 1) comprises rhomboidal cells similar to the Neuroform stent (Boston Scientific, Inc.). The second stent (stent 2) was constructed with hexagonal cells with the same amount of metal as the first stent. The placement of the stents into the vascular model is a complicated problem. For this purpose, the skeleton of the parent vessel was first extracted using a technique for skeletonization of tetrahedral grids.[143] Then a cylinder was generated along this skeleton and allowed to inflate until it contacted the arterial walls. Then the stent was mapped to this cylinder and allowed to deform under internal elastic forces and contact forces with the vessel wall. Once the stents were deployed inside the vascular model, the "pre-stent" mesh was adaptively refined around the stent wires and thus two new "post-stent" grids were obtained, one for each stent design. Flow simulations for the "post-stent" cases were performed with the embedded grids approach under the same flow conditions as in the "pre-stent" case. Figure 25 shows volume renderings of the 3DRA images from two viewing points (a and b) and the corresponding anatomical models (c and d). The two stents after deployment into the anatomical model are shown in Fig. 25(e) and (f).

Visualizations of the flow dynamics before and after deployment of the two stents are presented in Fig. 26. These visualizations reveal a small region of inflow into the aneurysm in the left side of the neck that impacts the body and dome of the aneurysm and disperses into a major vortex structure (Fig. 26(a)). A region of relatively elevated wall shear stress in the body of the aneurysm can be observed in Fig. 26(d). Both stents produced some changes in the intra-aneurysmal flow structure. Stent 1 deviated the inflow jet towards the dome of the aneurysm

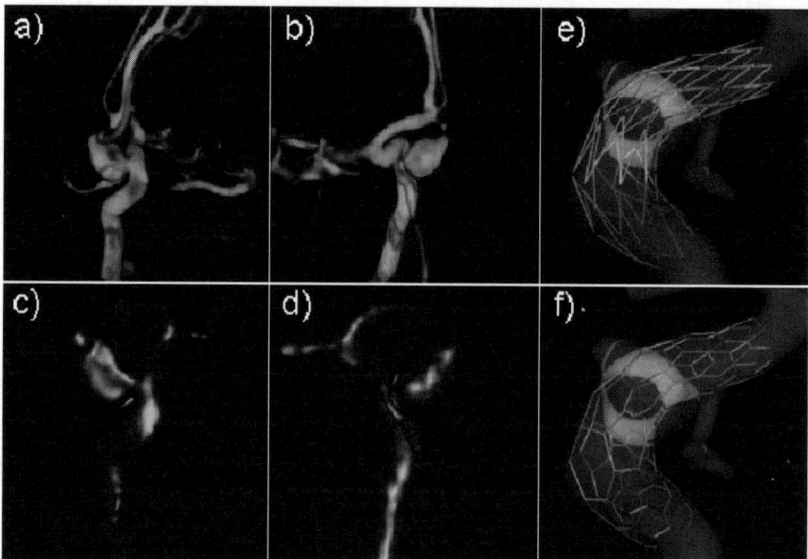

Fig. 25. Image-based vascular model of a cerebral aneurysm and simulated stents: (a) 3D rotational angiography image (front view), (b) 3D rotational angiography image (back view), (c) vascular model (front view), (d) vascular model (back view), (e) simulated stent #1 (Neuroform), (f) simulated stent #2 (hexagonal cells).

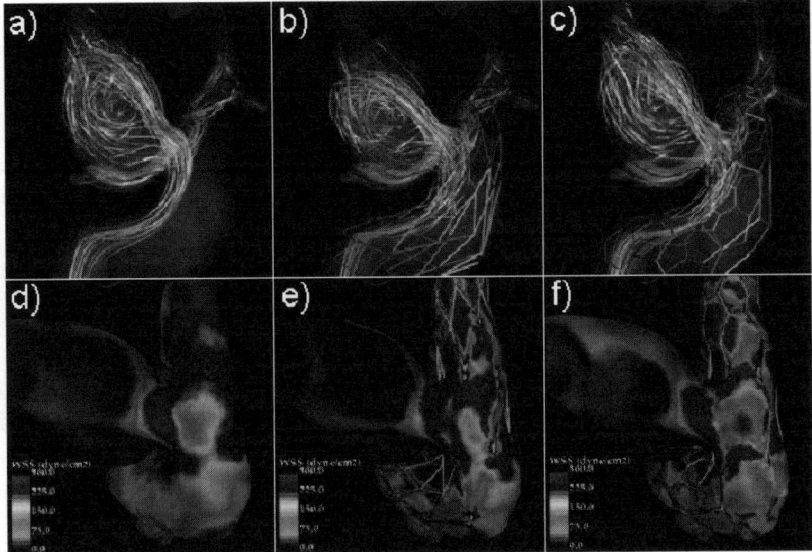

Fig. 26.   Hemodynamics visualization before and after stent deployment: (a) flow pattern before stenting, (b) flow pattern after stent #1 deployment, (c) flow pattern after stent #2 deployment, (d) wall shear stress before stenting, (e) wall shear stress after stent #1 deployment, (f) wall shear stress after stent #2 deployment.

(Fig. 26(b)). A second vortex structure formed in the superior part of the inflow jet. The wall shear stress pattern remained relatively unchanged, although smaller values were observed in the body of the aneurysm (Fig. 26(e)) compared to the pre-stent distribution (Fig. 26(d)). On the other hand, stent 2 deviated the inflow jet towards the aneurysm body, increasing the flow velocity and shear stress in the superior lobulation (Fig. 26(c) and (f)). The flow alterations produced by both stents were not dramatic. The reason is that only one stent wire crossed the small inflow zone of this aneurysm blocking or dispersing the inflow jet. Therefore, if this particular patient was to be treated with only a stent, a better design is needed. More wires across the inflow jet need to be placed. One possibility would be to design a new stent with wires oriented more perpendicularly to the vessel axis. Nevertheless, this example shows that personalized analysis of hemodynamics are feasible using the grid embedding techniques previously described, and that these analyses could be used for selecting the best treatment option for individual patients.

4.5. *Models of aneurysm coiling*

The final example corresponds to simulations of the blood flow in cerebral aneurysms after deployment of coils. These calculations are useful to better understand the underlying mechanisms that make these devices work, and also in order to study the role of hemodynamic forces in the process of coil recompaction or recanalization.

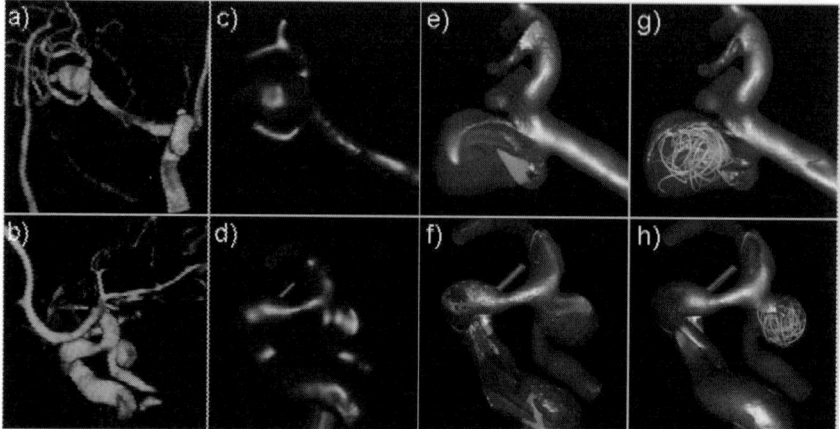

Fig. 27.　Examples of aneurysm coiling simulations: (a,b) 3D rotational angiography images, (c,d) vascular models, (e,f) iso-velocity surface before coiling, (g,h) iso-velocity surface after coiling.

Two aneurysms were selected from our database of cerebral aneurysms. One was located in the right middle cerebral aneurysm (MCA) and the other in the right ICA at the origin of the posterior communicating artery (PCoA). Patient-specific anatomical models were constructed from 3DRA images, as explained before. Figure 27 shows the 3DRA images ((a) and (b)) and the corresponding anatomical models ((c) and (d)) for both aneurysms. Pre-coiling hemodynamic simulations were carried out under pulsatile flow conditions. Then, simulated coils were deployed in the sac of each aneurysm, and new hemodynamic simulations were carried out with the mesh embedding technique. The coils were simulated as beads of spheres and had a length of 20 cm and a thickness of 0.01 cm. The inflow jets before coiling at peak systole are visualized as iso-velocity surfaces in Fig. 27(e) and (f). Both aneurysms exhibit relatively large inflow jets impacting on the superior part of the aneurysm body. Corresponding visualizations after coiling are presented in Fig. 27(g) and (h). These visualizations show how the coil mass blocks the inflow jet changing its size, concentration and orientation. Although these simulations represent the initial stages of the coiling procedure (after deployment of only one coil), they can be useful for better understanding how these devices work as well as investigating the effects of incomplete coiling of aneurysms and relating hemodynamic patterns to clinical outcomes including coil recannalization.

5.　Conclusions

The simulation of blood flows past endovascular devices in patient-specific geometries is important for understanding the alterations in the flow patterns induced by these devices and their interaction with the vessel wall biology and biomechanics. This information is useful not only for improving the design of these devices, but also for selecting the best treatment for each patient. In the former case, idealized models and simulations may be sufficient since one is interested in the general characteristics of the devices, while in the latter case the simulations must be made patient-specific. The use of computational models to personalize and plan surgical and endovascular interventions is an example of the predictive power of computer simulations that cannot be replaced by advances in medical imaging. Even if new imaging techniques were developed to accurately quantify blood flow patterns and wall shear stress *in vivo*, computational technologies provide the extra possibility of asking what-if questions, and exploring their answers using virtual models such as those presented here.

In addition to difficulties associated with constructing anatomical models from medical images, the simulation of subject-specific flows with endovascular devices adds the extra complexity of generating geometrical models and grids of the vasculature and the devices at the same time. In these cases, generating body conforming meshes is a formidable task. The use of adaptive surface merging techniques allows us to separate the problem into different components that can be modeled individually and then fused together. This strategy simplifies somewhat the geometric modeling for the body conforming approach, but meshing the resulting domain remains a challenging problem. On the other hand, adaptive unstructured grid embedding and immersive techniques are promising for the calculation of hemodynamics past endovascular devices in patient-specific anatomies because they can deal with the high degrees of geometric complexity required by these applications. These techniques combines the advantages of unstructured body conforming grids for representing the blood vessels, and the flexibility of embedded or immersed methods to deal with objects of arbitrary shape immersed in the blood stream.

The ability of simulating blood flows past endovascular devices such as stents and coils in patient-specific anatomies using embedded and immersive techniques was illustrated with a number of examples. Although these examples dealt with hemodynamics in cerebral aneurysms, the simulation techniques have a wide variety of applications to other vascular problems such as heart valves, disturbances in the flow field induced by a catheter used for measurement of differential pressures across a stenosis, brain cooling with endovascular catheters for stroke treatment, etc. The numerical examples presented here also show that the embedding and immersive methods can yield results that closely match those obtained with body conforming grids, provided that the grids are adequately refined around the devices. Grid refinement is a fully automated procedure and thus it does not add any extra burden to the modeler. Obviously, the meshes after refinement are mush larger than those used to compute the flows without any device, but this complication affects the embedded and immersive as well as the body conforming approaches. Another advantage of the embedded/immersive approach is that they could be used in much the same way for simulations that involve dynamic adjustment/moving of the endovascular devices. In these situations, the grid needs to be cut and adaptively refined after each re-positioning of the devices, but this procedure is fully automated. Body fitted grids will require re-computing the geometry of the vasculature intersected by the devices and re-generating the volumetric grid, which is extremely more complicated.

Acknowledgments

We thank Philips Medical Systems and the American Heart Association for financial support.

References

1. W. E. Stehbens, Intracranial aneurysms, in *Pathology of the Cerebral Blood Vessels* (The C. V. Mosby Company, St. Louis, MO, 1972), pp. 351–470.
2. B. Weir, Unruptured intracranial aneurysms: a review. *J. Neurosurg.* **96** (2002) 3–42.
3. G. N. Foutrakis, H. Yonas and R. J. Sclabassi, Saccular aneurysm formation in curved and bifurcation arteries. *AJNR Am. J. Neuroradiol.* **20** (1999) 1309–1317.
4. F. Tomasello, D. D'Avella, F. M. Salpietro and M. Longo, Asymptomatic aneurysms. Literature meta-analysis and indications for treatment. *J. Neurosurg. Sci.* **42**(1) (1998) 47–51.
5. H. R. Winn, J. A. Jane, J. Taylor, D. Kaiser and G. W. Britz, Prevalence of asymptomatic incidental aneurysms: review of 4568 arteriograms. *J. Neurosurg.* **96**(1) (2002) 43–49.
6. F. H. Linn, G. J. Rinkel, A. Algra and J. van Gijn, Incidence of subarachnoid hemorrhage: role of region, year and rate of computed Tomography: a meta-analysis. *Stroke* **27**(4) (1996) 625–629.
7. M. Kaminogo, M. Yonekura and S. Shibata, Incidence and outcome of multiple intracranial aneurysms in a defined population. *Stroke* **34**(1) (2003) 16–21.
8. C. Kim, J. Cervos-Navarro, C. Patzold, Y. Tokuriki, Y. Takebe and K. Hori, *In vivo* study of flow pattern at human carotid bifurcation with regard to aneurysm development. *Acta Neurochir (Wien)* **115**(3–4) (1992) 112–117.
9. K. N. T. Kayembe, M. Sasahara and F. Hazama, Cerebral aneurysms and variations of the circle of Willis. *Stroke* **15** (1984) 846–850.
10. N. F. Kassell, J. C. Torner, E. C. J. Haley, J. A. Jane, H. P. Adams and G. L. Kongable, The international cooperative study on the timing of aneurysm surgery. Part 1: Overall management results. *J. Neurosurg* **73**(1) (1990) 18–36.
11. H. Nishioka, J. C. Torner, C. J. Graf, N. F. Kassell, A. L. Sahs and L. C. Goettler, Cooperative study of intracranial aneurysms and subarachnoid hemorrhage: a long-term prognostic study. II. Ruptured intracranial aneurysms managed conservatively. *Arch. Neurol.* **41**(11) (1984) 1142–1146.
12. P. M. White and J. M. Wardlaw, Unruptured intracranial aneurysms. *J. Neuroradiol* **30**(5) (2003) 336–350.
13. A. Molyneux, R. Kerr, I. Stratton, P. Sandercock, M. Clarke, J. Shrimpton and R. Holman, International Subarachnoid Aneurysm Trial (ISAT) Collaborative Group. International Subarachnoid Aneurysm Trial (ISAT) of neurosurgical clipping versus endovascular coiling in 2143 patients with ruptured intracranial aneurysms: a randomised trial. *Lancet* **360**(9342) (2002) 1267–1274.

14. A. J. Ringer, D. K. Lopes, A. L. Boulos, L. R. Guterman and L. N. Hopkins, Current techniques for endovascular treatment of intracranial aneurysms. *Semin. Cerebrovasc. Dis. Stroke* **1**(1) (2001).

15. C. W. Kerber and C. B. Heilman, Flow in experimental berry aneurysms: method and model. *AJNR Am. J. Neuroradiol.* **4**(3) (1983) 374–377.

16. C. W. Kerber, S. G. Imbesi and K. Knox, Flow dynamics in a lethal anterior communicating artery aneurysm. *AJNR Am. J. Neuroradiol.* **20**(10) (1999) 2000–2003.

17. Y. P. Gobin, J. L. Counard and P. Flaud, *In vitro* study of haemodynamics in a giant saccular aneurysm model: influence of flow dynamics in the parent vessel and effects of coil embolization. *Neuroradiology* **36**(7) (1994) 530–536.

18. S. K. Kyriacou and J. D. Humphrey, Influence of size, shape and properties on the mechanics of axisymmetric saccular aneurysms. *J. Biomech.* **29**(8) (1996) 1015–1022.

19. H. V. Ortega, Computer simulation helps predict cerebral aneurysms. *J. Med. Eng. Technol.* **22**(4) (1998) 179–181.

20. M. H. Buonocore, Visualizing blood flow patterns using streamlines, arrows and particle paths. *Magn. Reson. Med.* **40**(2) (1998) 210–226.

21. H. G. Boecher-Schwarz, K. Ringel, L. Kopacz, A. Heimann and O. Kempski, *Ex vivo* study of the physical effect of coils on pressure and flow dynamics in experimental aneurysms. *AJNR Am. J. Neuroradiol.* **21**(8) (2000) 1532–1536.

22. C. Groden, J. Laudan, S. Gatchell and H. Zeumer, Three-dimensional pulsatile flow simulation before and after endovascular coil embolization of a terminal cerebral aneurysm. *J. Cereb. Blood Flow Metab.* **21**(12) (2001) 1464–1471.

23. R. W. Metcalfe, The promise of computational fluid dynamics as a tool for delineating therapeutic options in the treatment of aneurysms. *AJNR Am. J. Neuroradiol.* **24**(4) (2003) 553–554.

24. B. B. Lieber, V. Livescu, L. N. Hopkins and A. K. Wakhloo, Particle image velocimetry assessment of stent design influence on intra-aneurysmal flow. *Ann. Biomed. Eng.* **30** (2002) 768–777.

25. M. Hirabayashi, M. Ohta and D. A. Rufenacht, Characterization of flow reduction properties in an aneurysm due to a stent. *Phys. Rev. E Stat. Nonlin. Soft. Matter. Phys.* **68**(2) (2003) 0219918.

26. C. N. Ionita, Y. Hoi, H. Meng and S. Rudin, Particle image velocimetry (PIV) evaluation of flow modification in aneurysm phantoms using asymmetric stents, in *SPIE Med. Imaging* (San Diego, California, 2004), pp. 14–19.

27. L. D. Jou, C. M. Quick, W. L. Young, M. T. Lawton, R. Higashida, A. Martin and D. Saloner, Computational approach to quantifying hemodynamic forces in giant cerebral aneurysms. *AJNR Am. J. Neuroradiol.* **24**(9) (2003) 1804–1810.

28. D. A. Steinman, J. S. Milner, C. J. Norley, S. P. Lownie and D. W. Holdworth, Image-based computational simulation of flow dynamics in a giant intracranial aneurysm. *AJNR Am. J. Neuroradiol.* **24**(4) (2003) 559–566.

29. J. R. Cebral, M. Hernandez and A. F. Frangi, Computational analysis of blood flow dynamics in cerebral aneurysms from CTA and 3D rotational angiography image data. in *Int. Con. Comput. Bioeng.* Vol. 1 (Zaragoza, Spain, 2003), pp. 191–198.

30. J. R. Cebral, M. Hernandez, A. F. Frangi, C. M. Putman, R. Pergolizzi and J. E. Burgess, Subject-specific modeling of intracranial aneurysms. in *SPIE Med. Imaging*, Vol. 5369 (San Diego, California, 2004), pp. 319–327.

31. J. R. Cebral, M. A. Castro, J. E. Burgess and C. M. Putman, Cerebral aneurysm hemodynamics modeling from 3D rotational angiography, in *IEEE Int. Symp. Biomed. Imaging* (Arlington, Virginia, 2004), pp. 944–947.

32. C. Mimata, M. Kitaoka, S. Nagashiro, K. Fyama, H. Hori, H. Yoshioka and Ushio, Differential distribution and expression of collagens in the cerebral aneurysmal wall. *ACTA Neuropath.* **94** (1997) 197–206.

33. P. Gaetani, F. Tartara, F. Tancioni, R. Rodriguez, Y. Baena, E. Casari, M. Alfano and V. Graziolo, Deficiency of total collagen content and of deoxypuridinoline in intracranial aneurysm walls. *FEBS Lett.* **404** (1997) 303–306.

34. H. M. Finlay, L. McCullough and P. B. Canham, Three-dimensional collagen organization of human brain arteries at different transmural pressures. *J. Vasc. Res.* **32** (1995) 301–312.

35. F. X. Schmid, K. Bielenberg, A. Schneider, A. Haussler, A. Keyser and D. Birnbaum, Ascending aortic aneurysm associated with bicuspid and tricuspid aortic valve: involvement and clinical relevance of smooth muscle cell apoptosis and expression of cell death- initiating proteins. *Eur. J. Cardio-Thoracic Surg.* **23**(4) (2003) 537–543.

36. S. Kondo, N. Hashimoto and H. Kikuchi, Apoptosis of medial smooth muscle cells in the development of saccular cerebral aneurysms in rats. *Stroke* **29** (1998) 181–189.

37. T. Sakaki, E. Kohumura, T. Kishiguchi, T. Yuguch, T. Yamashita and T. Hayakawa, Loss and apoptosis of smooth muscle cells in intracranial aneurysms. Studies with in situ DNA end labeling and antibody against single-stranded DNA. *ACTA Neurochir.* **139** (1997) 469–474.

38. R. W. Thomson, S. Liao and J. A. Curc, Vascular smooth muscle cell apoptosis in abdominal aortic aneurysms. *Coron. Artery Dis.* **8** (1997) 623–631.

39. H. Nakatani, N. Hashimoto and Kang, Cerebral blood flow patterns at major vessel bifurcations and aneurysms in rats. *J. Neurosurg.* **74** (1991) 258–262.

40. C. F. Gonzalez, Y. I. Choi and V. Ortega, Intracranial aneurysms: flow analysis of their origin and progression. *AJNR Am. J. Neuroradiol.* **13** (1992) 181–188.

41. A. C. Burleson, C. M. Strother and V. T. Turitto, Computer modeling of intracranial saccular and lateral aneurysms for the study of their hemodynamics. *Neurosurg.* **37** (1995) 774–784.

42. H. Tenjin, F. Asakura and Y. Nakahara, Evaluation of intraaneurysmal blood velocity by time-density curve analysis and digital subtraction angiography. *AJNR Am. J. Neuroradiol.* **19** (1998) 1303–1307.

43. H. Ujiie, H. Tachibana and O. Hiramtsu, Effects of size and shape (aspect ratio) on the hemodynamics of saccular aneurysms: a possible index for the surgical treatment of intracranial aneurysms. *Neurosurg.* **45** (1999) 119–130.

44. S. Tateshima, Y. Murayama and J. P. Villablanca, Intraaneurysmal flow dynamics study featuring an acrylic aneurysm model manufactured using computerized tomography angiogram as a mold. *J. Neurosurg.* **95**(6) (2001) 1020–1027.

45. T. Satoh, K. Onoda and S. Tsuchimoto, Visualization of intraaneurysmal flow patterns with transluminal flow images of 3D MR angiograms in conjunction with aneurysmal configurations. *AJNR Am. J. Neuroradiol.* **24** (2003) 1436–1445.

46. T. M. Liou and S. N. Liou. A review of *In vitro* studies of hemodynamic characteristics in terminal and lateral aneurysm models, in *National Scientific Council ROC(B).* Vol. **23**(4) (1999), pp. 133–148.

47. S. Tateshima, Y. Murayama, J. P. Villablanca, T. Morino, K. Nomura, K. Tanishita and F. Vinuela, *In vitro* measurement of fluid-induced wall shear stress in unruptured cerebral aneurysms harboring blebs. *Stroke* **34**(1) (2003) 187–192.

48. S. Tateshima, F. Vinuela, J. P. Villablanca, Y. Murayama, T. Morino, K. Nomura and K. Tanishita, Three-dimensional blood flow analysis in a wide-necked internal carotid artery-ophthalmic artery aneurysm. *J. Neurosurg.* **99**(3) (2003) 526–533.

49. M. P. Arroyo and C. A. Greated, Stereoscopic particle image velocimetry. *Measure. Sci. Techno.* **2** (1991) 1181–1186.

50. P. J. Yim, J. R. Cebral, A. Weaver, R. J. Lutz, O. Soto, G. Boudewijn, B. Vasbinder, V. H. Ho and P. L. Choyke, Estimation of the differential pressure at renal artery stenoses. *Magn. Reson. Med.* **51** (2004) 969–977.

51. P. J. Yim, J. R. Cebral, Y. Zhang, R. J. Lutz and P. L. Choyke, Evaluation of magnetic resonance angiography for measuring arterial wall shear stress. *Ann. Biomed. Eng.* **28** (2000) S–59.

52. S. Tateshima, J. Grinstead, S. Sinha, Y. Nien, Y. Murayama, J. P. Villablanca, K. Tanishita and F. Vinuela, Intra-aneurysmal flow visualization by phase contrast magnetic resonance imaging: feasibility *In vitro* study using a geometrically-realistic aneurysm model. *J. Neurosurg.* **100** (2004) 1041–1048.

53. T. Hassan, M. Ezura, E. V. Timofeev, T. Tominaga, T. Saito, A. Takahashi, K. Takayama and T. Yoshimoto, Computational simulation of therapeutic parent artery occlusion to treat giant vertebrobasilar aneurysm. *AJNR Am. J. Neuroradiol.* **25**(1) (2004) 63–68.

54. J. R. Cebral, M. A. Castro, O. Soto, R. Löhner and N. Alperin, Blood flow models of the circle of Willis from magnetic resonance data. *J. Eng. Math.* **47**(3–4) (2003) 369–386.

55. J. R. Cebral, M. A. Castro, J. E. Burgess, R. Pergolizzi, M. J. Sheridan and C. M. Putman, Characterization of cerebral aneurysm for assessing risk of rupture using patient-specific computational hemodynamics models. *AJNR Am. J. Neuroradiol.* **26** (2005) 2550–2559.

56. C. A. Taylor and M. T. Draney, Computational techniques in therapeutic decision-making. *Comput. Assisted Surg.* **4** (1999) 231–247.

57. J. R. Cebral and R. Löhner, Efficient simulation of blood flow past complex endovascular devices using an adaptive embedding technique. *IEEE Trans. Med. Imaging* **24**(4) (2005) 468–477.

58. J. R. Cebral, M. A. Castro, S. Appanaboyina, C. M. Putman, D. Millan and A. F. Frangi, Efficient pipeline for image-based patient-specific analysis of cerebral aneurysm hemodynamics: Technique and sensitivity. *IEEE Trans. Med. Imaging* **24**(1) (2005) 457–467.

59. J. R. Cebral and R. Löhner, From medical images to anatomically accurate finite element grids. *Int. J. Num. Methods Eng.* **51** (2001) 985–1008.

60. J. Beutel and M. Sonka, *Handbook of medical imaging, Volume 2: Medical image processing and analysis* (SPIE Press monograph vol. PM80, 2000).

61. J. Weickert, Anisotropic diffusion in image processing. *ECMI Series* (Stutgart, Germany, Teubner-Verlag, 1998).

62. A. F. Frangi, Multiscale vessel enhancement filtering. *Lect. Notes Comput. Sci.* **1496** (1998) 130–137.

63. J. A. Sethian, *Level set methods and fast marching methods: evolving interfaces in computational geometry, fluid mechanics, computer vision and materials sciences.* Vol. 3 (Cambridge monographs on applied and computational mathematics, Cambridge University Press, 1998).

64. Y. Chen, S. Thiruenkadam, H. Tagare, F. Huang, D. Wilson and E. Geiser, On the incorporation of shape priors into geometric active contours, in *IEEE Workshop on Variational and Level Set Methods.* (2001) pp. 145–152.

65. M. Hernandez and A. F. Frangi, Non-parametric geodesic active regions: method and evaluation for cerebral aneurysms segmentation in 3DRA and CTA. *Med. Image Anal.* **11**(3) (2006) 224–241.

66. P. J. Yim, G. Boudewijn, B. Vasbinder, V. B. Ho and P. L. Choyke, Isosurfaces as deformable models for magnetic resonance angiography. *IEEE Trans. Med. Imaging* **22**(7) (2003) 875–881.

67. P. J. Yim, J. R. Cebral, R. Mullick and P. L. Choyke, Vessel surface reconstruction with a tubular deformable model. *IEEE Trans. Med. Imaging* **20**(12) (2001) 1411–1421.

68. P. J. Yim, B. Vasbinder, V. H. Ho and P. L. Choyke. A Deformable isosurface and vascular applications. in *SPIE Med. Imaging*, Vol. 4684 (San Diego, California, 2002), pp. 1390–1397.

69. P. J. Yim, K. DeMarco, M. A. Castro and J. R. Cebral, Characterization of shear stress on the wall of carotid artery using magnetic resonance imaging and computational fluid dynamics. *Studies Health Technol. Informat.* **113** (2005) 412–442.

70. J. R. Cebral, C. M. Putman, R. Pergolizzi, J. E. Burgess and P. J. Yim, Multi-modality image-based models of carotid artery hemodynamics. in *SPIE Med. Imaging*. Vol. 5369 (San Diego, California, 2004), pp. 529–538.

71. J. R. Cebral, M. A. Castro, D. Millan, A. F. Frangi and C. M. Putman, Pilot clinical investigation of aneurysm rupture using image-based computational fluid dynamics models. in *SPIE Med. Imaging*, Vol. 5746 (San Diego, CA, 2005), pp. 245–256.

72. J. R. Cebral, R. Löhner, P. L. Choyke and P. J. Yim, Merging of intersecting triangulations for finite element modeling. *J. Biomech.* **34** (2001) 815–819.

73. M. A. Castro, C. M. Putman and J. R. Cebral, Patient-specific computational modeling of cerebral aneurysms with multiple avenues of flow from 3D rotational angiography images. *Acad. Radiol.* **13**(7) (2006) 811–821.

74. G. Taubin, A signal processing approach to fair surface design, in *Computer Graphics*. (1995) pp. 351–358.

75. R. Löhner, Regridding surface triangulations. *J. Comput. Phys.* **126** (1996) 1–10.

76. R. Löhner, Automatic unstructured grid generators. *Finite Elem. Analy. Design* **25** (1997) 111–134.

77. S. J. Owen, A survey of unstructured mesh generation technology. in *7th International Meshing Roundtable* (Sandia National Laboratory, 1998), pp. 239–267.

78. R. Löhner, *Applied CFD Techniques* (John Wiley & Sons, 2001).

79. R. Löhner, Extensions and improvements of the advancing front grid generation technique. *Comput. Methods Appl. Mech. Eng.* **5** (1996) 119–132.

80. J. Mazumdar, *Biofluid Mechanics* (Singapore: World Scientific, 1992).

81. R. Löhner, C. Yang, E. Oñate and S. Idelssohn, An unstructured grid-based, parallel free surface solver. *Appl. Num. Math.* **31** (1999) 271–293.

82. M. D. Gunzburger, Mathematical aspects of finite element methods for incompressible viscous flows, in *Finite Elements: Theory and Application*, H. A. V. Dwoyer, ed., (Springer-Verlag, 1987), pp. 124–150.

83. M. Fortin and F. Thomasset, Mixed finite element methods for incompressible flow problems. *J. Comput. Phys.* **31** (1979) 113–145.

84. A. Soulaimani, M. Fortin, Y. Ouellet, G. Dhatt and F. Bertrand, Simple continuous pressure elements for two- and three-dimensional incompressible flows. *Comp. Methods Appl. Mech. Eng.* **62** (1987) 47–69.

85. F. Thomasset, *Implementation of Finite Element Methods for Navier-Stokes Equations* (Springer-Verlag, 1981).

86. C. Taylor and P. Hood, A numerical solution of the Navier-Stokes equations using the finite element method. *Comp. Fluids* **1** (1973) 73–100.

87. R. Löhner, *A fast finite element solver for incompressible flows.* Vol. AIAA-90-0398 (Reno, Nevada, 1990).
88. L. P. Franca, T. J. R. Hughes, A. F. D. Loula and I. Miranda. A new family of stable elements for the Stokes problem based on mixed Galerkin/least-squares finite element formulation, in *7th Int. Conf. Finite Elements Flow Problems.* (Huntsville, Alabama, 1989).
89. T. E. Tezduyar, R. Shih, S. Mittal and S. E. Ray, Incompressible flow computations with stabilized bilinear and linear equal-order interpolation velocity-pressure elements, *Report UMSI 90* (1990).
90. L. P. Franca and S. L. Frey, Stabilized finite element methods: II. The incompressible Navier-Stokes equations. *Comp. Methods Appl. Mech. Eng.* **99** (1992) 209–233.
91. A. J. Chorin, Numerical solution of the Navier-Stokes equations. *Math. Comp.* **22** (1968) 745–762.
92. J. Kim and P. Moin, Application of a fractional-step method to incompressible Navier-Stokes equations. *J. Comput. Phys.* **59** (1985) 308–323.
93. T. Hino, Computation of free surface flow areound an advancing ship by the Navier-Stokes equations, in *5th Int. on Conf. Numerical Ship Hydrodynamics* (Hiroshima, Japan, 1989).
94. P. M. Gresho, C. D. Upson, S. T. Chan and R. L. Lee, Recent progress in the solution of the time-dependent, three-dimensional, incompressible Navier-Stokes equations, in *4th Int. Symp. Finite Element Methods Flow Problems* (Tokio, Japan, 1982).
95. J. Donea, S. Giuliani, H. Laval and L. Quartapelle, Solution of the unsteady Navier-Stokes equations by a fractional step method. *Comp. Methods Appl. Mech. Eng.* **30** (1982) 53–73.
96. J. D. Huffenus and D. Khaletzky, A finite element method to solve the Navier-Stokes equations using the method of characteristics. *Int. J. Num. Methods Eng.* **4** (1984) 247–269.
97. T. C. Jue, B. Ramaswamy and J. E. Akin, Finite element simulation of 2D Bernard convection with gravity modulation. *FED* **123** (1991).
98. A. T. Patera, A spectral element method for fluid dynamics: laminar flow in a channel expansion. *J. Comput. Phys.* **54** (1984) 468–488.
99. P. Wesseling, *Principles of Computational Fluid Dynamics* (Springer, 2001).
100. D. Martin and R. Löhner, *An Implicit Linelet-Based Solver for Incompressible Flows.* Vol. AIAA-92-0668, (Reno, Nevada, 1992).
101. R. Ramamurti, W. C. Sandberg and R. Löhner, Simulation of flow about flapping airfoils using a finite element incompressible flow solver. *AIAA J.* **39**(2) (2001) 253–260.
102. R. Codina, Pressure stability in fractional step finite element methods for incompressible flows. *J. Comput. Phys.* **170** (2001) 112–140.
103. Y. Saad, *Iterative Methods for Sparse Linear Systems* (Boston, Massachusetts, PWS Pub. Co., 1996).
104. O. Soto, R. Löhner and F. Camelli, A linelet preconditioner for incompressible flow solvers. *Int. J. Heat Fluid Flow* **13**(1) (2003) 133–147.
105. J. Waltz and R. Löhner, *A Grid Coarsening Algorithm for Unstructured Multigrid Applications*, Vol. AIAA-00-0925 (Reno, Nevada, 2000).
106. J. Alonso, L. Martinelli and A. Jameson. *Multigrid Unsteady Navier-Stokes Calculations with Aeroelastic Applications*, Vol. AIAA-95-0048 (Reno, Nevada, 1995).
107. O. Soto, R. Löhner, J. R. Cebral and R. Codina, A time-accurate implicit monolithic finite element scheme for incompressible flow problems, in *ECCOMAS CFD*, (Swansea, Wales, U. K., 2001).

108. H. Luo, J. D. Baum and R. Löhner, A fast matrix-free implicit method for compressible flows on unstructured grids. *J. Comput. Phys.* **146** (1998) 664–690.

109. D. Sharov, H. Luo, J. D. Baum and R. Löhner, Implementation of unstructured grid GMRES+LU-SGS method on shared-memory, cache-based parallel computers, in *AIAA Aerospace Science Meeting.* Vol. AIAA-00-0927 (Reno, Nevada, 2000).

110. P. Neofitou and D. Drikakis, Non-Newtonian modeling effects on stenotic channel flows, in *ECCOMAS CFD* (Swansea, Wales, U.K., 2001).

111. K. Perktold and G. Rappitsch, Computer simulation of arterial blood flow. vessel diseases under the aspect of local hemodynamics. *Biological Flows* (Plenum Press, 1995), pp. 83–114.

112. J. R. Womersley, Method for the calculation of velocity, rate of flow and viscous drag in arteries when the pressure gradient is known. *J. Physiol.* **127** (1955) 553–563.

113. C. A. Taylor, T. J. R. Hughes and C. K. Zarins, Finite element modeling of blood flow in arteries. *Comput. Methods Appl. Mech. Eng.* **158** (1998) 155–196.

114. I. E. Vignon-Clementel, A. C. Figueroa, K. E. Jansen and C. A. Taylor, Outflow boundary conditions for three-dimensional finite element modeling of blood flow and pressure in arteries. *Comput. Methods Appl. Mech. Eng.* **195** (2006) 3776–3796.

115. M. S. Olufsen, C. S. Peskin, W. Y. Kim, E. M. Pedersen, A. Nadim and J. Larsen, Numerical simulation and experimental validation of blood flow in arteries with structured-tree outflow conditions. *Ann. Biomed. Eng.* **28** (2000) 1281–1299.

116. L. Formaggia, F. Nobile, A. Quarteroni and A. Veneziani, Multiscale modeling of the circulatory system: a preliminary analysis. *Report EPFL/DMA 6. 99, Visualization in Science,* (1999).

117. J. R. Cebral, P. J. Yim, R. Löhner, O. Soto and P. L. Choyke, Blood flow modeling in carotid arteries using computational fluid dynamics and magnetic resonance imaging. *Acad. Radiol.* **9** (2002) 1286–1299.

118. S. Z. Zhao, X. Y. Xu, A. D. Hughes, S. A. Thom, A. V. Stanton, B. Ariff and Q. Long, Blood flow and vessel mechanics in a physiologically realistic model of a human carotid arterial bifurcation. *J. Biomech.* **33** (2000) 975–984.

119. L. Dempere-Marco, E. Oubel, M. A. Castro, C. M. Putman, A. F. Frangi and J. R. Cebral, Estimation of wall motion in intracranial aneurysms and its effects on hemodynamic patterns. in *Medical Image Computing and Computer Assisted Intervention (MICCAI)* (Copenhagen, Denmark, 2006).

120. L. Dempere-Marco, E. Oubel, A. F. Frangi, C. M. Putman, M. A. Castro and J. R. Cebral, Wall motion and hemodynamics of intracranial aneurysms. in *World Congress on Biomechanics* (Munich, Germany, 2006).

121. A. S. Anayiotos, S. A. Jones, D. P. Giddens, S. Glasgov and C. K. Zarins, Shear stress in a compliant model of the human carotid bifurcation. *J. Biomech. Eng.* **116** (1994) 98–106.

122. M. Shojima, M. Oshima, K. Takagi, R. Torii, M. Hayakawa, K. Katada, A. Morita and T. Kirino, Magnitude and role of wall shear stress on cerebral aneurysm: computational fluid dynamic study of 20 middle cerebral artery aneurysms. *Stroke* **35**(11) (2004) 2500–2505.

123. C. A. Taylor and M. T. Draney, Experimental and Computational Methods in Cardiovascular fluid Mechanics. *Ann. Rev. Fluid Mechan.* **36** (2004) 197–231.

124. J. R. Cebral, R. Löhner, O. Soto, P. L. Choyke and P. J. Yim, Image-based finite element modeling of hemodynamics in stenosed carotid artery. in *SPIE Med. Imaging,* Vol. 4683 (San Diego, California, 2002), pp. 297–304.

125. R. Löhner, Robust, vectorized search algorithms for interpolation on unstructured grids. *J. Comput. Phys.* **118** (1995) 380–387.

126. F. Calamante, P. J. Yim and J. R. Cebral, Estimation of bolus dispersion effects in perfusion MRI using image-based computational fluid dynamics. *NeuroImage* **19** (2003) 342–352.

127. M. D. Ford, G. R. Stuhne, H. N. Nikolov, D. F. Habets, S. P. Lownie, D. W. Holdsworth and D. A. Steinman, Virtual angiography for visualization and validation of computational models of aneurysm hemodynamics. *IEEE Trans. Med. Imaging* **24**(12) (2005) 1586–1592.

128. V. Interrante and C. Grosch, Strategies for effectively visualizing 3D flow with volume LIC, in *Visualization'97*, (1997) pp. 421–424.

129. V. Interrante and C. Grosch, Visualizing 3D flow. *IEEE Comput. Graph. Appl.* **18**(4) (1998) 49–53.

130. L. Chen, I. Fujishiro and Y. Suzuki, Comprehensible volume LIC rendering based on 3D significance map, *Report GeoFEM. 2001-012, Research Organization for Information Science and Technology* (Tokyo, Japan, 2001), (http://geofem. tokyo. rist. or. jp/report_common/GeoFEM01_012. pdf)

131. R. B. Pember, J. B. Bell, P. Colella, W. Y. Crutchfield and M. L. Welcome, An adaptive Cartesian method for unsteady compressible flow in irregular regions. *J. Comput. Phys.* **120** (1995) 278.

132. A. M. Landsberg and J. P. Boris, *The Virtual Cell Embedding Method: A Simple Approach for Gridding Complex Geometries*, Vol. AIAA-97-1982 (Reno, Nevada, 1997).

133. M. J. Aftosmis, M. J. Berger and G. Adomavicius, *A Parallel Multilevel Method for Adaptively Refined Cartesian Grids with Embedded Boundaries*, Vol. AIAA-00-0808 (Reno, Nevada, 2000).

134. R. J. LeVeque and Z. Li, The immersed interface method for elliptic equations with discontinuous coefficients and singular sources. *SIAM J. Num. Anal.* **31** (1994) 1019–1044.

135. C. S. Peskin, The immersed boundary method. *Acta Numerica* **11** (2002) 479–517.

136. J. D. Baum, E. Mestreau, H. Luo and R. Löhner, Modeling structural response to blast loading using a coupled CFD/CSD methodology, in *Des. An. Prot. Struct. Impact/Impulsive/ Shock Loads (DAPSIL)* (Tokyo, Japan, 2003).

137. J. vande Voord, J. Vierendeels and E. Dick, Flow simulation in rotary volumetric pumps and compressors with the ficticiuous domain method. *J. Comp. Appl. Math.* **168** (2004) 491–499.

138. J. Mohd-Yusof, Development of immersed boundary methods for complex geometries, *Report Center for Turbulence Research, Annual Research Briefs* (1998).

139. B. K. Cook and R. P. Jensen, Dicrete element methods. *ASCE* (2002).

140. R. Löhner and E. Oñate, A general advancing front technique for filling space with arbitrary objects. *Int. J. Num. Methods Eng.* **61** (2004) 1977–1991.

141. B. Fornberg, A numerical study of steady viscous flow past a circular cylinder. *J. Fluid Mech.* **98** (1980) 819–855.

142. G. R. Stuhne and D. A. Steinman, Finite element modeling of the hemodynamics of stented aneurysms. *J. Biomech. Eng.* **126**(3) (2004) 382–387.

143. J. R. Cebral and R. Löhner, Flow visualization on unstructured grids using geometrical cuts, vortex detection and shock surfaces, in *AIAA Aerospace Sciences Meeting*, Vol. AIAA-01-0915 (Reno, Nevada, 2001).

CHAPTER 3

ON MODELING SOFT BIOLOGICAL TISSUES
WITH THE NATURAL ELEMENT METHOD

M. DOBLARÉ*, B. CALVO, M. A. MARTÍNEZ, E. PEÑA,
A. PÉREZ DEL PALOMAR and J. F. RODRÍGUEZ

Group of Structural Mechanics and Materials Modeling
Aragón Institute of Engineering Research (I3A)
University of Zaragoza, María de Luna
3 E-50018 Zaragoza, Spain
*mdoblare@unizar.es

While finite elements has been considered during the last decades as the universal tool to perform simulations in biomechanics, a recently developed wide family of methods, globally coined as meshless methods, has emerged as an attractive choice for an increasing variety of engineering problems. They present some key advantages such as the absence of a mesh in the traditional sense, particularly important in domains of very complex geometry, a less sensitivity to the nodal distribution and therefore to the implicit mesh distorsion what is especially interesting to handle problems under finite strains and large displacements in a Lagrangian framework. Here, we analyze the convenience and possible advantages of using meshless methods in numerical simulations of soft biological tissues. Biological tissues are usually nonlinear, anisotropic, inhomogeneous, viscoelastic, and undergo large deformations, so these methods seem to be an appealing possibility for this type of applications. In particular, we discuss the use of one of these methods, the so-called natural element method that has specific and important features as interpolatory character, easy handling of geometry, and essential boundary conditions via the so-called alpha-NEM extension, well-defined mathematical properties and a simple computer implementation. Different examples are solved using this approach including the human cornea, the temporo-mandibular joint, knee ligaments, and the passive behavior of the heart.

Keywords: Meshless methods; natural element method; soft tissues; human joints; cornea; heart.

1. Introduction

Numerical simulation plays a fundamental role in many branches of science. Computational biomechanics is one of these branches in which the numerical simulation of very complex processes takes place. Simulation of soft organs and bony structures deals with complex geometries, large deformations and involved models of constitutive behavior. The appearance of the finite element method (FEM) in the fifties allowed to perform such simulations in that field.[1] However, the method relies on the proper discretization of the geometry, an aspect which might become cumbersome with actual geometries.[2] In this regard, mesh generation in a general three-dimensional model is far from being completely automatized and the development of an specific finite element model usually takes a large amount of user time, and indeed when the modeled organ suffers large deformations, a remeshing strategy is frequently required in order to avoid numerical errors that can break out the simulation.[3]

In the last years (especially after the appearance of the pioneer work of Nayroles et al.[4]) we have assisted to the rapid growth of a new family of numerical methods globally coined as meshless or mesh-free. They are mainly based on Galerkin schemes, although there also exist collocation-based approaches. Their main advantage is less dependence of the nodal distribution, which makes them very adequate for large strain problems. These methods have been named in many different ways according to their applications, as for example: smooth particle hydrodynamics (SPH),[5] particle in cell (PIC),[6] element free galerkin (EFG),[7,8] reproducing kernel particle methods (RKPM),[9,10] hp-Clouds[11] and partition of unity FEM.[12] Duarte,[13] Belytschko et al.,[14] Li and Liu[15] review their main properties and the advantages and drawbacks of their application to each type of problem.

Despite these advantages, they still have some drawbacks. One example is the non-interpolating character of the shape functions that makes the imposition of essential (Dirichlet) boundary conditions both cumbersome and inaccurate. This is true even after imposing the "exact" value of boundary conditions at the nodes using (for example) Lagrange multipliers or penalty approaches.[7,11] Another aspect is the use of an appropriate numerical integration scheme, although different stabilization and correction techniques have been proposed to enhance consistency and improve accuracy.[16]

One of newest meshless methods in the field of solid mechanics is the natural element method (NEM).[17-19] It is based on a Galerkin approximation built over the well-known natural neighbor interpolation.[20] It uses the concepts of Delaunay triangulation[21] and Dirichlet tessellation[22] to construct the shape functions, which are defined over the convex hull of the set of points that defines the domain under study. Sukumar[23-25] was the first to apply NEM in 2D solid mechanics, demonstrating its interesting properties like interpolating behavior, the linear consistency and smoothness of the shape functions and the capability of exactly reproducing essential boundary conditions along convex boundaries.

Cueto et al.[26] proposed a modification to generalize this property to non-convex boundaries. They showed that the definition of the shape functions over an appropiate α-shape of the domain permits the description of the problem only in terms of nodes and to get the desired interpolating behavior over any type of boundary. This property is essential for piece-wise homogeneous domains where a non-convex domain is always found. In a recent work of Cueto et al.[27] all these features of the α-NEM have been extended to three dimensions.

Some meshless methods mentioned above have been used on large deformation problems.[28] The application of SPH to non-linear impacts has been studied in

Johnson *et al.*[29] Bonet *et al.*[30] employed SPH to simulate metal forming processes. Chen *et al.*[31] applied RKPM to the large deformation analysis of path-independent and path-dependent non-linear materials like rubber and elasto-plastic metals. Other interesting work is presented in Jun *et al.*[32] where an explicit formulation and an stabilized nodal integration scheme were used in the context of large deformation problems.

This paper exposes the capabilities of NEM in simulating large deformations of non-linear biological tissues and organs. It is organized as follows. Section 2 reviews the continuum mechanics basis of hyperelastic material. Section 3 overview the NEM implementation, describing the standard and non-standard Natural Neighbor Interpolation for two and three-dimensions, as well as the implementation of the formulation for large deformations within NEM. Section 4 shows some applications of this method in simulating a number of biological tissues and organs as the human cornea, the temporo-mandibular joint, knee ligaments, and the passive behavior of the heart. The paper closes with some concluding remarks in Sec. 5.

2. Mechanical Behavior of Biological Soft Tissues

Many biological tissues such as ligaments or blood vessels are subjected to large deformations with negligible volume changes, that is, only quasi-isochoric ($J \approx 1$) motions are possible. These materials can be seeing as a network of collagenous fibres or muscular tissue embedded in a high compliant matrix (i.e. a ground substance made of proteoglycans, water, collagen and glycoproteins).[33] Therefore, most fibrous soft tissues are assumed to be continuous fiber reinforced and sometimes layered materials. When the reinforcement is only due to one family of fibers (it has a single preferred direction), it is usually modeled as *transversely isotropic hyperelastic material*.[34] On the other hand, when two or more families of fibers are present, the tissue is modeled as a *fully anisotropic hyperelastic material*.[35]

The basic continuum mechanics formulation for this class of materials is given as follows. Let $\mathbf{x} = \chi(\mathbf{X}, t)\colon \Omega_0 \times \mathbb{R} \to \mathbb{R}^3$ denote the motion mapping and let $\mathbf{F}$ be the associated deformation gradient. Here $\mathbf{X}$ and $\mathbf{x}$ define the respective positions of a particle in the reference Ω_0 and current Ω configurations such as $\mathbf{F} = d\mathbf{x}/d\mathbf{X}$. Further, let $J \equiv det\mathbf{F}$ be the jacobian of the motion. To properly define volumetric and deviatoric responses in the nonlinear range, we introduce the following kinematic decomposition:[36]

$$\mathbf{F} = J^{\frac{1}{3}}\bar{\mathbf{F}}, \qquad \bar{\mathbf{F}} = J^{-\frac{1}{3}}\mathbf{F} \tag{1}$$

$$\mathbf{C} = \mathbf{F}^T\mathbf{F}, \qquad \bar{\mathbf{C}} = J^{-\frac{2}{3}}\mathbf{C} = \bar{\mathbf{F}}^T\bar{\mathbf{F}} \tag{2}$$

The term $J^{\frac{1}{3}}\mathbf{I}$ is associated with volume-changing deformations, while $\bar{\mathbf{F}}$ is associated with volume-preserving deformations. We shall call $\bar{\mathbf{F}}$ and $\bar{\mathbf{C}}$ the modified deformation gradient and the modified right Cauchy-Green tensors, respectively.

The direction of a fiber at a point $\mathbf{X} \in \Omega_0$ is defined by a unit vector field $\mathbf{m}_0(\mathbf{X})$. It is usually assumed that, under deformation, the fiber moves with the material points of the continuum body. Therefore, the stretch of the fiber, λ, defined as the ratio between its lengths at the deformed and reference configurations, can be expressed as

$$\lambda \mathbf{m}(\mathbf{x}, t) = \mathbf{F}(X, t)\mathbf{m}_0(\mathbf{X}), \qquad \lambda^2 = \mathbf{m}_0 \mathbf{F}^T \mathbf{F} \mathbf{m}_0 = \mathbf{m}_0 \mathbf{C} \mathbf{m}_0, \qquad (3)$$

where $\mathbf{m}$ is the unit vector of the fiber in the deformed configuration. For a second family of fibers characterized by the unit vector field $\mathbf{n}_0(\mathbf{X})$, the kinematics is analogous to that defined in Eq. (3).

To characterize isothermal processes, we postulate the existence of a unique decoupled representation of the strain-energy density function $\Psi(\mathbf{C}, \mathbf{m}_0, \mathbf{n}_0)$.[37] Based on the kinematic assumption Eq. (1) and following Spencer[38] it can be shown that the integrity bases for the three symmetric second order tensors $\bar{\mathbf{C}}, \mathbf{m}_0 \otimes \mathbf{m}_0, \mathbf{n}_0 \otimes \mathbf{n}_0$ are given in terms of eight invariants. Therefore, we can express Ψ as

$$\begin{aligned}
\Psi &= \Psi_{vol}(J) + \Psi_{dev}(\bar{\mathbf{C}}, \mathbf{m}_0 \otimes \mathbf{m}_0, \mathbf{n}_0 \otimes \mathbf{n}_0), \\
&= \Psi_{vol}(J) + \Psi_{dev}(\bar{I}_1, \bar{I}_2, \bar{I}_4, \bar{I}_5, \bar{I}_6, \bar{I}_7, \bar{I}_8, \bar{I}_9),
\end{aligned} \qquad (4)$$

with

$$\begin{aligned}
&\bar{I}_1 = tr\bar{\mathbf{C}}, \quad \bar{I}_2 = \frac{1}{2}((tr(\bar{\mathbf{C}})^2 - tr\bar{\mathbf{C}}^2), \\
&\bar{I}_4 = \mathbf{m}_0 \bar{\mathbf{C}} \mathbf{m}_0, \quad \bar{I}_5 = \mathbf{m}_0 \bar{\mathbf{C}}^2 \mathbf{m}_0, \quad \bar{I}_6 = \mathbf{n}_0 \bar{\mathbf{C}} \mathbf{n}_0, \\
&\bar{I}_7 = \mathbf{n}_0 \bar{\mathbf{C}}^2 \mathbf{n}_0, \quad \bar{I}_8 = \mathbf{m}_0 \bar{\mathbf{C}} \mathbf{n}_0, \quad \bar{I}_9 = (\mathbf{n}_0 \mathbf{m}_0)^2.
\end{aligned} \qquad (5)$$

$\bar{I}_1$ and $\bar{I}_2$ are the first two strain invariants of the symmetric modified Cauchy-Green tensor, $\bar{\mathbf{C}}$. The pseudo-invariants $\bar{I}_4, \ldots, \bar{I}_9$ characterize the anisotropy constitutive response of the fibers, $\bar{I}_4$ and $\bar{I}_6$ have a clear physical meaning since they are the squares of the stretches along the two families of fibers. In order to reduce the number of material parameters and to work with physically motivated invariants, we shall omit the dependency of the free energy Ψ on $\bar{I}_5, \bar{I}_7, \bar{I}_8$ and $\bar{I}_9$. This hypothesis is commonly used in biomechanical modeling.[39]

The stress response is then obtained from the derivatives of the stored-energy function, getting

$$\mathbf{S} = 2\frac{\partial \Psi}{\partial \mathbf{C}} = \mathbf{S}_{vol} + \mathbf{S}_{dev} = Jp\mathbf{C}^{-1} + J^{-\frac{2}{3}} DEV(\bar{\mathbf{S}}), \qquad (6)$$

where p is the hydrostatic pressure, $\bar{\mathbf{S}}$ the modified second Piola-Kirchhoff stress tensor

$$p = \frac{d\Psi_{vol}(J)}{dJ}, \qquad \bar{\mathbf{S}} = 2\frac{\partial \Psi_{dev}(\bar{\mathbf{C}}, \mathbf{m}_0, \mathbf{n}_0)}{\partial \bar{\mathbf{C}}}, \qquad (7)$$

and $DEV(\cdot)$ the material deviator operator

$$DEV(\cdot) = (\cdot) - \frac{1}{3}[(\cdot) : \bar{\mathbf{C}}]\bar{\mathbf{C}}^{-1}. \tag{8}$$

The Cauchy stress tensor $\boldsymbol{\sigma}$ is $1/J$ times the push-forward of $\mathbf{S}$ ($\boldsymbol{\sigma} = J^{-1}\boldsymbol{\chi}_*(\boldsymbol{S})$), that is, $\sigma_{ij} = J^{-1}F_{iI}F_{jJ}S_{IJ}$, so, from Eq. (6), we obtain

$$\boldsymbol{\sigma} = p\mathbf{1} + \frac{2}{J}dev\left[\bar{\mathbf{F}}\frac{\partial\Psi_{iso}(\bar{\mathbf{C}}, \mathbf{m}_0, \mathbf{n}_0)}{\partial\bar{\mathbf{C}}}\bar{\mathbf{F}}^T\right] \tag{9}$$

with $\mathbf{1}$ the second-order identity tensor and dev the deviator operator in the spatial description[40]

$$dev(\cdot) = (\cdot) - \frac{1}{3}[(\cdot) : \mathbf{1}]\mathbf{1}. \tag{10}$$

With the second Piola-Kirchhoff defined in Eq. (6), explicit expressions for the elastic tensor, $\mathbb{C}$, can be readily defined as

$$\mathbb{C} = 2\frac{\partial\mathbf{S}(\mathbf{C})}{\partial\mathbf{C}} = \mathbb{C}_{vol} + \mathbb{C}_{dev} = 2\frac{\partial\mathbf{S}_{vol}}{\partial\mathbf{C}} + 2\frac{\partial\mathbf{S}_{dev}}{\partial\mathbf{C}} \tag{11}$$

where $\mathbb{C}_{vol}$ and $\mathbb{C}_{dev}$ are given by[40]

$$\mathbb{C}_{vol} = 2\mathbf{C}^{-1} \otimes \left(p\frac{\partial J}{\partial\mathbf{C}} + J\frac{\partial p}{\partial\mathbf{C}}\right) + 2Jp\frac{\partial\mathbf{C}^{-1}}{\partial\mathbf{C}}$$

$$= J\tilde{p}\mathbf{C}^{-1} \otimes \mathbf{C}^{-1} + 2Jp\mathbb{I}_{C^{-1}} \tag{12}$$

$$\mathbb{C}_{dev} = -\frac{4}{3}J^{-\frac{4}{3}}\left(\frac{\partial\Psi_{dev}}{\partial\bar{\mathbf{C}}} \otimes \bar{\mathbf{C}}^{-1} + \bar{\mathbf{C}}^{-1} \otimes \frac{\partial\Psi_{dev}}{\partial\bar{\mathbf{C}}}\right)$$

$$+ \frac{4}{3}J^{-\frac{4}{3}}\left(\frac{\partial\Psi_{dev}}{\partial\bar{\mathbf{C}}} : \bar{\mathbf{C}}\right)\left(\mathbb{I}_{\bar{C}^{-1}} + \frac{1}{3}\bar{\mathbf{C}}^{-1} \otimes \bar{\mathbf{C}}^{-1}\right) + J^{-\frac{4}{3}}\bar{\mathbb{C}}_{\bar{w}}, \tag{13}$$

where,

$$\bar{\mathbb{C}}_{\bar{w}} = 4\frac{\partial^2\Psi_{dev}}{\partial\bar{\mathbf{C}}\partial\bar{\mathbf{C}}} - \frac{4}{3}\left[\left(\frac{\partial^2\Psi_{dev}}{\partial\bar{\mathbf{C}}\partial\bar{\mathbf{C}}} : \bar{\mathbf{C}}\right) \otimes \bar{\mathbf{C}}^{-1} + \bar{\mathbf{C}}^{-1} \otimes \left(\frac{\partial^2\Psi_{dev}}{\partial\bar{\mathbf{C}}\partial\bar{\mathbf{C}}} : \bar{\mathbf{C}}\right)\right]$$

$$+ \frac{4}{9}\left(\bar{\mathbf{C}} : \frac{\partial^2\Psi_{dev}}{\partial\bar{\mathbf{C}}\partial\bar{\mathbf{C}}} : \bar{\mathbf{C}}\right)\bar{\mathbf{C}}^{-1} \otimes \bar{\mathbf{C}}^{-1} \tag{14}$$

with $\mathbb{I}_{C^{-1}} = \frac{\partial\mathbf{C}^{-1}}{\partial\mathbf{C}} = -\frac{1}{2}(C_{IK}^{-1}C_{JL}^{-1} + C_{IL}^{-1}C_{JK}^{-1})$. For convenience, we have introduced the scalar function $\tilde{p}$, defined by

$$\tilde{p} = p + J\frac{dp}{dJ} \tag{15}$$

with the constitutive equation for p given in Eq. (7).

The elasticity tensor in the spatial description or the *spatial tensor of elasticities*, denoted by $\mathbb{c}$, is defined as the push-forward of $\mathbb{C}$ times a factor J^{-1}, so that

$$\mathbb{c} = J^{-1}\boldsymbol{\chi}_*(\mathbb{C}) = \mathbb{c}_{vol} + \mathbb{c}_{dev}. \qquad (16)$$

3. The Natural Element Implementation

A deep study of the application of the NEM to elastostatics has been carried out by Sukumar *et al.*[23-25] Recently, the extension to elastodynamics has also been presented.[41] This section is devoted to give some key details concerning the implementation of the NEM for elastostatics applications.

3.1. *Natural neighbor interpolation*

The NEM is based on the Natural Neighbor interpolation scheme[20,42] that relies on the concepts of Delaunay triangulations and Dirichlet tesselations[21,22] of a set of nodes (See Fig. 1).

For a given node n_I, the associated Voronoi cell is composed of all the points that are closer to the node n_I than to any other node. Formally,

$$T_I = \{\boldsymbol{x} \in \mathbb{R}^3 : d(\boldsymbol{x}, \boldsymbol{x}_I) < d(\boldsymbol{x}, \boldsymbol{x}_J) \,\forall\, J \neq I\}, \qquad (17)$$

where T_I is the Voronoi cell and $d(\cdot, \cdot)$ represents the Euclidean distance. In a similar way, the second order Voronoi cell is defined as the locus of the points, where the closest node is n_I and the second closest node is n_J:

$$T_{IJ} = \{\boldsymbol{x} \in \mathbb{R}^3 : d(\boldsymbol{x}, \boldsymbol{x}_I) < d(\boldsymbol{x}, \boldsymbol{x}_J) < d(\boldsymbol{x}, \boldsymbol{x}_K) \,\forall\, J \neq I \neq K\}. \qquad (18)$$

Thus, if a new node is added to a given cloud of points the Voronoi cells will be altered. Sibson[42] defined the natural neighbor coordinates of a point $\boldsymbol{x}$ with respect to one of his neighbors I as the ratio of the cell T_I that is transferred to T_x when adding $\boldsymbol{x}$ to the initial cloud of points to the total area of T_x. In other words, if $k(\boldsymbol{x})$ and $k_I(\boldsymbol{x})$ are the Lebesgue measures of T_x and T_{xI} respectively, the natural

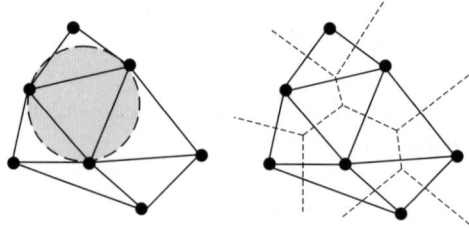

Fig. 1.   Delaunay triangulation and Voronoi diagram of a cloud of points.

neighbor coordinates of x with respect to the node I is defined as

$$\phi_I(x) = \frac{\kappa_I(x)}{\kappa(x)}. \tag{19}$$

In Fig. 2 this relationship may be written as

$$\phi_1(x) = \frac{A_{abfe}}{A_{abcd}} \tag{20}$$

It is straightforward to prove that NE shape functions form a partition of unity.

The NEM has some important properties, such as the interpolatory character of the shape functions, the linear consistency of the interpolant and the partition of unity property. In other words, the natural neighbor interpolant can exactly reproduce a linear or constant displacement field.[24] Another important property of the interpolant described above is its ability to reproduce a linear interpolant along convex boundaries (the corresponding proof for two dimensions can be found in Sukumar *et al.*[23,24] where the extension to 3D is straightforward). This is not true in the general case of non-convex boundaries, where contributions of interior points are not negligible. Sukumar[23] reported errors of about 2% using non-uniform distributions of points, finer near the boundary.

Recently, a modification of the way in which the natural neighbor interpolant is built has been proposed in order to achieve linear interpolation also over non-convex boundaries.[26] In most meshless methods, simulations are performed without employing an explicit definition of the boundary of the domain. However, it is possible to rigorously extract the *shape* of a set of points by invoking the concept of α-shape of the cloud.[26,43] Cueto *et al.*[26] demonstrated that the linear interpolation property over convex boundaries can be extended to non-convex ones if the cloud of points has sufficient density to obtain enough detail to accurately describe the boundary and if the natural neighborhood is limited to the case in which two nodes belong to the same triangle (tetrahedron) in a certain α-complex. This means that

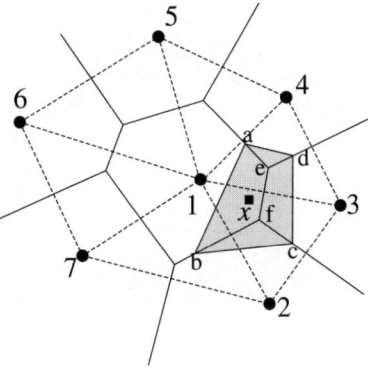

Fig. 2.   Definition of the natural neighbor coordinates of a point x.

the Voronoi cells are no longer the basis for the computation of the shape function. Instead, we consider a cell

$$T_I = \{\boldsymbol{x} \in \mathbb{R}^3 : d(\boldsymbol{x}, n_I) < d(\boldsymbol{x}, n_J) \ \forall J \neq I \wedge \sigma_T \in \mathcal{C}_\alpha(N)\} \tag{21}$$

$\mathcal{C}_\alpha(N)$ stands for an appropriate α-complex, where σ_T is the k-simplex that forms n_I, n_J and any of the other point in the set N.

The shape function thus obtained is shown in Fig. 3.[28] Note that since the only modification is the the number of natural neighbors at a given point, taking into account geometrical information given by the α-shape of the cloud, basic properties of the shape functions (such as continuity and the local coordinate property) are not modified or lost. See Cueto et al.[27] for more details on this topic.

3.2. Computation of the natural neighbor shape functions

NE shape functions are usually computed using Watson's algorithm.[44] To our knowledge, this algorithm is only defined in two-dimensions. In addition, it fails when computing values at points lying at a Voronoi edge. In this work, and for the computation of the three-dimensional shape functions, we preferred to use the algorithm from Lasserre.[45] This algorithm has been designed to compute volumes of polyhedra in $\mathbb{R}^n$, and has been successfully applied by Braun and Sambridge[18] to compute natural neighbor coordinates in NEM applications.

Lasserre's algorithm begins by expressing the volume of a convex polyhedron in the form of a set of inequalities in $\mathbb{R}^n$ that may be written as

$$\{\boldsymbol{x} | \boldsymbol{A}\boldsymbol{x} \leq \boldsymbol{b}\}, \tag{22}$$

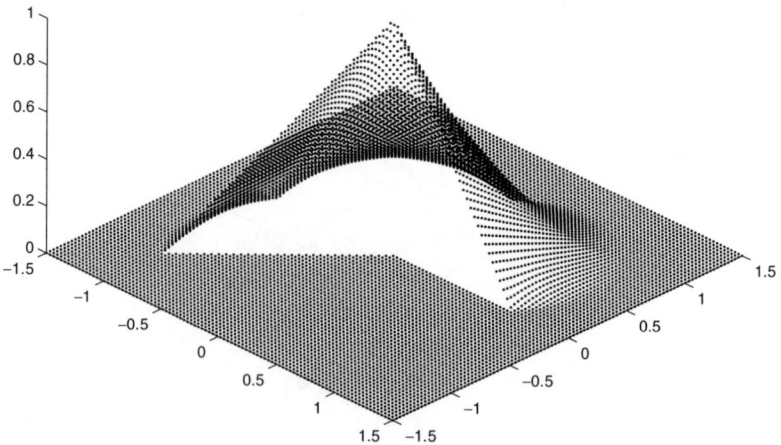

Fig. 3.   Linear interpolation along non-convex boundaries.

where x represents a point in $\mathbb{R}^n$, A is a $m \times n$ matrix, and b is a column vector of dimension m (number of constraints defining the volume). The volume enclosed by the polytope is then

$$V = V(n, A, b), \qquad (23)$$

where the i-th face of the polytope is given by:

$$\{x | (a_i \cdot x) = b_i, Ax \leq b\}, \qquad (24)$$

where a_i represents the i-th column of A. Its volume, in $\mathbb{R}^{n-1}$ space is denoted by:

$$V_i \equiv V_i(n - 1, A, b). \qquad (25)$$

A traditional way of computing the volume of the polytope is:

$$V(n, A, b) = \frac{1}{n} \sum_{i=1}^{m'} d(p, H_i) \times V_i(n - 1, A, b), \qquad (26)$$

where p is a fixed point in space, m' the minimum number of restrictions that define the polytope (no redundant restrictions are considered) and $d(p, H_i)$ the distance from point p to the hyperplane H_i given by the i-th restriction defining the volume.

Lasserre presented this algorithm in a recursive way, so the volume is computed in the form of a binary tree, beginning with dimension n and leading to the computation of n lengths in $\mathbb{R}$. This volume can then be computed by:

$$V(n, A, b) = \frac{1}{n} \sum_{i=0}^{m} \frac{b_i}{|a_{it}|} V'_{it}(n - 1, \overline{A}_{i,t}, \overline{b}_t). \qquad (27)$$

In this expression $\overline{A}_{i,t}$ represents the reduced matrix, obtained from A by elimination of the t-th variable, by means of the equation $a_i x = b_i$; $\overline{b}_t$ is the reduced vector after this elimination and a_{it} the t-th element of a_i. V'_{it} represents the volume in dimension $n - 1$ obtained with the reduced matrix $\overline{A}_{i,t}$ and the reduced vector $\overline{b}_t$. In the work of Braun and Sambridge[18] the value of t is chosen such that

$$|a_{it}| = \max_j |a_{ij}| \qquad (28)$$

This algorithm is defined over the whole space $\mathbb{R}^n$, no matter where the nodes or the integration points are located. However, it is considerably slower than Watson's algorithm (more expensive than traditional FE shape function computation). This computational cost has been established by Braun and Sambridge in a factor of about two versus the Watson's algorithm.

3.3. Natural element formulation

In the context of two- and three-dimensional solid mechanics, the unknown variable
(the displacement field in the standard displacement method) is thus approximated
in the form:

$$u^h(x) = \sum_{I=1}^{n} \phi_I(x) u_I \tag{29}$$

where u_I is the vector of nodal displacements and n the number of natural neighbors
of each point x. This leads to a C^0 interpolation scheme, although it is also possible
to build a C^1 approach.[25]

We introduce a natural element approximation both for the displacements,
like in Eq. (29) and for the space of admissible variations. This approximation
is defined as

$$\delta u = \sum_{k=1}^{n} \phi_k \delta u_k, \quad \delta u_k \in \mathbb{R}^3, \tag{30}$$

where ϕ_k are the shape functions defined by Eq. (20) and n is the number of natural
neighbors of the point at which the approximate function is computed. This is a
standard Galerkin approach.

Let φ_{t_n} a known solution at the pseudo-time increment t_n. We look for the
solution at t_{n+1}, $\varphi_{t_{n+1}} = \varphi_{t_n} + \Delta u_{t_{n+1}}$. The starting point is the consistent
linearization of the generalized displacement model about φ_{t_n}. The solution for
$\Delta u_{t_{n+1}}$ is iteratively computed using a Newton approach.

$$\Delta u_{t_{n+1}}^{(k+1)} = \Delta u_{t_{n+1}}^{(k)} + \Delta(\Delta u)_{t_{n+1}}^{(k+1)} \tag{31}$$

where $\Delta(\Delta u)^{(k+1)}$ are the displacement increments in iteration $k+1$ and represent
the degrees of freedom of the linearized algebraic system

$$\sum_{j=1}^{m} (^M K +^G K)_{ij} \Delta(\Delta u)_j^{(k+1)} = (^{ext}F -^{int}F)_i, \quad i = 1, \ldots, m, \tag{32}$$

where the subscript t_{n+1} has been omitted, m is the total number of points of the
problem, and $^M K$ and $^G K$ are the material and geometric part of the consistent
tangent stiffness matrix respectively. They are defined as

$$^M K_{ij} = \sum_{t=1}^{Nt} \int_{\Omega_t} B_i^T \mathbb{C} B_j J dV \tag{33}$$

$$^G K_{ij} = \sum_{t=1}^{Nt} \int_{\Omega_t} \hat{B}_i^T \sigma \hat{B}_j J dV, \tag{34}$$

where B are the spatial derivatives of the shape functions, $J = det F$, Ω_t is the
volume of each tetrahedron of the Delaunay tetrahedrisation and N_t, the total

number of tetrahedra. A complete Hammer quadrature have been employed in each Delaunay cell, with three and four points for the $2-D$ and $3-D$ cases, respectively, is also possible. A stabilized conforming nodal integration scheme for this method.[46]

Finally, the current configuration is updated after each iteration as:

$$\varphi_{t_{n+1}}^{(k+1)} = \varphi_{t_n}^{(k)} + \triangle \mathbf{u}_{t_{n+1}}^{(k+1)} \tag{35}$$

4. Examples

4.1. *Biomechanical modeling of human cornea*

The cornea is one of the components of the eye that helps to focus light to create the virtual image on the retina. It works much like the lens of a camera that focuses light to create image in the film. The pass of light through the cornea is known as refraction. Usually, the shape of the cornea is not perfect and the image on the retina is out-of-focus (blurred) or distorted. These imperfections in the focusing power of the eye are called refractive errors.

Surgical procedures whose aim is to improve focusing power of the eye are collectively known as refractive surgery. Their goal is to create emmetropia by altering the shape of the cornea. Several surgical techniques have been developed to treat different refractive errors. Photorefractive keratectomy (PRK) and the more up-to-date laser *in situ* keratomileusis (LASIK) correct myopia and hyperopia, whereas astigmatic disorders are corrected by techniques such as arcuate keratotomy (AK) or limbal relaxing incisions (LRI), among others.

The problem is to define those parameters that influence the surgery outcome, i.e. laser and geometric parameters concerning both incision and ablation. For this reason, the understanding of the biomechanical response of the cornea before and after surgery is of great clinical importance, with the final aim of providing information to the surgeons, regarding optimal surgical parameters.[47]

The biomechanical response of the cornea plays a significant role in the final corneal curvature and hence, in the success of refractive surgery. We postulate that the anisotropy in lamellae orientation also results in a mechanical anisotropy.

The cornea solid geometry is possible for each specific patient, by defining the global geometric parameters: thickness, diameter and radius of the inner and outer corneal curvatures, Fig. 4. The geometrical model of the healthy cornea in our case was approximated, however, by an axially-symmetric geometry around the optical axis, Fig. 4(a). As a first approach, the human cornea was represented by a 3-D spherical section of the Gullstrand eye (radius, $R = 7.86$ mm, base diameter $\phi = 11.5$ mm). The 3-D spherical section was limited by areas of different radii with origin the optical axis. This approach leads to different thicknesses of the cornea at the centre (0.55 mm) and near the limbus (0.65 mm).

Cornea was considered to be composed of an anisotropic material through the specification of two preferred material directions in terms of two local vectors defined

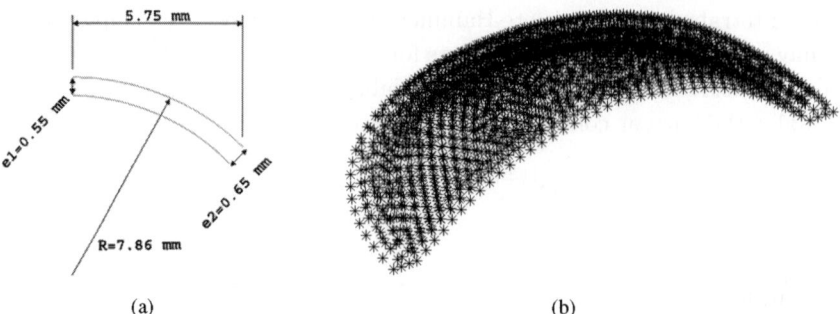

Fig. 4.   Geometrical parameters and natural element mesh of the human cornea. (a) Spherical section of the Gullstrand eye. (b) Cloud of points.

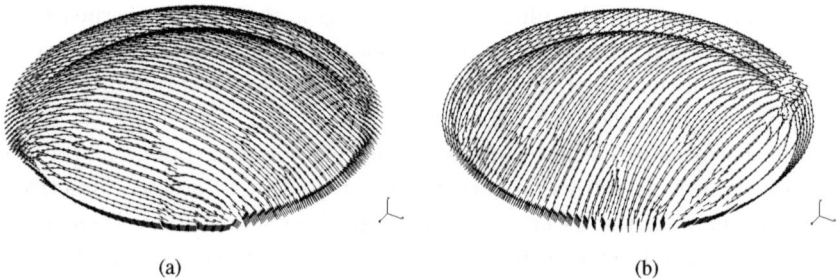

Fig. 5.   Fibril distribution in the finite element model of the human cornea. (a) Nasal-temporal direction. (b) Superior-inferior direction.

at each nodal point. Two fibril directions were defined:[48] one family along the nasal-temporal direction and another along the superior-inferior direction, Fig. 5. The circumferential fibril distribution in the limbus provides a large stiffness and therefore the limbus was considered fixed with zero displacement in all degrees of freedom. Radial symmetric intraocular pressure (IOP) was introduced as a surface load on the inner endothelium. Physiological IOP has an average value of around 15.7 mm Hg, and may vary from 14 to 18 mm Hg. In our model, the cornea was loaded with an IOP of 2.0×10^{-3} MPa (equivalent to 15 mm Hg).[49]

For the purposes of this model, the elastic response of the tissue will be assumed to arise from the resistance of the collagen fibrils and the matrix, that is, from a unique strain energy function defined as in Eq. (43). Following other authors,[78] we have considered

$$\Psi_{vol} = \frac{1}{D}(Ln(J))^2 \tag{36}$$

which quasi-enforces the null volumetric change depending on the value of the penalty coefficient $1/D$. As well as corneal stroma, arteries are also formed of a ground substance reinforced with collagen fibrils oriented in two preferred directions. Therefore, it is possible to use the same type of constitutive models. We have applied

Holzapfel's constitutive model[35] initially developed to model arterial tissue to model corneal behavior. However, the parameters that appear in the definition of the strain energy function are completely different in both cases.

$$\Psi_{iso} = \frac{C_1}{2}(\bar{I}_1 - 3) + \frac{C_2}{2}(\bar{I}_2 - 3)$$
$$+ \frac{k_1}{2k_2}\{\exp[k_2(\bar{I}_4 - 1)^2] - 1\} + \frac{k_1}{2k_2}\{\exp[k_2(\bar{I}_6 - 1)^2] - 1\}. \quad (37)$$

The two preferred orientation directions are included in the anisotropic part of the strain energy function Eq. (37), and are represented by the invariants $\bar{I}_4$ and $\bar{I}_6$. The isotropic part includes both ground substance and randomly oriented fibrils, and is represented by invariants $\bar{I}_1$ and $\bar{I}_2$.

We employed a non-linear regression method to obtain the material constants, and used data from the membrane inflating tests performed on fresh, intact human corneas by Bryant and MacDonnell.[51] The material constants obtained are shown in Table 1.

Figure 6(a) shows the vertical displacement distribution in the human cornea for the IOP value here considered. The maximal displacement took place at the apex. There appeared a slightly higher displacement at the bottom surface where the IOP was applied. The displacement distribution had almost spherical symmetry despite the fibril distribution was not. With the deformed geometry it is possible to compute the new curvature and to study the influence of elastic behavior.

The maximal principal stress took place at the bottom surface of the limbus, Fig. 6(b). The stress distribution was slightly more unsymmetrical than strains.

Table 1.   Material parameters for the anisotropic fibered material.

C_1 (MPa)	D (MPa^{-1})	C_2 (MPa)	k_1 (MPa)	k_2	k_3 (MPa)	k_4
0.005	13.3333	0.0	0.004852	102.643	0.004852	102.643

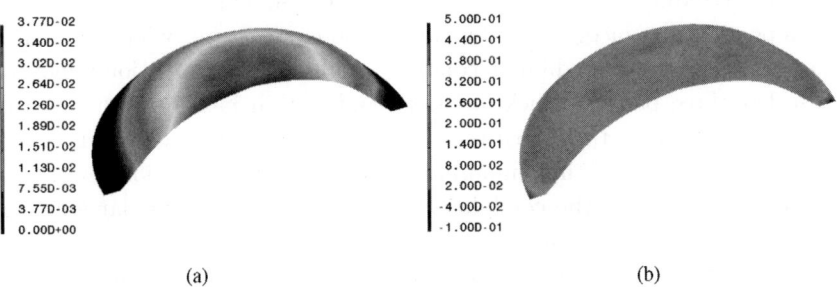

(a)   (b)

Fig. 6.   Results in the healthy human cornea. (a) Vertical displacements (mm). (b) Maximal principal stress (MPa).

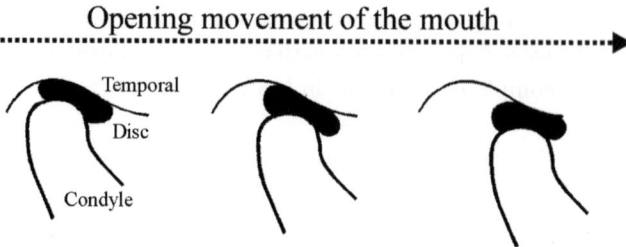

Fig. 7.   Schematic description of the opening movement.

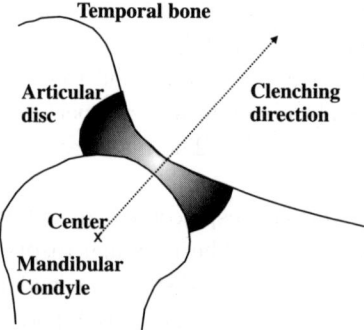

Fig. 8.   Schematic diagram of the imposed displacement direction (lateral view).

4.2. Temporomandibular disc

The temporomandibular joint (TMJ) is one of the most frequently used joints in the body, allowing us to talk, chew, yawn, swallow and sneeze and it is susceptible to all the conditions that affect other joints in the body, including ankylosis, arthritis, trauma, dislocations, developmental anomalies and neoplasms. The TMJ enables the frictionless movement between the temporal bone and the mandible. Between the condylar process of the mandible and the glenoid fossa of the temporal bone, it lies an interposed fibrocartilaginous disc. It provides a stable platform for the rotational and gliding movements of the joint and also acts as a shock absorber.[52] This component is a biconcave, fibrocartilaginous structure, which provides the gliding surface for the mandibular condyle, resulting in smooth joint movement. The disc has three parts: a thick anterior band, a thin intermediate zone, and a thick posterior band. In the closed position of the mouth, the condyle is separated from the articular fossa of the temporal bone by the thick posterior band, while in the mouth open position the condyle is separated from the articular eminence of the temporal bone by the thin intermediate zone.

In spite of the great combination of movements that the human jaw can perform, the response of the articular disc during clenching is the joint movement most extensively studied to date.[53,54] This is not only due to its simplicity since the condyle does not rotate and only compress the disc against the temporal, but for its correlation with the response of the disc in some pathologic situation like in bruxism.

The developed geometrical model of the joint was built from nuclear magnetic resonance (NMR) and computerized tomography (CT) images, which were obtained from a 65 years old asymptomatic male subject. The contours of the cranium (temporal bone) and the mandible were obtained from the CT scan (Figs. 9(a) and 9(b)), while soft tissues contours were constructed from the NMR images (Fig. 9(c)). In this joint, bones were considered to be rigid also. Therefore, in order to create the rigid surfaces for the mandible and the temporal bone, a surface tesselation (STL) of these bone components was created and then meshed automatically in the commercial package I-DEAS v.9. The articular disc was manually created, its contours were detected semiautomatically by means of a custom-design code, that allows the user to identify different components through a grey scale. These contours were approximated by splines, from which the volume of the disc was created and then filled with a cloud of nodes.

As mentioned before, bones were treated as rigid surfaces and the goal of the work was to analyze the response of the disc during clenching. This fibrocartilaginous component is an aneural and avascular tissue which distributes

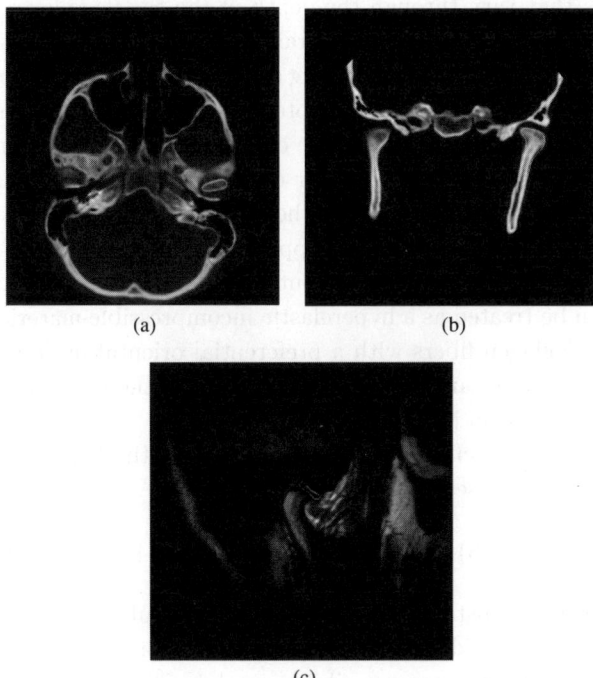

(a)   (b)

(c)

Fig. 9. Computerized tomography and magnetic resonance images of the skull. (a) Axial CT. (b) Coronal CT. (c) Sagittal NMR.

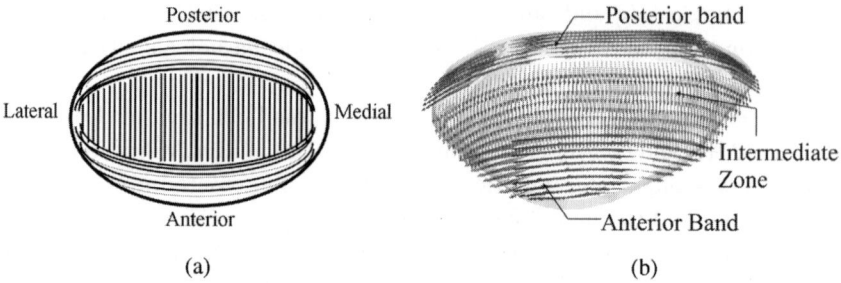

Fig. 10. (a) Schematic diagram of fibres distribution in the articular disc (viewed from top).
(b) Collagen fibres distribution in the cloud of nodes.

the loads transmitted in articular joints across the underlying bony structures.[55]
Articular cartilages in conjunction with synovial liquid provide a powerful
lubrication mechanism that produces very low wear rates and low frictional
coefficients.[56,57] Cartilage can be considered a composite material composed by
an organic solid matrix saturated with water. In normal tissue, the water phase
averages from 65% to 80% of the total weight. The dominant load-bearing structural
components of the solid matrix by composition are collagen molecules and negatively
charged proteoglycans (PGs). Collagen, on average, constitutes nearly 75% of the
dry tissue's weight; it assembles to form fibres with a preferential orientation and
with dimensions that vary through the depth of the cartilage layer.[58] This fibrous
network plays an important role in the reinforcement and mechanical stability of
cartilage, by resisting swelling or stretching of the tissue.[59,60] The ground substance,
that consists of proteoglycans, glycoproteins and water, provides the cartilage
strength to compressive stresses. Because of the relatively low permeability of the
cartilage's porous-permeable extracellular matrix, the fluid pressurization built up
in the cartilage contributes to most of the load bearing capacity of the tissue.[58]
For the case of clenching, the load is applied very fast and then due to its low
permeability, the liquid can not squeeze out of the matrix, therefore, in this specific
case, the disc can be treated as a hyperelastic incompressible material with a strong
reinforcement of collagen fibers with a preferential orientation in each part. Thus,
fibers were oriented in an anteroposterior direction in the intermediate zone, while
in a mediolateral direction in both bands.

The strain energy function chosen to characterize the hyperelastic behavior of
the disc was earlier proposed by,[35]

$$\Psi = c_1(\widetilde{I_1} - 3) + \frac{k_1}{2k_2}\{\exp[k_2(\widetilde{I_4} - 1)^2] - 1\} + \frac{1}{D}(J - 1)^2 \tag{38}$$

where c_1 is a material constant related to the ground substance, $k_1 > 0$ and $k_2 > 0$
are the parameters which identify the exponential behavior due to the presence of
collagen fibres, and D is the compressibility modulus.[61]

The simulation started with the jaw in closed position, followed by a
displacement of the mandible against the temporal bone in a direction corresponding

to the estimated direction of the joint reaction force.[62] This direction was similar to that obtained by Breul *et al.*[63] An imposed displacement of 0.2 mm applied in 1s in the direction defined above was introduced (Fig. 8).

In Fig. 11 the geometry (rigid surface elements) and a detail of the α-shape of the disc from the cloud of nodes are depicted, as well as its displacement under the clenching load.

The stress distribution can be seen in Figs. 12 and 13. One of the advantages of the natural element method is that the discontinuities that arise in the finite element method due to irregularities in the mesh can be avoided. It can be seen how the stress distributions are smooth along the top and bottom surfaces. As can be seen in Fig. 12, the maximum principal stresses were located at the posterior band of the disc where the disc tries to open as it is compressed. However, the maximum compressive stresses were located in the intermediate zone (both in the bottom and top surfaces) of the disc (Fig. 13).

4.3. Passive modeling of heart

The primary function of the heart is to pump blood through the body, delivering nutrients and removing wastes from each of the organs, and transporting hormones and other messengers between various regions of the body.[64] The heart is divided by the interventricular septum in left and right parts. These parts are also divided

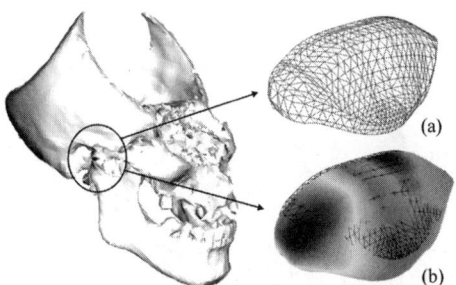

Fig. 11.   Finite element mesh of the rigid surfaces of the bone. (a) α-shape of the cloud of nodes. (b) Deformed plot of the disc.

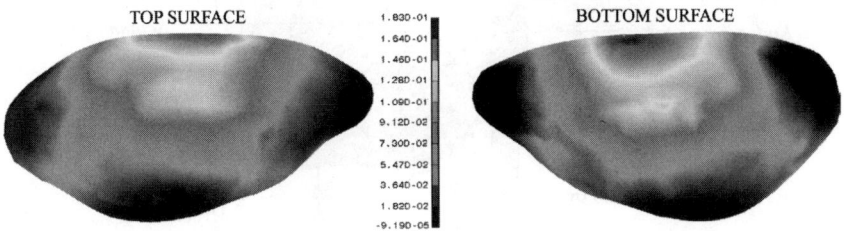

Fig. 12.   Maximum principal stresses in the articular disc.

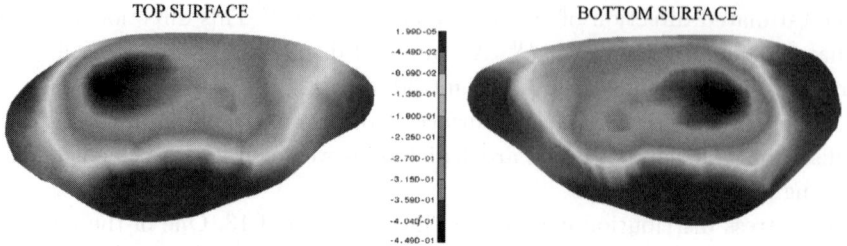

TOP SURFACE   BOTTOM SURFACE

Fig. 13.   Minimum principal stresses in the articular disc.

horizontally by the fibrous skeleton of the heart or basal skeleton leading to four separate chambers. The upper chambers are the left and right atria, while the lower chambers correspond to the left and right ventricles as shown in Fig. 14.

Between the cavities of the atria and ventricles lie atrioventricular valves: on the right, the tricuspid valve, and on the left the mitral valve. Semilunar valves separate, on the other hand, the outflow tracts of each ventricle and its great artery, the pulmonary artery and the aorta. Atria are smaller in size and thinner than ventricles and work as low pressure blood reservoirs for the ventricles. The ventricles, the predominant pumping chambers, develop much higher pressure than the atria having much thicker muscular walls, specially the left ventricle which has approximately three times the mass and two times the thickness of the right ventricle. The cavity of the left ventricle resembles an ellipsoid or elongated cone in

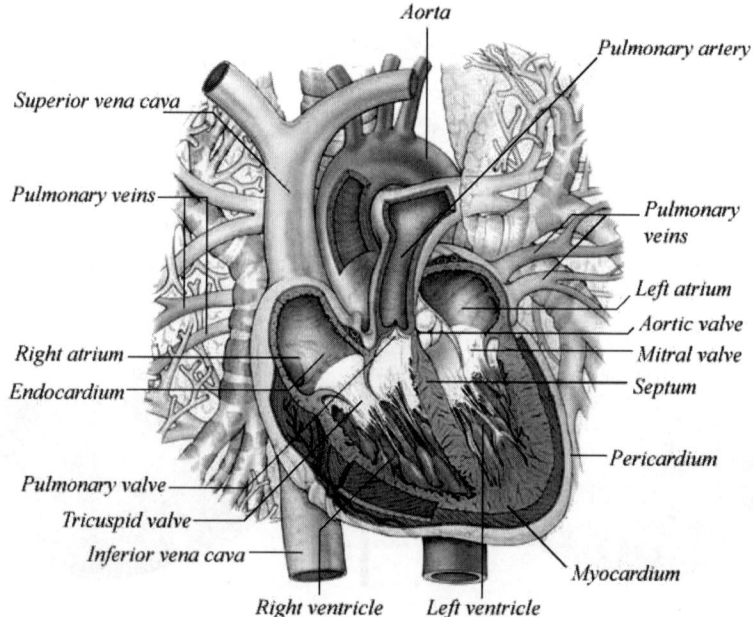

Fig. 14.   Longitudinal cross section of the heart.

which both the inflow and outflow tracts are adjacent. In contrast, the right ventricle pumps at lower pressure (about one seventh the pressure of the left ventricle) and has a crescentic cross section forming a shallow U which warps around the left ventricle. Both ventricles are separated by the interventricular septum which usually functions as part of the left ventricle. The papillary muscles are attached to the mitral and aortic valves through fibrous cords (chordae tendinae) arising form the inner walls of the right and left ventricles. These muscles contract during systole preventing the valve leaflets to move backward (prolapse) into the atria in late systole, when intraventricular pressure reaches its maximum. Semilunar valves are similar in structure and functioning to the atrioventricular valves. These valves prevent the backflow to the ventricles once the blood has reached the great arteries.

The walls of the heart are organized in several layers: the epicardium that covers the outer surface of the heart, inner surfaces of the atria and ventricles are lined with the endocardium, and the myocardium which lays in between. The ventricular myocardium, the large mass of cardiac muscle that lays between the epicardium and endocardium, consists of overlapping sheets of muscle bundles running from the base of the pulmonary artery to the aorta describing a double helix in the space and defining to chambers, the left and right ventricles.[65] Myocardial is composed of contractile cylindrical muscle cells (myocites) with lengths between 80 and 100 m and diameters ranging from 10 to 20 m. These muscle fibers are bound together by endomysial collagen defining branching sheets through out the wall, which interconnect by perymisial collagen which allows each sheet to slide with respect to each other with minimal resistance. These sheets are generally oriented normal to the ventricle free wall. Therefore, a fully characterization of the cardiac microstructure requires defining a set of orthogonal directions: a fiber direction $\mathbf{f}$, a sheet direction $\mathbf{s}$, and a sheet normal direction $\mathbf{b}$ as has been proposed by LeGrice et al.[66] (see Fig. 15).

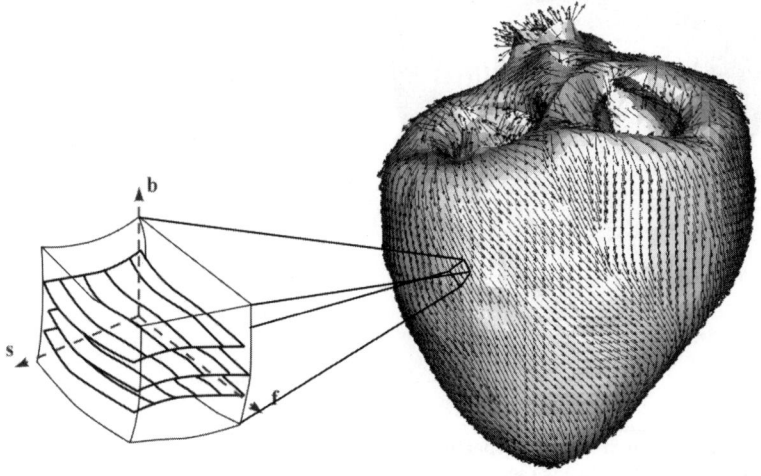

Fig. 15. Structure of the myocardium.

The ventricular geometry and myocardial fiber angles of the heart model correspond to a 26 Kg pig.[67,68] The data was obtained from the Bioengineering Research Group at the University of Auckland.[a] Contour splines were created from points on the external surfaces of the heart. These splines were used to defined epicardial and endocardial surfaces and then the heart volume. This operation was entirely conducted in the commercial package I-DEAS v.9. The heart volume was automatically filled with a cloud of nodes with the software HARPOON v.2.0.

The fiber structure of the heart was interpolated from the measured points[67] to the model by first identifying the closest N_n measured points to each point in the cloud, and then using the following interpolating function

$$\mathbf{n} = \frac{\sum_{i=1}^{N_n} (\prod_{k=1, k \neq i}^{N_n} d_k) \mathbf{m}^{(i)}}{\sum_{i=1}^{N_n} \prod_{k=1, k \neq i}^{N_n} d_k}, \tag{39}$$

where d_k is the distance from the kth measured point to the current model point, and $\mathbf{m}^{(i)}$ is the fiber orientation at the ith measured point. The interpolated field so obtained was smoothed further using the surface normals. Figure 16 shows the fiber distribution for the model.

In order to model the cardiac cycle, the material model must contemplate the active behavior of the tissue at the same time that it accounts for the anisotropy of the underlying material. The activation of the muscle fibers changes the properties of the material at the same time that contracts the muscle itself. Therefore, most models of activation consider two transformations. The first one changing the

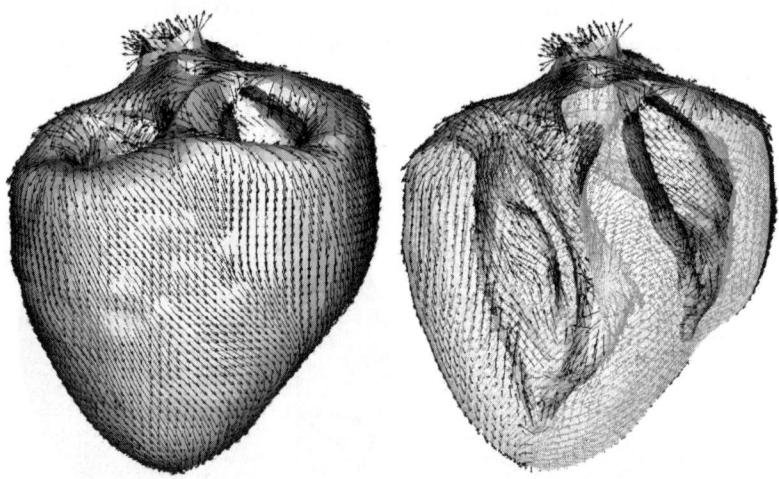

Fig. 16. Fiber architecture in the pig heart.

[a]Bioengineering Research Group, Departments of Engineering Science and Physiology, University of Auckland. URL: http://www.esc.auckland.ac.nz/Groups/Bioengineering/CMISS/.

material properties without changing the geometry, and a second transformation contracting the muscle without changing the geometry. Bourdarias *et al.*[69] have proposed a model for the myocardium based on the model by Lin and Yin.[70] However, we should point that, if passive behavior of the heart is being modeled, an anisotropic SEF of the form Eq. (38) can be used for the myocardium. For the active behavior, the strain energy functions proposed by Bourdarias *et al.* and Lin and Yin have the form

$$\Psi^f_{act}(\mathbf{C}) = a^a_1(\bar{I}_1 - 3)(\bar{I}_4 - 1) + a^a_2(\bar{I}_1 - 3)^2 + a^a_3(\bar{I}_4 - 1)^2, \tag{40}$$

for the Bourdarias *et al.*[69] model and

$$\Psi^f_{act}(\mathbf{C}) = a^a_1(\bar{I}_1 - 3)(\bar{I}_4 - 1) + a^a_2(\bar{I}_1 - 3)^2 + a^a_3(\bar{I}_4 - 1)^2 + a^a_4(\bar{I}_4 - 1), \tag{41}$$

for the Lin and Yin[70] model. The main difference between both models lies in the fact that the model proposed by Bourdarias *et al.* introduces the muscle contraction directly in the definition Cauchy stress as

$$\boldsymbol{\sigma} = p\mathbf{1} + \frac{2}{J}dev\left[\bar{\mathbf{F}}\frac{\partial\Psi(\bar{\mathbf{C}},\mathbf{n}_0)}{\partial\bar{\mathbf{C}}}\bar{\mathbf{F}}^T\right] + \beta(t)T^{(0)}\lambda^2\mathbf{n}\otimes\mathbf{n}, \tag{42}$$

where λ is the actual elongation of the muscle fiber, $T^{(0)}$ is a constant, and $\mathbf{n}$ the current fiber direction.

For the calculations that follow, model Eq. (38) has been used, with constants $c_1 = 0.4607$, $k_1 = 2.4619$, and $k_2 = 4.6996$. These constants where obtained by fitting tensile data reported by Nash and Hunter.[71]

Boundary condition corresponding to a passive inflation during vetricular diastole were imposed to the model presented here. Different internal pressures were applied to the inner endocardial surfaces of each cavity, 3.0 kPa (22.5 mm Hg) for the left ventricle and 0.6 kPa (4.5 mm Hg) for the right one. Null displacements were imposed in nodes near to the base of each ventricle, modeling the influence of the heart valves during distole.

Figure 17 shows the maximal principal stretches in the heart model, with a maximum of 11% in the medial zone of the left ventricle. Maximal principal stress took place also in this part of the left ventricle, Fig. 18, with a maximum value of 12 MPa. The two contours present very smooth distribution as a consequence of the low dependence of the NEM on the location of the cloud of points.

4.4. Human knee ligaments

Although the knee may look like a simple joint, it is however, one of the more complex. Moreover, the knee is more likely to be injured than any other joint in the body. The knee is essentially made up of four bones: femur, tibia, patella and fibula; four ligaments: anterior and posterior ligaments (ACL, PCL) and lateral and medial collateral ligaments (LCL and MCL), patellar tendon (PT), articular

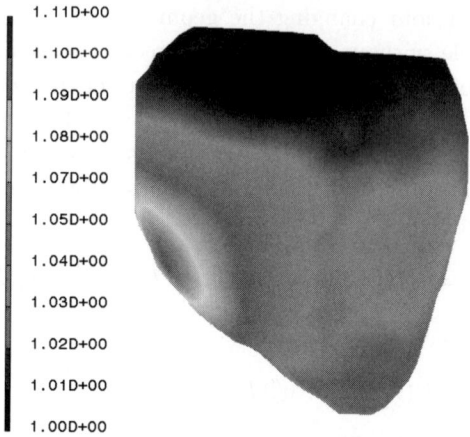

1.11D+00
1.10D+00
1.09D+00
1.08D+00
1.07D+00
1.05D+00
1.04D+00
1.03D+00
1.02D+00
1.01D+00
1.00D+00

Fig. 17.   Maximal principal stretches in the heart.

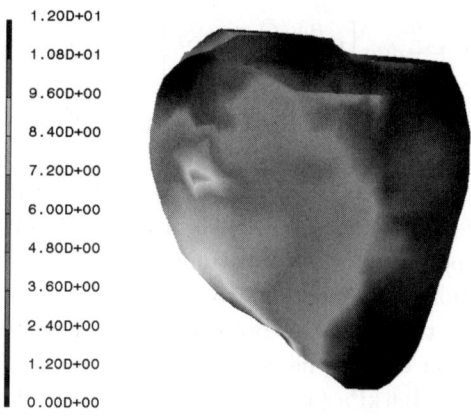

1.20D+01
1.08D+01
9.60D+00
8.40D+00
7.20D+00
6.00D+00
4.80D+00
3.60D+00
2.40D+00
1.20D+00
0.00D+00

Fig. 18.   Maximal principal stress in the heart.

cartilage and menisci . The human knee joint compliance and stability required for optimal daily functions are provided by several components like menisci, cartilage, ligaments and muscle forces that allow complex mechanical responses to different types of physiological loads.

Because of the relative incongruence of the articular surfaces, ligaments play an important role in providing passive stability to the joint. For the development of adequate diagnostic and surgical procedures, it is essential to understand the role of individual ligament as motion restraints.[72] The primary role of the ligaments that surround the knee is to provide stability to the joint throughout its range of motion. Each ligament plays a role in providing stability in more than one degree of freedom as well as restraining knee motion in response to externally applied loads. Overall joint stability depends on the contributions of the individual ligaments as well as interaction between them.

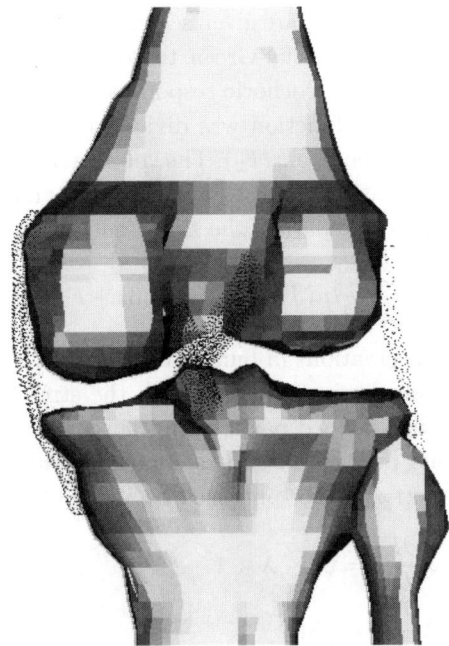

Fig. 19.   Natural element model of the human knee.

A detailed model of the human knee is shown in Fig. 19. The model includes realistic hard and soft tissue geometries for all the major structures. The surface geometries of the femur, fibula, tibia and patella were reconstructed from a set of CT scans, while the knee ligament were obtained from MNR data (anterior cruciate ligament, posterior cruciate ligament, lateral collateral ligament and medial collateral ligament).[73]

Cross-sectional contours were manually digitized from these images and the curves imported into the commercial code I-DEAS. The external surfaces were created by extrusion and a regularly distributed cloud of points was generated inside this volume. The femur and tibia were considered as rigid bodies, so only the external surfaces were meshed with rigid shell elements. On modeling ligaments, two important assumptions were made. First, no difference in the material behavior between the ligament body and its insertion were considered. Second, material characteristics depending on time, such as viscoelasticity, creep and relaxation were neglected[74] due again to the high ratio between the viscoelastic time constant of the material and the loading time of interest in this study. A transversely isotropic hyperelastic model was used including the effect of one family of fibers, usually applied to ligaments.[75]

We postulated the existence of a unique decoupled representation of the strain-energy density function Ψ such as

$$\Psi = \Psi_{vol}(J) + \Psi_{iso}(\bar{\mathbf{C}}, \mathbf{a}_0 \otimes \mathbf{a}_0) \tag{43}$$

where $\Psi_{vol}(J)$ and $\Psi_{iso}(\bar{\mathbf{C}}, \mathbf{a}_0 \otimes \mathbf{a}_0)$ are given scalar-valued functions of the Jacobian $J = det\mathbf{F}$ and the modified Cauchy-Green tensor $\bar{\mathbf{C}} = J^{\frac{2}{3}}\mathbf{C}$ respectively, that describe the volumetric and the isochoric responses of the material. The isochoric part Ψ_{iso} of the strain-energy function was divided in an isotropic part (F_1) and other depending on the collagen fibers (F_2). The volumetric part Ψ_{vol} was considered in a standard manner for quasi-incompressible materials, and a Neo-Hookean model was considered for the isotropic part of the strain-energy function. We had in turn

$$\Psi = \frac{1}{2D}ln(J)^2 + C_1(\bar{I}_1 - 3) + F_2(\lambda) \tag{44}$$

Following physical observations in human ligaments, we assumed that collagen fibers do not support compressive loads. Second, the stress–strain relation curves for ligaments have two well-defined parts: an initial curve with increasing stiffness (toe region) and a second part with stiffness almost constant (linear region).[76] We used the free-energy function earlier proposed by Weiss *et al.*[77]

$$\lambda\frac{\partial F_2}{\partial \lambda} = 0 \quad \lambda < 1$$
$$\lambda\frac{\partial F_2}{\partial \lambda} = C_3(e^{C_4(\lambda-1)} - 1) \quad \lambda < \lambda^* \tag{45}$$
$$\lambda\frac{\partial F_2}{\partial \lambda} = C_5\lambda + C_6 \quad \lambda > \lambda^*$$

where C_1 is the Neo-Hookean constant and D the inverse of the bulk modulus $k = 1/D$ which was chosen for all the ligaments as $k/C_1 = 1000$. We used with the average constants obtained by Gardiner and Weiss[78] for the MCL in their experimental data. The LCL constants were assumed to be identical to those of the MCL. The uniaxial stress–strain curves obtained by Butler *et al.*[79] for ACL, PCL and PT were fit with those obtained by Weiss's getting the associated constants that have been included in Table 2.

The ligaments were attached to the tibia at the distal end and to the femur in its proximal end (Fig. 20). A prescribed displacement and rotation history corresponding to the flexion motion of the knee was applied to the femur until a rotation of 60°. Figure 20 shows the maximum principal stress contour for a 60° flexion angle. A significant tensile stress appeared in the posterior part of the

Table 2. Material parameters for the ligaments.

	C_1 (MPa)	C_2 (MPa)	C_3 (MPa)	C_4	C_5 (MPa)	λ^*	D (MPa^{-1})
MCL	1.44	0.0	0.57	48.0	467.1	1.063	0.00126
LCL	1.44	0.0	0.57	48.0	467.1	1.063	0.00126
ACL	1.95	0.0	0.0139	116.22	535.039	1.046	0.00683
PCL	3.25	0.0	0.1196	87.178	431.063	1.035	0.0041
PT	2.75	0.0	0.065	115.89	777.56	1.042	0.00484

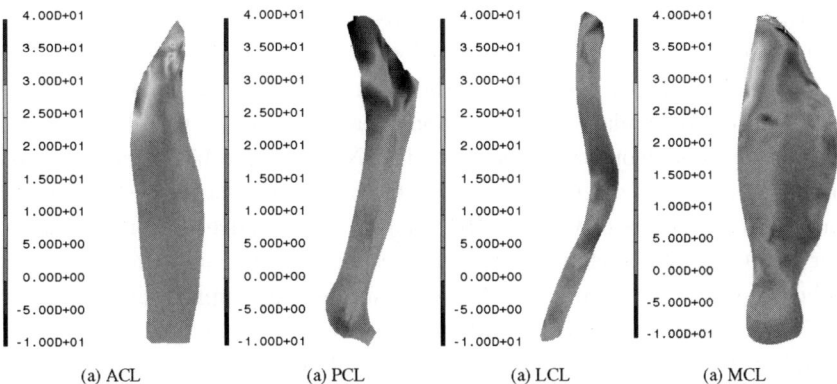

Fig. 20.   Maximal principal stresses in the ligaments in response to a knee flexion of 60° (MPa).

ACL. The obtained results also showed that the PCL was mainly in compression. The LCL is mainly relaxed during this movement. The anterior load produced in the MCL a stress distribution similar to a beam flexion problem, with tension in the anterior-distal and the posterior-proximal parts of the MCL.

5. Conclusions

The main objective of this work is to present the possible advantages of using meshless methods in simulations of biomechanics problems, specifically in application to modeling of living soft tissues. This family of methods present some appealing characteristics comparing to the well-known FEM.[2] They avoid the difficult task of mesh generation in very complex geometries, such as the case of living tissues. A finite element meshing process can be very costly depending on the complexity of the geometry, but a volume reconstruction approach and distribution of points inside this volume is relatively simple. Meshless methods appear to be an efficient alternative to FEM for this type of problems.

Biomechanics of living soft tissues usually involves several geometric non-linearities such us large displacements and strains, as well as material non-linearities. Soft tissues can be seeing as a network of fibre collagenous or muscular tissue embedded in a high compliant matrix. Therefore, most fibrous soft tissues are modeled as continuum hyperelastic fiber reinforced and sometimes layered material. This type of problems are usually associate with mesh distortions.[28] In the NEM there is virtually no limitation to "mesh" distortions, showing that results are much less dependent on the regularity of the nodal distribution than FEMs. Compared to the finite element method, NEM is better at handling large deformation without any special numerical treatment because it is less dependent on the original mesh. From these results, NEM appears to be an efficient alternative to FEM for large deformation problems, especially when using a total Lagrangian description.[28]

Natural Neighbor Galerkin methods present some advantages with respect to other meshless methods for its application in biomechanics framework. On one hand, Natural Neighbor Galerkin methods are strictly interpolant and thus are very well suited to simulate piece-wise homogeneous domains with high accuracy.[80] On the other, the geometrical basis of the NEMs, that has been pointed out, is specially important when dealing with biomechanical structures obtained after volume reconstructions of CT or MRI images, for instance. Recent works by the authors in other fields such as fluid mechanics have leaded us to think that Natural Neighbor Galerkin techniques are able to be successfully applied also in other fields within Biomechanics, such as blood flow, blood-vessel interaction and others.

Four examples have been presented that show the wide range of problems where NEMs can be applied to. First, the numerical simulation of refractive procedures in the human cornea. The objective is to analyze those parameters that influence the surgery outcome. The biomechanical response of the cornea plays a significant role in the final corneal curvature and hence, in the success of refractive surgery. The second example corresponds to the simulation of the motion of the temporomandibular joint, and concretely the stress analysis in the fibrocartilaginous disc. The passive inflation during vetricular diastole of a pig heart is also presented. Fiber distribution of the cardiac tissue must be taken into account to model the anisotropy of the underlying material. As a final example, a numerical simulation of the flexion motion of the human knee is also presented, studying the stress distribution appearing in the main ligaments of the joint, ACL, PCL, MCL and LCL.

Acknowledgments

The authors gratefully acknowledge the support of the Spanish Education and Science Ministry (CYCIT DPI2003-09110-C02-01, DPI2004-07410-C03-01 and FIS2005-05020-C03-03) and the Spanish Ministry of Health through the National Network IM3 (Molecular and Multimodal Medical Imaging, Cardiovascular modeling, PI052006).

References

1. M. A. Crisfeld. *Non-Linear Finite Element Analysis of Solids and Structures* (Wiley, New York, 1996).
2. M. Doblaré, E. Cueto, B. Calvo, M. A. Martínez, J. M. García and J. Cegoñino, On the employ of meshless methods in biomechanics. *Comput. Methods Appl. Mech. Eng.* **194** (2005) 801–821.
3. M. Papadrakakis and B. H. V. Topping (eds). *Advances in Non-Linear Finite Element Methods* (Civil-Comp Ltd., Edinburgh, 1994).
4. B. Nayroles, G. Touzot and P. Villon, Generalizing the finite element method: Diffuse approximation and diffuse elements. *Comput. Mech.* **10** (1992) 307–318.

5. J. J. Monaghan. Why particle methods work. *SIAM J. Sci. Stat. Comput.* **3**(4) (1982) 422–433.

6. D. Sulsky, S. J. Zhou and H. L. Schreyer, Application of a particle-in-cell method to solid mechanics. *Comp. Phys. Commun.* **87** (1994) 179–196.

7. T. Belytschko, Y. Y. Lu and L. Gu, Element-free Galerkin methods. *Int. J. Num. Methods Eng.* **37** (1994) 229–256.

8. Y. Y. Lu, T. Belytschko and L. Gu, A new implementation of the element free Galerkin methods. *Comp. Methods Appl. Mech. Eng.* **113** (1994) 397–414.

9. W. K. Liu, S. Jun, S. Li, J. Adee and T. Belytschko, Reproducing kernel particle methods. *Int. J. Num. Methods Eng.* **38** (1995) 1655–1679.

10. W. K. Liu, S. Jun and Y. F. Zhang, Reproducing kernel particle methods. *Int. J. Num. Methods Fluid* **20** (1995) 1081–1106.

11. C. A. M. Duarte and J. T. Oden, An H-p Adaptive Method using Clouds. *Comput. Methods Appl. Mech. Eng.* **139** (1996) 237–262.

12. I. Babuška and J. M. Melenk, The partition of Unity Method. *Int. J. Num. Methods Eng.* **40** (1997) 727–758.

13. C. A. M. Duarte. *A Review of Some Meshless Methods to Solve Partial Differential Equations.* (TICAM, University of Texas at Austin, 1995), pp. 95–106.

14. T. Belytschko, Y. Krongauz, D. Organ, M. Fleming and P. Krysl, Meshless methods: an overview and recent developments. *Comput. Methods Appl. Mech. Eng.* **139** (1998) 3–47.

15. S. Li and W. K. Liu, Meshfree and particle method and their applications. *Appl. Mech. Rev.* **55** (2002) 1–34.

16. J.-S. Chen, C.-T. Wu, S. Yoon and Y. You, A stabilized conforming nodal integration for Galerkin mesh-free methods. *Int. J. Num. Methods Eng.* **50** (2001) 435–466.

17. L. Traversoni. Natural neighbor finite elements. *Intl. Conf. Hydraulic Eng. Software. Hydrosoft Proc.* (Computational Mechanics publications, 1994), pp. 291–297.

18. J. Braun and M. Sambridge, A numerical method for solving partial differential equations on highly irregular evolving grids. *Nature* **376** (1995) 655–660.

19. M. Sambridge, J. Braun and H. McQueen, Geophysical parametrization and interpolation of irregular data using natural neighbors. *Geophys. J. Int.* **122** (1995) 837–857.

20. R. Sibson. Interpreting multivariate data. V. Barnett, Ed. *A Brief Description of Natural Neighbor Interpolation* (John Wiley, 1981), pp. 21–36.

21. B. Delaunay, Sur la Sphère Vide. A la memoire de Georges Voronoi. Izvestia Akademii Nauk SSSR, *Otdelenie Matematicheskii i Estestvennyka Nauk.* **7** (1934) 793–800.

22. G. M. Voronoi, Nouvelles applications des paramètres continus à la théorie des formes quadratiques. Deuxième Memoire: Recherches sur les parallélloèdres Primitifs. *J. Reine Angew. Math.* **134** (1908) 198–287.

23. N. Sukumar, B. Moran and T. Belytschko, The natural element method in solid mechanics. *Int. J. Num. Methods Eng.* **43**(5) (1998) 839–887.

24. N. Sukumar, *The Natural Element Method in Solid Mechanics* (Northwestern University, Evanston, Illinois, 1998).

25. N. Sukumar and B. Moran, C^1 Natural neighbor interpolant for partial differential equations. *Num. Methods Partial Diff. Eqns.* **15**(4) (1999) 417–447.

26. E. Cueto, M. Doblaré and L. Gracia, Imposing essential boundary conditions in the natural element method by means of density-scaled α-shapes. *Int. J Num Methods Eng.* **49**(4) (2000) 519–546.

27. E. Cueto, B. Calvo and M. Doblaré, Modeling three-dimensional piece-wise homogeneous domains using the α-shape based natural element method. *Int. J. Num. Methods Eng.* **54** (2002) 871–897.

28. B. Calvo, M. A. Martinez and M. Doblaré, On solving hyperelasticity with the Natural Element Method. *Int. J. Num. Methods Eng.* **62** (2005) 159–185.

29. G. R. Johnson, E. H. Petersen and R. A. Stryk, Incorporation of an SPH option in the EPIC code for a wide range of high velocity impact computations. *Int. J. Impact Eng.* **14** (1993) 385–394.

30. J. Bonet and S. Kulasegaram, Correction and stabilization of smooth particle hydrodynamics methods with applications in metal forming simulations. *Int. J. Num. Methods Eng.* **47** (2000) 1189–1214.

31. J. S. Chen, C. Pan, C. T. Wu and W. K. Liu, Reproducing kernel particle methods for large deformation Aanalysis of nonlinear structures. *Comput. Methods Appl. Mech. Eng.* **139** (1996) 195–227.

32. S. Jun, W. K. Liu and T. Belytschko, Explicit reproducing kernel particle methods for large deformation problems. *Int. J. Num. Methods Eng.* **41** (1998) 137–166.

33. Y. C. Fung. *Biomechanics: Mechanical Properties of Living Tissue* (Springer, New York, 1993).

34. J. A. Weiss, B. N. Maker and S. Govindjee, Finite element implementation of incompressible, transversely isotropic hyperelasticity. *Comput. Methods Appl. Mech. Eng.* **135** (1996) 107–128.

35. G. A. Holzapfel. *Nonlinear Solid Mechanics. A Continuum Approach for Engineering* (Wiley, Chichester, 2000).

36. P. J. Flory, Thermodynamic relations for high elastic materials. *Trans. Faraday Soc.* **57** (1961) 829–838.

37. J. C. Simo and R. L. Taylor, Consistent tangent operators for rate-independent elastoplasticity. *Comput. Methods Appl. Mech. Eng.* **48** (1985) 101–118.

38. A. J. M. Spencer. *Continuum Mechanics* (Longman Scientific & Technical, Essex, 1980).

39. G. A. Holzapfel, Biomechanics of soft tissue in *Handbook of Materials Behavior Models*, J. Lemaitre, ed., Vol. III (Academic Press, 2001), pp. 1057–1073.

40. J. C. Simo and T. J. Hughes. *Computational Inelasticity* (Springer-Verlag, New York, 1998).

41. D. Bueche, N. Sukumar and B. Moran, Dispersive properties of the natural element method. *Comput. Mech.* **25**(2/3) (2000) 207–219.

42. R. Sibson, A vector identity for the Dirichlet Tesselation. *Math. Proc. Cambridge Philosophical Soc.* **87** (1980) 151–155.

43. H. Edelsbrunner and E. Mücke, Three dimensional alpha shapes. *ACM Trans. Graph.* **13** (1994) 43–72.

44. D. Watson, Nngridr. *An Implementation of Natural Neighbor Interpolation* (Published by the author, 1994).

45. J. B. Lasserre, An analytical expression and an algorithm for the volume of a convex polyhedron in $\mathbb{R}^n$. *J. Optim. Theory Appl.* **39**(3) (1983) 363–377.

46. D. Gonzalez, E. Cueto, M. A. Martinez and M. Doblare, Numerical integration in Natural Neighbor Galerkin methods. *Int. J. Num. Methods Eng.* **60**(12) (2004) 2077–2104.

47. P. Pinsky and V. Datye, A microstructurally-based finite element model of the incised human cornea. *J. Biomech.* **10** (1991) 907–922.

48. K. Meek and R. Newton, Organization of collagen fibrils in the corneal stroma in relation to mechanical properties and surgical practice. *J. Refrac. Surg.* **15** (1999) 695–699.

49. V. Alastrue, B. Calvo, E. Peña and M. Doblare, Biomechanical modeling of refractive corneal surgery. *ASME J. Biomech. Eng.* **128** (2006) 150–160.

50. J. Gardiner and J. Weiss, Subjet-specific finite element analysis of the human medial collateral ligament during valgus knee loading. *J. Orthop. Res.* **21** (2003) 1098–1106.
51. M. Bryant and P. McDonnell, Constitutive laws for biomechanicalmodeling of refractive surgery. *J. Biomech. Eng.* **118** (1996) 473–481.
52. J. C. Nickel and K. R. McLachlan, In vivo measurement of the frictional properties of the temporomandibular joint disc. *Arch. Oral. Biol.* **39**(4) (1994) 323–331.
53. K. Nagahara, S. Murata, S. Nakamura and T. Tsuchiya, Displacement and stress distribution in the temporomandibular joint during clenching. *Angle Orthodon.* **69** (1999) 372.
54. M. Beek, J. H. Koolstra, L. J. van Ruijven and T. M. G. J. van Eijden, Three-dimensional finite element analysis of the human temporomandibular joint disc. *J. Biomech.* **33** (2000) 307–316.
55. C. Wang, C. T. Hung and V. C. Mow, An analysis of the effects of depth-dependent aggregate modulus on articular cartilage stress-relaxation behavior in compression. *J. Biomech.* **34** (2001) 75–84.
56. G. A. Ateshian, W. H. Warden, J. J. Kim, R. P. Grelsamer and V. C. Mow, Finite Deformation biphasic material properties of bovine articular cartilage from confined compression experiments. *J. Biomech.* **30** (1997) 1157–1164.
57. G. A. Ateshian, H. Q. Wang and W. M. Lai, The role of interstitial fluid pressurization and surface porosities on the boundary friction of articular cartilage. *J. Tribol.* **120** (1998) 241–248.
58. V. C. Mow and X. E. Guo, Mechano-electrochemical properties of articular cartilage: their inhomogeneities and anisotropies. *Ann. Rev. Biomed. Eng.* **4** (2003) 175–209.
59. A. Maroudas, Balance between swelling pressures and collagen tension in normal and degenerate cartilage. *Nature* **260** (1976) 808–809.
60. W. L. Hukins, R. M. Aspden and Y. E. Yarker, Fiber reinforcement and mechanical stability in articular cartilage. *Eng. Med.* **13** (1984) 153–156.
61. A. Pérez-Palomar and M. Doblaré, The effect of collagen reinforcement in the behavior of the temporomandibular joint disc. *J. Biomech.* **39** (2006) 1075–1085.
62. J. H. Koolstra and TMGJ Van Eijden. Application and validation of a three-dimensional mathematical model of the human masticatory system in vivo. *J. Biomech.* **25** (1992) 175–187.
63. R. Breul, G. Mall, J. Landgraf and R. Scheck, Biomechanical analysis of stress distribution in the human temporomandibular joint. *Ann. Anatomy.* **182** (1999) 55–60.
64. A. M. Katz. *Physiology of the Heart.* Third edition (Lippincott Williams and Wilkins, 2001).
65. F. Torrent-Guasp, M. Kocica, A. Corno, M. Komeda, F. Carreras, A. Flotats, J. Cosin and H. Wen, Towards new understanding of the heart structure and function. *Eur. J. Cardio-Thoracic Surg.* **27**(2) (2005) 191–201.
66. I. J. LeGrice, B. H. Smaill, L. Z. Chai, S. G. Edgar, J. B. Gavin and P. J. Hunter, Laminar structure of the heart: ventricle myocyte arrangement and connective tissue architecture in the dog. *Am. J. Physiol.* **269** (Hear Circ. Physiology 38) (1995) H571–H582.
67. C. Stevens, An anatomically based computational study of cardiac mechanics and myocardial infarction. PhD Thesis (The University of Auckland, 2002).
68. C. Stevens, E. Remme, I. LeGrice and P. Hunter, Ventricular mechanics in diastole: material parameter sensitivity. *J. Biomech.* **36** (2002) 737–748.
69. C. Bourdarias, S. Gerbi and J. Ohayon, A three dimensional finite element meted for biological active soft tissue. Formulation in cylindrical polar coordinates. *ESAIM: Math. Modeling Num. Analy.* **37**(4) (2003) 725–739.

70. D. H. S. Lin and F. C. P. Yin, A multiaxial constitutive law for mammalian left ventricular myocardium in steady-state barium contracture or tetanus. *ASME J. Biomech. Eng.* **120** (1998) 504–517.
71. M. P. Nash and P. J. Hunter, Computational mechanics of the heart. From tissue structure to ventricular function. *J. Elasticity.* **61** (2000) 113–141.
72. L. Blankevoort and R. Huiskes, Ligament-bone interaction in a three-dimensional model of the knee. *ASME J. Biomech. Eng.* **113** (1991) 263–269.
73. E. Peña, B. Calvo, M. A. Martinez and M. Doblaré, A three-dimensional finite element analysis of the combined behavior of ligaments and menisci in the healthy human knee joint. *J. Biomech.* **39** (2006) 1686–1701.
74. J. A. Weiss and J. C. Gardiner, Three-dimensional deformation and stress distribution in an analytical/computational model of the anterior cruciate ligament. *J. Biomech.* **33** (2001) 1069–1077.
75. S. Hirokawa and R. Tsuruno, Computational modeling of ligament mechanics. *Critical Rev. Biomed. Eng.* **29** (2000) 1–70.
76. A. Viidik, Structure and function of normal and healing tendons and ligaments in *Biomecanics of Diarthorial Joints*, V. C. Mow, A. Ratchiffe and S. L.-Y. Woo ed., (Springer-Verlag, 1990), pp. 3–38.
77. J. A. Weiss, B. N. Maker and S. Govindjee, Finite element implementation of incompressible, transversely isotropic hyperelasticity. *Comput. Methods Appl. Mech. Eng.* **135** (1996) 107–128.
78. J. C. Gardiner and J. A. Weiss, Subjet-specific finite element analysis of the human medial collateral ligament during valgus knee loading. *J. Orthop. Res.* **21** (2003) 1098–1106.
79. D. L. Butler, M. Y. Sheh, D. C. Stouffer, V. A. Samaranayake and M. S. Levy, Surface strain variation in human patellar tendon and knee cruciate ligaments. *ASME J. Biomech. Eng.* **39** (1990) 38–45.
80. E. Cueto, N. Sukumar, B. Calvo, M. A. Martínez, J. Cegoñino and M. Doblaré, Overview and recent developments in Natural Neighbor Galerkin methods. *Arch. Comput. Method Eng.* **10** (1990) 307–387.

CHAPTER 4

TECHNIQUES IN COMPUTER-AIDED DIAGNOSIS AND THEIR APPLICATION IN CLINICAL INVESTIGATION OF BRONCHIAL SYSTEMS

C. I. FETITA*, A. SARAGAGLIA, M. THIRIET, F. PRÊTEUX and P. A. GRENIER

Institut National des Télécommunications
ARTEMIS Department, 9 rue Charles Fourier, 91011 Evry, France
*catalin.fetita@int-evry.fr

Respiratory diseases constitute a major preoccupation for the medical community, due to their worldwide extent, their high incidence in the industrialized countries and an important mortality rate. In this context, early diagnosis is the key issue for the patient healthcare policy. After its introduction in clinical routine during the last decade, helical computed tomography (CT) became rapidly the recomended imaging technique for assessing airway disease. With the advent of multidetector row CT (MDCT), high resolution images of the airways were possible to be acquired throughout the whole thorax, in a single breath hold. But the advantage to benefit of high-quality data for pulmonary investigation was counterbalanced by the large amount of data the clinician had to deal with. Computer-aided diagnosis (CAD) techniques are now proposed in routine investigation. This paper aims at presenting an overview of the advances in the CAD techniques designed for bronchial systems analysis. According to their investigation ability, both basic and advanced methods are addressed throughout this presentation. From direct visualization, to complex segmentation, interaction, navigation, simulation and quantification issues, the challenges raised by the airway pathology investigation are discussed and various solutions are presented and illustrated.

Keywords: Pulmonary airways; 3D segmentation; medial axis; mesh modeling; airflow simulation; airway reactivity; bronchus wall remodeling; computer-aided diagnosis; multidetector CT.

1. Introduction

Airway diseases represent one of the main causes of death, after cardiovascular diseases and cancers. Their prevalence continued to increase in the last decade, particularly in the industrialized countries. Of various origins — infectious, inflammatory, cicatriceal, congenital — airway diseases induce morphological changes of the respiratory system leading to functional disorders. Such diseases can be either focal or diffuse and may affect both large and small airways.

While different investigation modalities were available in clinical routine, such as functional respiratory investigations, chest radiography, fiberoptic bronchoscopy, only the introduction of the computed tomography (CT) in the last decade made it possible to provide a non-invasive, local investigation of the airways. The continous development of the CT technology led today to the helical multidetector row scanners (MDCT) able to acquire high-resolution volumetric images of airways throughout the whole thorax in a single breath hold, in about 10 s. Such image data is able to depict even minor intra- and extraluminal pathology in the trachea and proximal bronchi and, combined with appropriate post-processing tools, allow to assess the extent of stenosis, bronchiectasis and small airway disease.

In this paper, we focus our attention on the MDCT investigation modality and on the associated computer-aided diagnosis (CAD) tools developed for airway analysis. Section 2 provides an insight into the MDCT scanning protocol which defines the image data quality and fixes the limits of the structure quantification accuracy. Several protocols are recommended according to the requested analysis. In the following, for the sake of clarity, Sec. 3 presents the anatomy and function of the bronchial system and discusses the main pathologies affecting its morphology. Such diseases raise several challenges in terms of assisted clinical diagnosis system design, which will constitute the guiding lines in the presentation of our survey. In this respect, Sec. 4 introduces the so-called basic CAD techniques relying uniquely on data rendering and visualization functionalities. Such techniques do not perform any data preprocessing in order to extract information on the bronchial structure. Instead, their analysis capability exploits the intrinsic tissue attenuation characteristics enclosed by the MDCT data. Originally contrasted data can be investigated via *cine-viewing* or *multiplanar reformation* techniques. 3D to 2D data projection via *volume rendering* offers additional functionalities for a global or local, external or endoluminal analysis of airways, where the original data contrast is modified by means of specific transfer functions and illumination models: *minimum intensity projection, maximum intensity projection, unshaded* and *shaded composite rendering*.

Going deeper into the bronchial systems investigation requires advanced CAD tools which are presented in the Sec. 5. Such tools rely on information extraction from the MDCT data, namely on the *3D segmentation* of the airway structure. Combined with volume rendering display facilities, a global analysis of the bronchial tree morphology becomes easily accessible to the clinician. Interaction and navigation capabilities are added via an *axis*-based description, making thus possible local assessment of airways: *morphometric measures, automated trajectory computation* for *virtual bronchoscopy* investigation, analysis of the *airway wall remodeling*. Patient-specific *3D mesh model synthesis* allows data exchange, preoperative planning, and functional simulation. Finally, such representation is also useful for leading research in quantitative studies for inhaled medication in asthma and other chronic obstructive pulmonary disease (COPD).

The development of CAD tools is performed in association with the imaging modality employed. It is thus essential to discuss in the following the MDCT data acquisition protocol and the influence of its parameters on the analysis performance which can be expected.

2. MDCT Scanning Protocol

In the following, the reader is supposed to be familiar with the basic principles of the computed tomography, namely image reconstruction from projections.[1,2] We shall thus focus on the particularities of the helical (spiral) CT and multidetector row spiral CT (MDCT).

The principle of the spiral CT consists of continuously moving the scanner table while the couple tube-detector turns around the patient.[3] Raw projection data is interpolated along a cross-section plane and an image of the anatomical tissues attenuation is reconstructed using classic algorithms (i.e., filtered backprojection). The advantage of spiral over conventional CT is a higher speed and the ability to reconstruct cross-section images at any longitudinal location, leading to true volumetric CT data (Fig. 1).

The key parameters influencing the image spatial resolution are: the X-ray beam collimation (responsible for partial volume effects), the pitch (ratio between the spiral repetition step and the collimation), the reconstruction interval between successive axial images, the field of view (in-plane reconstruction diameter), the reconstruction matrix (image size in pixels) and the reconstruction kernel (the frequency filter involved in the filtered backprojection algorithm).

When using state-of-the-art single detector spiral CT scanners with a rotation period less than one second (0.5–0.8 s), it was shown that an acceptable compromise was reached in clinical routine for a pitch value of 1.5 to 2, 3 to 5 mm slice thickness, and 30–40% overlaping in axial image reconstruction.[4–6]

Multidetector row CT (MDCT) uses several detectors illuminated simultaneously by the X-ray beam in order to accelerate the acquisition process for thin collimations. For example, a 16-detector row CT scanner makes it possible to explore the entire thorax in less than 10 s using a beam collimation from 0.625 mm to 1.5 mm. Reconstruction of overlapped axial images will generate isotropic or near isotropic data with voxel volume of around $0.5 \times 0.5 \times 0.5$ mm^3 when using a 512×512 matrix. This is of outmost importance for the 3D post-processing tools

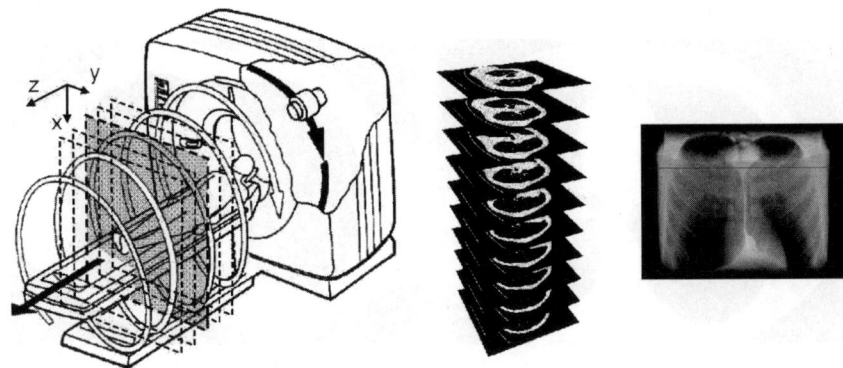

Fig. 1. Principle of volumetric image acquisition in spiral CT. Cross-section images are reconstructed in the axial (*x-y*) plane at the desired sampling interval along the *z*-axis leading to volumetric image data.

developed for airway investigation.[7] Another advantage of the MDCT scanners is
their ability to propose retrospective changes of the effective slice thickness of which
the optimal value is equal to half the chosen collimation. This feature is particularly
helpful in daily practice because it does not impose additional acquisitions if higher
image resolution is requested in the z-axis for CAD analysis.

During the acquisition, it is mandatory for the patient to remain motionless
and hold his breath, in order to avoid respiratory motion artifacts which will make
the acquired data useless (Fig. 2). For specific analysis purposes requiring repeated
MDCT scanning in identical conditions, a spirometric system may be used in order
to control the lung volume during acquisition.

The dynamic range of the MDCT data covers 2000 values, calibrated with
respect to the attenuation coefficient of the water and known as Hounsfield Units
(HU):

$$1\,\mathrm{HU} = 1000\frac{\mu - \mu_w}{\mu_w},\tag{1}$$

where μ and μ_w denote the tissue and water density, respectively. By consequent,
there is a linear correlation between anatomical tissue density and the CT data
values. A value of $-1000\,\mathrm{HU}$ corresponds to air, $0\,\mathrm{HU}$ to water, and $1000\,\mathrm{HU}$ to
calcified bone. Due to the restricted perception range of the human eye (256 gray
levels), the whole range of Hounsfield Units cannot be displayed without significant
loss of information. In this respect, the radiologists use a sliding value window for
displaying only the tissues which density lie in the given interval. The HU values
in the display window are converted into 256 levels (0–255), while those lying
outside the window are saturated (0 beneath the inferior limit, and 255 above
the superior limit). The clinical window setting for airway investigation ranges
from -1000 to $200\,\mathrm{HU}$. Using such window setting, bronchi are displayed as dark
zones (airway lumen) surrounded by white or light gray closed contours (airway
wall), Fig. 2(a). Their appearance depends on the subdivision generation, image
acquisition protocol, and the orientation with respect to the axial plane.

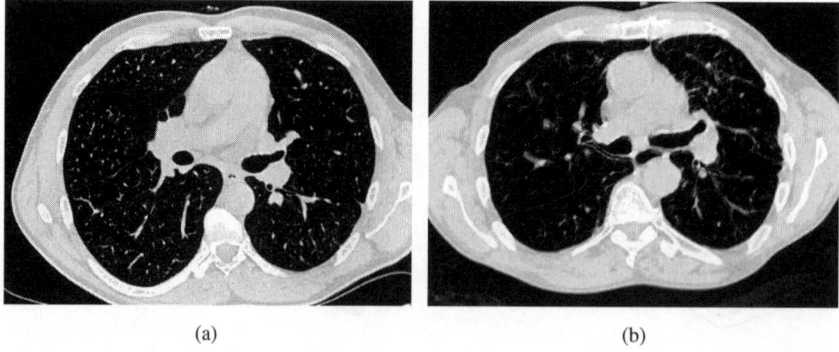

(a)   (b)

Fig. 2.   MDCT images acquired at the same anatomical level in two patients: (a) respecting breath
hold constraint and (b) during respiration, which results in motion artifacts.

To summarize, an MDCT protocol recommended for developing CAD functionalities will consider the following parameters:

- 0.625–0.75 mm X-ray beam collimation;
- overlapping in reconstruction of axial images;
- dedicated reconstruction kernel ensuring a good compromise between (high) level of detail and (low) level of noise in the image. The scanners manufacturers generally provide their proprietary designed filter for lung investigation (usually called "lung kernel");
- 512 × 512 reconstruction matrix or larger (768 × 768, 1024 × 1024);
- field-of-view focused on one lung or on the two lungs when using a larger reconstruction matrix.

3. Physiopathology of the Airways

The respiratory tract ensures the oxygen supply to, and certain toxic evacuation from blood. From a functional point of view, air volumes are moved on a well vascularized lung surface where gas-blood exchanges take place. The respiratory tract is composed of the upper airways and the tracheobronchial tree. The upper airways include the nose, the pharynx and the larynx and have a role of air humidification, heating, purification and transport. The tracheobronchial tree is a ramified air dispatching system, which superior part — trachea, bronchi and bronchioles — conveys the air to and from the alveolar ducts, specialized in gas exchange. The current MDCT imaging systems are able to depict airway structures down to 1 mm diameter (trachea and bronchi). Bronchioles of lumen diameter and wall thickness inferior to 1 mm and 0.1 mm, respectively, are below the MDCT resolution.

The morphological description of the tracheobronchial tree is important for understanding the analysis techniques developed and to evaluate their diagnosis value.

The trachea is a semi-rigid tubular structure of 10–12 cm long and 2–3 cm diameter. Its wall contains 16 to 20 U-shape cartilageneous rings, which extremities are connected by a fibro-elastic membrane with smooth muscle. The air column of the trachea is easily recognizable on CT images due to the high contrast with the adjacent dense mediastinal tissue, Fig. 3. Trachea subdivides into two main bronchi, RMB and LMB, supplying the right and the left lungs, respectively (Fig. 4). The main bronchi branch off in lobar bronchi (three for the right lung — RULB, RMLB, RILB, and two for the left lung — LULB, LILB), which at their turn split recursively into segmental, subsegmental, and so on. Their spatial orientation and associated nomenclature is given in Fig. 4, according to Naidich *et al.*[8]

Pulmonary airways are affected by various pathologies, noticeable with MDCT, which induce morphological changes and functional disorders. According

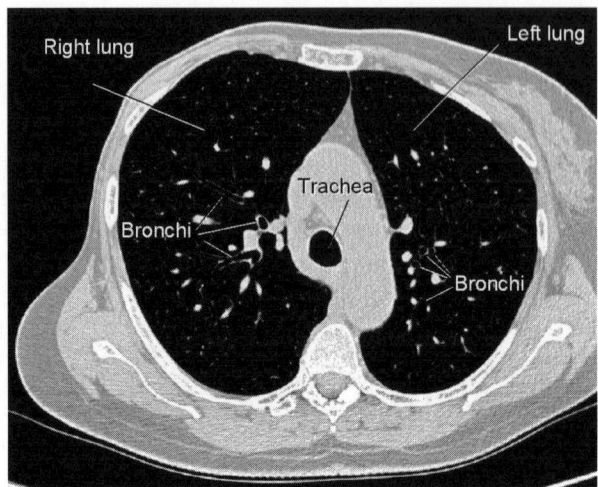

Fig. 3. MDCT axial image illustrating cross sections of the trachea and of some apical bronchi.

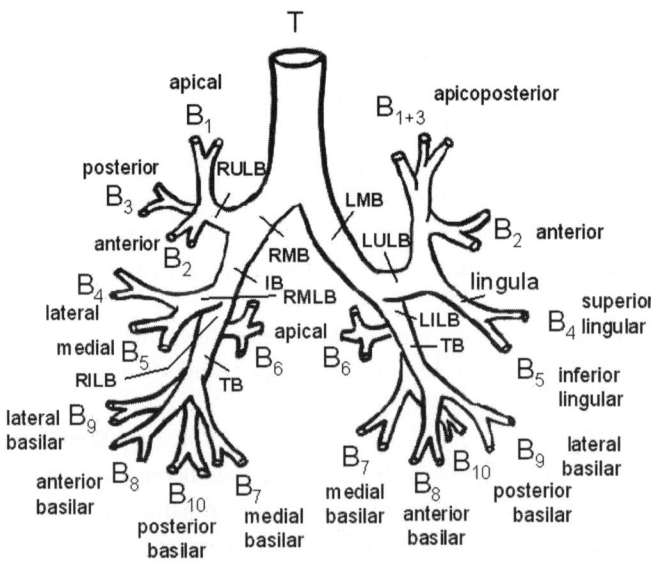

Fig. 4. Frontal view representation of the tracheobronchial tree up to the subsegmental level (4th order subdivision). T-trachea, RMB-right main bronchus, LMB-left main bronchus, IB-intermediate bronchus, RULB-right upper lobe bronchus, LULB-left upper lobe bronchus, RMLB-right middle lobe bronchus, RILB-right inferior lobe bronchus, LILB-left inferior lobe bronchus, TB-truncus basalis. Nomenclature from Naidich.[8]

to their impact on the airway morphology, such pathologies can be classed as follows:

- **stenosis**, characterized by a narrowing of the bronchus lumen, usually caused by bronchial tumours, a foreign body-associated inflammation or a mucous plug. On occasion, it is due to inflammatory or post-traumatic bronchial lesions;[9]
- **airway fistula**, which is an abnormal communication between oesophagus and airways, pleural cavity, pericardial cavity or great thoracic vessel;[10]
- **bronchial dehiscence**, seen as bronchial wall defect associated with extraluminal air collections;[11]
- **congenital abnormalities**, referring to anomalies of the bronchial branching pattern such as ectopic bronchi, supernumerary anomalous bronchus, bronchial atresia and lobar hypoplasia;[12,13]
- **bronchiectasis**, which is a chronic irreversible dilatation of diseased bronchi manifested under three forms: (a) *cylindrical bronchiectasis*, with a smooth dilatation of the affected bronchi, which do not taper normally toward the periphery,[14] (b) *varicose bronchiectasis* showing irregularity and beading of the affected bronchi with destruction and loss of the bronchial lumen peripherally[15] and (c) *cystic bronchiectasis*, characterized by increasing dilatation of bronchi toward the periphery, with ballooning, and a loss of bronchial subdivisions;[15]
- **chronic obstructive pulmonary disease (COPD)**, involving intrathoracic airways are manifested such as bronchial wall thickening,[16] saber-sheath trachea[17] and expiratory airway collapse due to abnormal flaccidity (tracheobronchomalacia);[18,19]
- **asthma**, known as a chronic inflammatory condition involving the airways, causes increases in the existing bronchial hyperresponsiveness consecutive to various stimuli.[20-23] The real current challenge for the MDCT in asthma is to visualize and quantify the airway lumen and wall in order to assess the extent of airway obstruction, the degree of inflammation in small airways, and to evaluate in vivo the airway wall remodeling.[24]

The diagnosis of such diseases with MDCT requires appropriate computer-assisted tools allowing data analysis from angles and perspectives other than those provided by the axial images. Such CAD tools may rely either on image visualization and 3D rendering techniques, applying directly to the original MDCT data, or combine both data preprocessing (for airway structure extraction) and visualization facilities.

The following sections present the different CAD approaches available in clinical routine or in medical research, and illustrate their ability to detect and analyze the mentioned pathologies, or to increase the diagnosis confidence.

4. Basic CAD Techniques Relying on MDCT Data Visualization and Rendering

This section introduces the different visualization modalities developed for MDCT data analysis, which do not require the separation (segmentation) of the airway structure from its anatomical environment. Such basic investigation modalities exploit the intrinsic contrast of the MDCT data related to anatomical density of the lung tissues. There are two major approaches for data investigation: (i) cross-section local analysis via 2D image interpolation from the volumetric data along section planes defined by the user, and (ii) global analysis via volume rendering techniques which perform volume data projection on an image plane according to specific ray composition and illumination models.

4.1. *Cross-section data imaging*

Cine-viewing is the simplest cross-section investigation modality exploiting the native axial CT images. It consists of displaying successive overlapped thin axial images on the same frame window, in the same manner as a video sequence. Such investigation mode allows the bronchial subdivisions to be followed from the segmental origin down to the smallest bronchi which can be.identified on CT images. In this way, the segmental and subsegmental distribution of any airway lesion can be easily monitored. Cine-viewing may also serve as a roadmap for planning an endoscopic intervention. Figures 5 and 6 illustrate two examples of several successive

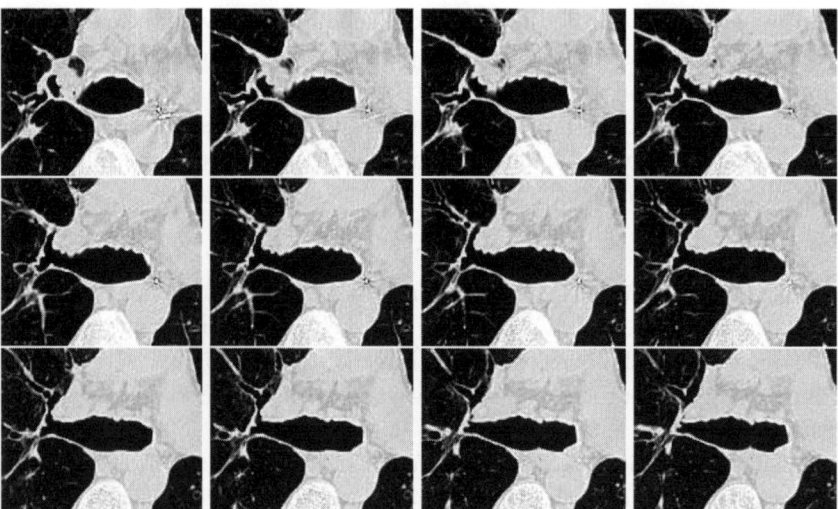

Fig. 5. Irregular contours of the internal wall of the RMB and RULB. Left to right and top to bottom: cine-viewing sequence monitoring the trachea subdivision into RMB and LMB, and the RMB subdivision into B_1, B_2, and B_3 segments.

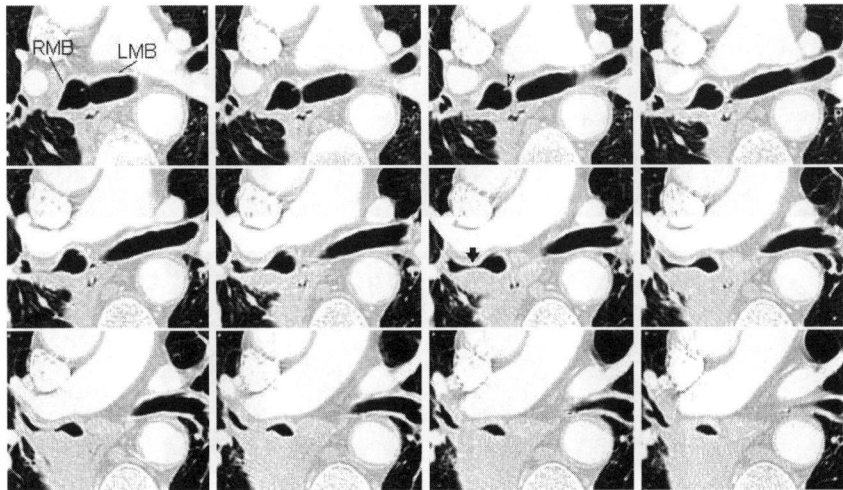

Fig. 6.   Bronchial stenosis in relation with lung carcinoma. Left to right and top to bottom: cine-viewing sequence monitoring the central airways subdivision (RMB and LMB). Note the epithelial tissue within the RMB lumen (white arrow head, 3rd image), the severe stenosis on the RULB (black arrow, 7th image) as well as the narrowing of the intermediate bronchus (IB).

axial images composing two cine-sequences which depict the central airways of pathologic subjects.

Multiplanar reformations (MPR) allow local investigation of the airways on cross-section images along planes interactively defined by the user. Cross-section images are created from the volumetric MDCT data by using linear interpolation. The MPR technique enhances the analysis of airway pathologies running in a plane other than the axial one.[25]

However, a single MPR image may not be sufficient to fully describe a pathology extent. Several multiplanar reformations of different obliquity, together with the native axial images are recommended for a confident analysis.[26] Figure 7 illustrate these aspects in the case of three studies: (a) a congenital malformation (ectopic bronchus associated with tracheal stenosis), (b) a bronchial stenosis in relation with a lung carcinoma and (c) a cystic bronchiectasis.

In the first two cases, the MPRs were obtained starting from the coronal plane[a] and performing slight rotations around the horizontal axis. In the last case, one axial and two oblique MPR images illustrate the bronchial dilatation, but they are insufficient to fully characterize the extent of the pathology.

It becomes obvious that the cross-section data imaging techniques are not adapted to the analysis of volumetric spatial information, the investigator being constrained to mentally reproduce the 3D relationships between the anatomical structures observed in 2D sections. The complement of the 3D information can be

---

[a]virtual plane crossing the head and the shoulders $((y - z)$ plane, *cf.* Fig. 1).

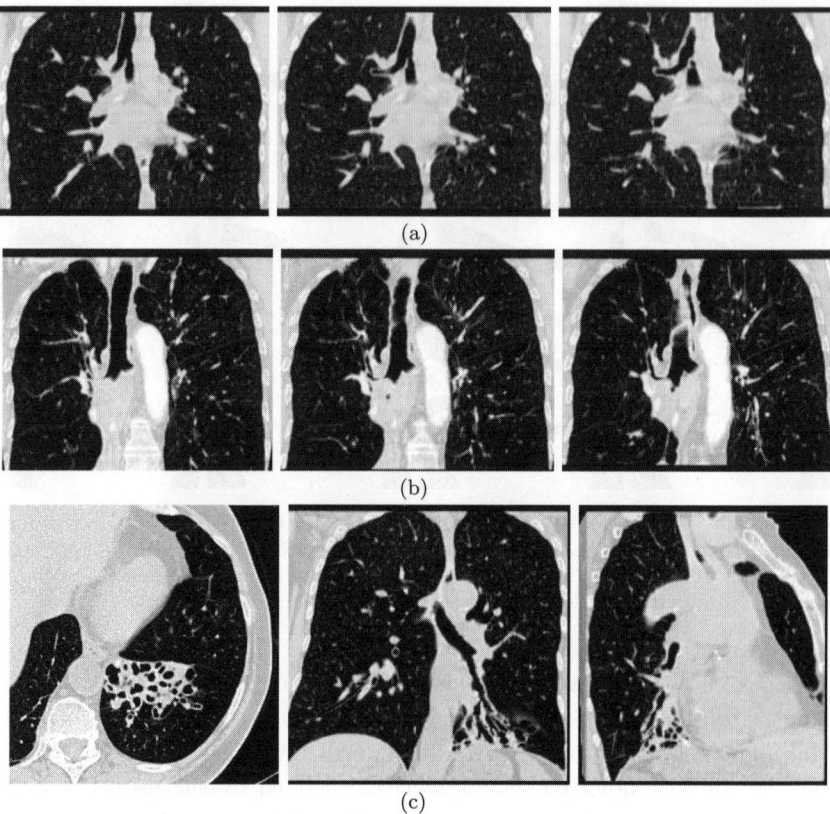

Fig. 7.   Clinical investigation using multiplanar reformations: (a) Congenital tracheal bronchus (RULB arising directly from trachea), (b) bronchial stenosis on the RULB in relation with a carcinoma and occlusion of the right IB (same subject as in Fig. 6), (c) varicose and cystic bronchiectasis in the basilar segments of the left lower lobe.

provided by using 3D rendering techniques which consider the whole or a part of the volume data in order to produce a projection image. The next section introduces the principle of the *volume rendering* and presents its application in computer-aided diagnosis.

4.2. *Volume rendering: a projective approach*

Volume rendering[27-30] produces projection images of an MDCT volume data according to the (virtual) camera projection geometry (paralel/divergent), its spatial orientation and the selected illumination model (Fig. 8). The principle consists of casting virtual rays from each point of the camera image plane, record the chain of the traversed elementary volumes composing the object (voxels) and compute the final color along the ray, which will be associated to the image point. The strength of such visualization approach is the ability to provide different models

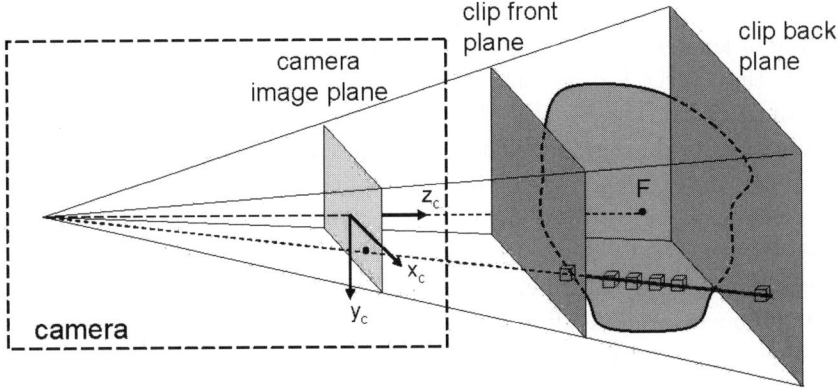

Fig. 8.   Principle of image formation in volume rendering.

for color composition along the ray which will produce different images for the same scene and will make possible anatomical structure discrimination with no need of previous segmentation.[31,32] The only spatial selection of the imaged data consists in interactiveley setting up two clipping planes, *clip front* and *clip back*, which limit the region of rendering. Only the volume data comprised between this clipping planes are taken into account during image projection.

Basically, two factors influence the image formation in volume rendering: the transfer function and the ray composition model. The transfer function defines a color and opacity table, indexed by the MDCT intensity values. In this way, the original intensity values along a projection ray are "encoded" into color/opacity values. The ray composition model uses the color/opacity provided by the transfer function in order to compute the final color of each image pixel. Three ray composition models apply for airway image analysis: minimum intensity, maximum intensity and composite rendering. They are detailed in the following.

4.2.1. *Minimum and maximum intensity projection (mIP/MIP)*

Minimum intensity projection (mIP) associates to an image point the minimum value encountered along its projection ray. The color transfer function used in this case is the identity function (for all three color planes), $f_R(x) = f_G(x) = f_B(x) = x$, while the opacity transfer function is ignored.

Due to the lower density of the airway lumen with respect to the surrounding tissues, the bronchi can be visualized with the mIP technique. Because of a small density difference with respect to the lung parenchyma (between 50 HU and 150 HU[33]), the image contrast is worse for distal bronchi than for the central airways. In addition, low-attenuated zones in the lung parenchyma (e.g. lung emphysema) may hide bronchi (Fig. 9(a)). Consequently, carefully selecting clipping planes and an appropriate view point is generally required for mIP rendering (Fig. 9(b)). Some examples of mIP images are illustrated in Fig. 9, where a gamma correction was applied in order to enhance the contrast between airways and lung parenchyma.

Note that several drawbacks limit the use of mIP in clinical routine:[6] underestimation of the bronchi diameters due to the partial volume effects, overestimation of high-grade stenoses which can be interpreted as bronchial occlusions (Fig. 9(d)), and missing of intraluminal growth of eccentric tumors.[24]

Maximum intensity projection (MIP) associates to an image point the maximum value encountered along its projection ray. The transfer functions are identical to those employed in mIP. MIP benefits in the display of the mucoid impactions seen in dilated bronchi, or in the display of the small centrilobular nodular and/or linear branching opacities expressing infectious or inflammatory bronchiolitis.[34]

4.2.2. Composite rendering

Composite rendering produces projection images by taking into account the contribution of all elementary volumes along the ray. Here, the color and opacity

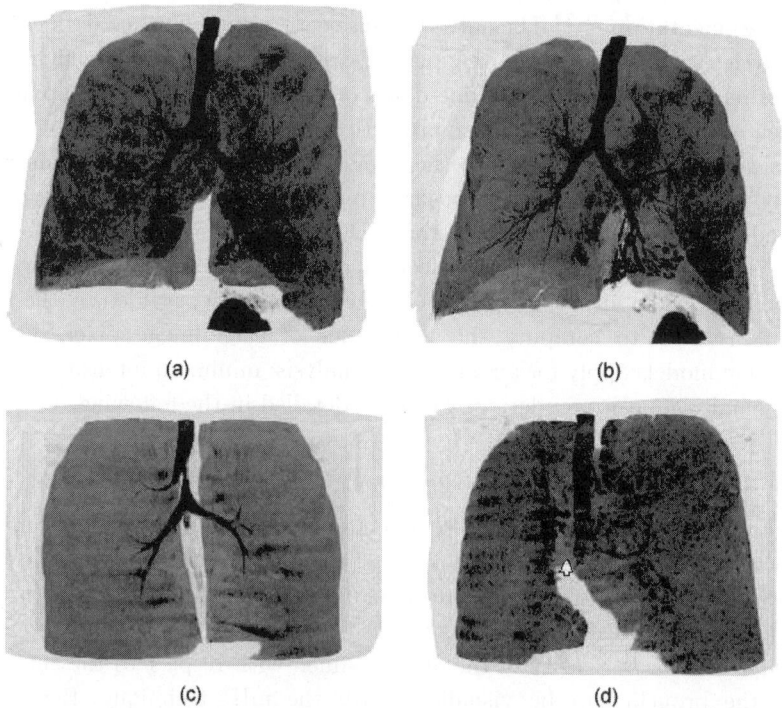

(a)   (b)

(c)   (d)

Fig. 9.   Minimum intensity projections of normal and pathologic airways. Setting clipping planes and view angle is often mandatory to avoid the superimposition of low-attenuated structures (a and b). Severe stenoses may be seen as total occlusions (d, arrow). (a) Bronchiectasis in the LIL bronchi (278 mm thick slab), case of Fig. 7(c). (b) Same as in (a), with 128 mm thick slab and 25° rotation. Airway structure becomes visible. (c) Ectopic bronchus with tracheal stenosis, case of Fig. 7(a). (d) Bronchial severe stenosis (RULB) and occlusion of the IB, case of Fig. 7(b).

transfer functions are set up according to the tissue densities which need to be highlighted. The color composition along the ray employs a weighted contribution of the elementary values derived from the Krueger's transport theory model.[35] The final color is recursively computed by moving from the back clipping plane to the front clipping plane and accumulating each point contribution in the following manner, Fig. 10. If $\mathbf{C}_n = (R, G, B)_n^T$ and α_n denote respectively the color vector and the opacity corresponding to the density of the nth elementary volume on the ray (according to the transfer functions), $\mathbf{I}_{n+1}$ the composite color computed from the back clipping plane to the $(n+1)$-th ray location, then, the composite color at the n-th position is given by:

$$\mathbf{I}_n = \alpha_n \mathbf{C}_n + (1 - \alpha_n)\mathbf{I}_{n+1}. \tag{2}$$

By setting the transfer functions in a manner that will associate the maximum light and opacity with the density values at lumen-wall tissue interface, images of the airways may be obtained as illustrated in Fig. 11. Note that the transfer functions are expressed in normalized values: the density range on the abscissa correspond to the $[-1000, 200]$ HU interval.

Composite volume rendering has also the ability to use surface shading modeling which provides a realistic visual effect when air-tissue interfaces are examined. Shaded volume rendering adds light reflectance properties in the illumination model described by Eq. (2). The color vector $\mathbf{C}_n$ derived from the color transfer function is here replaced by a weighted sum of three color components: *ambient* — $\mathbf{C}_a$, *diffuse* — $\mathbf{C}_d$ and *specular* — $\mathbf{C}_s$ which are defined in the following (Fig. 12). The ambient component models the incident light scattered by all surrounding objects. If $\mathbf{L}_c$ and $\mathbf{O}_c$ denote the light source and object colors respectively (Fig. 12(a)), the ambient component is a constant given by:

$$\mathbf{C}_a = \mathbf{L}_c \otimes \mathbf{O}_c, \tag{3}$$

where $\otimes$ stands for the tensor product. The diffuse component defines the color at a point on the object surface according to the light source direction vector $\mathbf{L}_n$ and

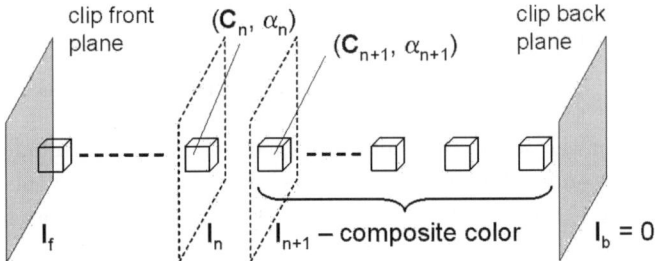

Fig. 10.   Illumination model in composite rendering.

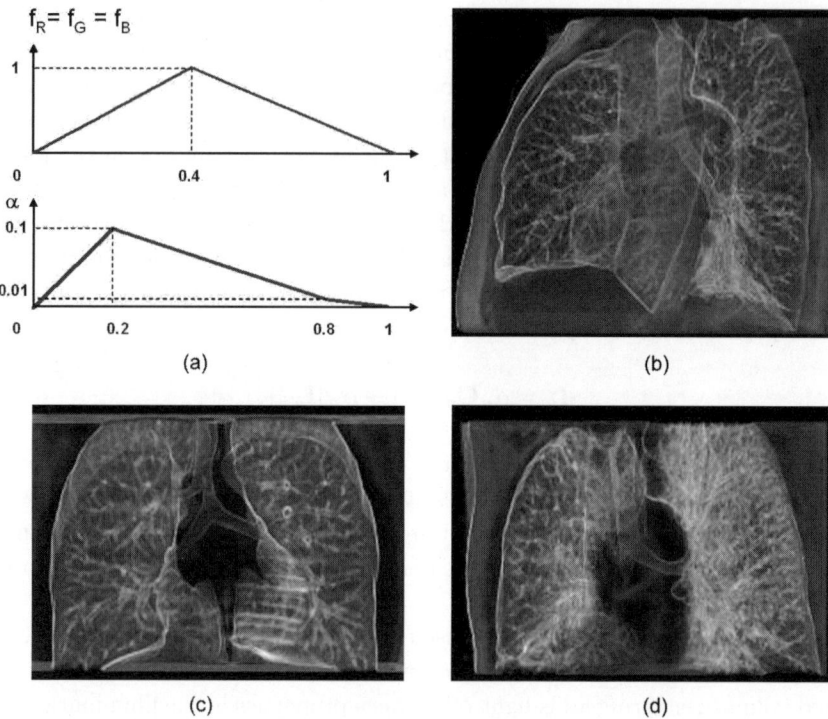

Fig. 11. Composite volume rendering of the subjects from Fig. 9. (a) Color/opacity transfer functions. (b) Bronchiectasis in the LIL bronchi. (c) Ectopic bronchus with tracheal stenosis. (d) Bronchial stenosis (RMB) and occlusion of the IB.

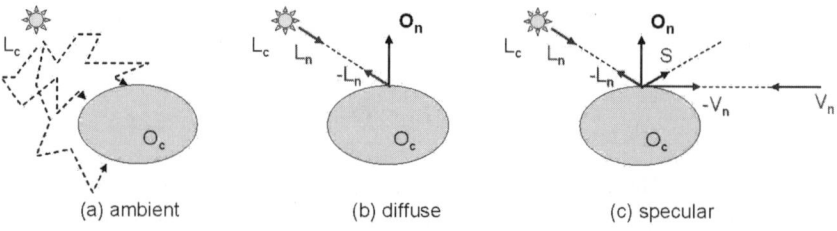

Fig. 12. Color components involved in shaded volume rendering.

the object surface normal $\mathbf{O}_n$ at that point (Fig. 12(b)):

$$\mathbf{C}_d = (\mathbf{L}_c \otimes \mathbf{O}_c) \, [\mathbf{O}_n \cdot (-\mathbf{L}_n)], \tag{4}$$

where · stands for the scalar product. The specular component models the direct reflections of the emitted light on a shiny surface and involves the light source direction vector $\mathbf{L}_n$, the object surface normal $\mathbf{O}_n$, and the camera view point $\mathbf{V}_n$ (Fig. 12(c)):

$$\mathbf{C}_s = (\mathbf{L}_c \otimes \mathbf{O}_c) \, [\mathbf{S} \cdot (-\mathbf{V}_n)]^{O_{sp}}, \tag{5}$$

where

$$S = 2\,[O_n \cdot (-L_n)]O_n + L_n \tag{6}$$

and O_{sp} denotes the specular power coefficient modeling the surface shiness.

Shaded volume rendering considers each elementary volume along a casted ray as a part of a tissue surface and computes the ambient, diffuse and specular values at each point where Eq. (2) is applied. In this respect, light source color L_c and spatial orientation L_n, as well as object surface normal O_n have to be evaluated. Note that the object color O_c represents the color returned by the color transfer function ($O_c = C_n$, according to Fig. 10). In medical imaging, a white light source is generally considered, $L_c = (1, 1, 1)^T$, placed inside the camera, $L_n = V_n$. The surface normal vector at a given point (x, y, z) is computed as the discrete 3D image gradient:

$$O_n(x, y, z) = \left(\frac{\partial F}{\partial x}, \frac{\partial F}{\partial y}, \frac{\partial F}{\partial z}\right)^T (x, y, z), \tag{7}$$

where the partial derivatives are computed in a discrete form:

$$\frac{\partial F}{\partial x}(x, y, z) = \frac{F(x + \Delta x, y, z) - F(x - \Delta x, y, z)}{2\Delta x} \tag{8}$$

$$\frac{\partial F}{\partial y}(x, y, z) = \frac{F(x, y + \Delta y, z) - F(x, y - \Delta y, z)}{2\Delta y} \tag{9}$$

$$\frac{\partial F}{\partial z}(x, y, z) = \frac{F(x, y, z + \Delta z) - F(x, y, z - \Delta z)}{2\Delta z} \tag{10}$$

where F denotes the native image intensity levels and Δx, Δy, Δz the spatial resolution of the MDCT data.

Summing up, in shaded volume rendering, the Eq. (2) of color composition along the ray becomes:

$$I_n = \alpha_n[w_a C_{a,n} + w_d C_{d,n} + w_s C_{s,n}] + (1 - \alpha_n)I_{n+1}, \tag{11}$$

where $C_{a,n}$, $C_{d,n}$, $C_{s,n}$ are respectiveley the ambient, diffuse and specular components computed at the n-th position along the ray, and w_a, w_d, w_s their corresponding weighting coefficients.

Due to the high contrast between the airway lumen and wall within proximal airways, shaded volume rendering can be applied to simulate endoluminal investigation of low-order subdivision bronchi. Such an investigation modality provides images similar to those observed with fiberoptic bronchoscopy and is known as *virtual bronchoscopy*. With the help of axial MDCT images, the radiologist can guide the virtual camera inside the airways to perform the analysis. Figures 13 and 14 shows virtual bronchoscopic images obtained in two patients, the former presenting a normal morphology of the proximal airways while the latter being affected by tracheobronchomalacia. The half-moon shape of the trachea and main

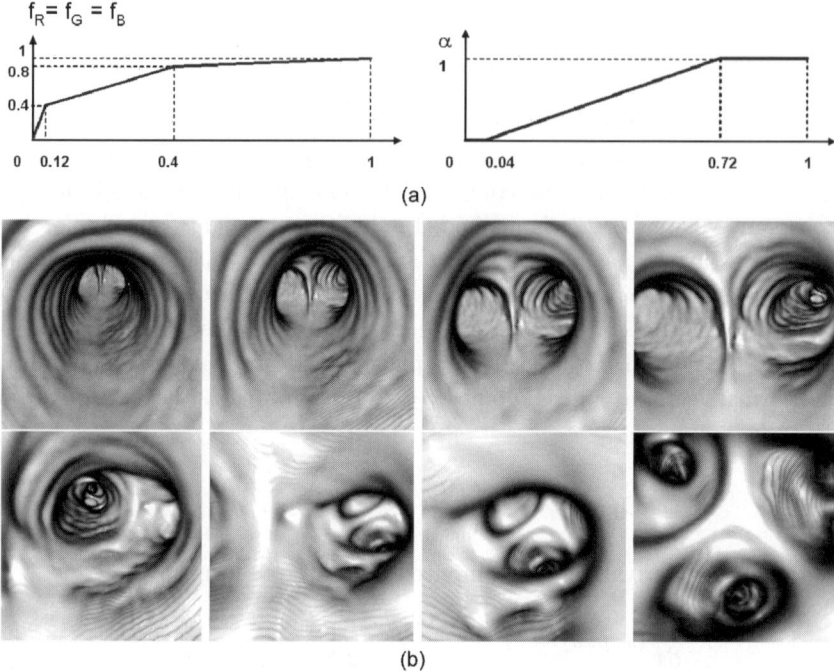

$f_R = f_G = f_B$

(a)

(b)

Fig. 13. Virtual bronchoscopy of normal airways: (a) Color/opacity transfer functions, (b) from left to right and top to bottom, endoscopic views from trachea through the RMB and RULB, up to the subdivision into B_1, B_2 and B_3. The surface folds on the lower part of the 6th and 7th views are due to partial volume effects and do not reflect an abnormality of the wall.

bronchi is clearly visible for the diseased airways (Fig. 14), which denotes an increase in compliance due to the loss of integrity of the wall's structural components.

Note that the choice of the opacity transfer function has the main impact on the final rendering. In virtual bronchoscopy, the interest is focused on the study of the inner airway wall surface, which means that a total opacity should be assigned to the native CT value corresponding to the wall and a zero opacity assigned to the air. This is not possible in practice due to the partial volume effects caused by X-ray beam collimation and spatial resolution. Such effects are even more pronounced for smaller airways. In this case, a threshold interval is chosen to define the zone between air and bronchus wall. In the example from Fig. 13, such interval was set to $[-950, -130]$ HU, which correspond to $[0.04, 0.72]$ in normalized values (reported to the $[-1000, 200]$ HU interval).

Note also the fine stripes on the relief surface. They appear like level-lines and are due to several factors: (1) the transition between (semi-)transparent and fully-opaque values according to the ray incidence on the surface, (2) the typical noise of CT images combined with partial volume effects and (3) the limited sampling resolution: angular, due to the aperture angle of the camera, in-plane (image

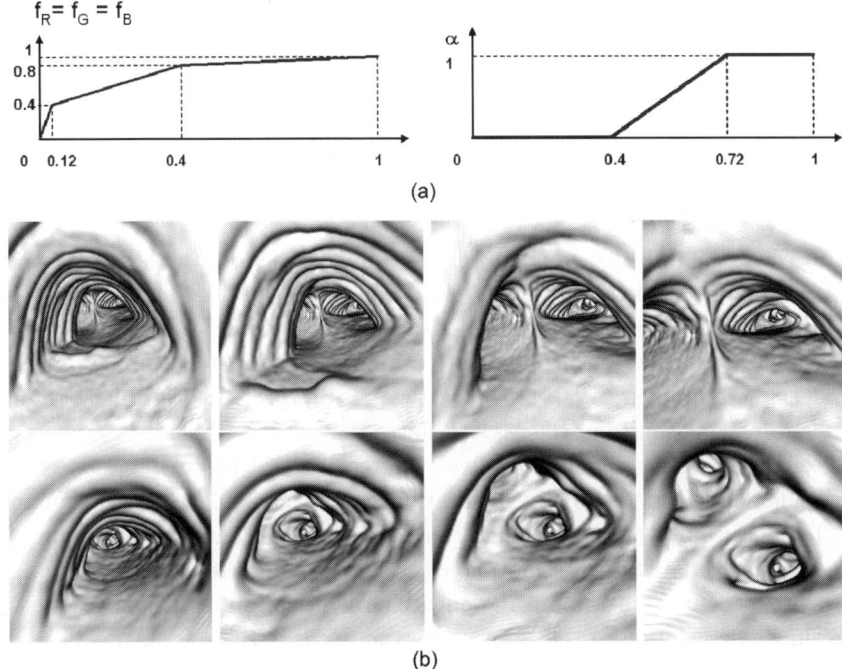

(a)

(b)

Fig. 14. Virtual bronchoscopy of airways affected by tracheobronchomalacia: (a) Color/opacity transfer functions, (b) from left to right and top to bottom, endoscopic views from trachea through the LMB, up to the subdivision into LULB and LILB.

resolution), and longitudinal (sampling interval along the casted rays). Conversely, the larger shadowed strips visible within the trachea are the cartilaginous rings.

Virtual bronchoscopy allows accurate reproduction of the major endoluminal abnormalities with an excellent correlation with fiberoptic bronchoscopy results regarding the location, severity and shape of airway narrowing.[36] In addition, an analysis beyond an obstructive lesion is possible with such a modality.

Despite these valuable abilities, virtual bronchoscopy remains very sensitive to partial volume effects and motion artifacts. An example of the influence of a partial volume effect can be seen in Fig. 13(b) as surface folds on the RULB visible on the lower side of the 6th and 7th images. Note also that virtual bronchoscopy is unable to identify mild stenosis, submucosal infiltration and superficial spreading tumors.[7,37]

Summing up, the basic CAD tools using the aforementioned visualization and rendering techniques provide some facilities for airway investigation but suffer from a common drawback: the difficulty to differentiate the bronchial tree from its environment. This limitation is particularly detrimental to the study of distal airways, which restricts the interest in using such techniques in clinical practice.

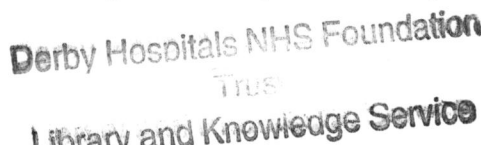

The solution consists in developing advanced CAD tools able to extract from the native MDCT data the information relative to the airways and to provide the associated facilities for interaction, navigation and analysis.

5. Advanced CAD Techniques Based on MDCT Data Segmentation and Interaction

The objective behind developing computer-aided diagnosis tools is not only to ensure a qualitative investigation of the airway tree but especially to provide a quantitative assessment of the disease. In this respect, MDCT data alone is no more enough to deliver such quantitative information. Instead, image processing approaches are implemented to extract and interpret the pertinent morpho-functional information from the MDCT data.

Depending on the required analysis degree, several processing steps have to be considered. First, the 3D segmentation of the airways from the volumetric MDCT data isolates the bronchial tree from its anatomical environment and allows a global analysis of its morphology. Local, quantitative information access requires to benefit from a more in-depth characterization of the airway network. An accurate description of the bronchial structure is derived from the airway axis computation which makes it possible to interact with, navigate within and locally quantify bronchial network. Finally, surface modeling of the segmented airways allows faster interactive analysis and data exchange for telemedecine applications, as well as realistic airflow simulation and particle deposition studies for inhaled therapy design. Recent research uses the surface modeling of the airway lumen to build-up a deformable model and develop a volumetric approach for airway wall segmentation and quantification.

5.1. *3D segmentation of the airways*

The techniques of airway segmentation from MDCT data rely on the morpho-physiological properties of bronchi interpreted in terms of image analysis. Note that airway segmentation generally refers to extracting the airway lumen or the inner airway wall surface. The segmentation of the outer surface of the bronchus wall is few addressed in the literature and will be discussed further in this paper.

Reffering to the segmentation approaches developed in the literature, three main classes can be observed: 2D/3D, fully-3D and mixed approaches. The 2D/3D techniques perform a 2D segmentation on each axial image of the CT dataset, then reconstruct the 3D geometry of the airways. Different methods, summarized in the following, were proposed to achieve these objectives.

The first techniques used thresholding to segment the 2D bronchial sections on each image, then kept only those components which presented a 3D connectivity with a defined subset (generally corresponding to the trachea). While such methods work well on *in vitro* data,[38] on clinical data they fail to provide acceptable results, mainly due to the impossibility to set-up a thresholding interval adapted for both large and small airways, or for airways running in the axial plane (the most affected by the partial volume effect). For these reasons, interactive procedures were developed,[37] where regions of interest are manually defined and the thresholding interval adjusted accordingly. Such methods are both inaccurate and tedious with respect to the large number of images produced by the current scanners (300 to 400 per thorax). Automated approaches were developed allowing bronchial contour detection on 2D images, then a 3D reconstruction under 3D connectivity constraints.[39] Tozaki *et al.* improve the 2D bronchial contour detection by employing several techniques: zero-crossing applied to the second derivative of the image,[40] Gaussian and mean curvature.[40] In the same class of approaches, Fetita *et al.* developed a 2D segmentation method combining bronchial lumen marking and contour extraction[41] using respectively the *connection cost* morphological operator and a constrained watershed.[42] The 3D reconstruction is performed by imposing the same connectivity constraints between the 2D segmented components on successive images. In addition, a 3D topological structure is built-up to guide the restoration of interrupted branches and to filter out the non-bronchial components. Fig. 15 shows an example of a 3D segmentation of bronchial tree using the latter 2D/3D technique.

With the development of multislice CT scanners, the volumetric CT data became quasi-isotropic in terms of 3D spatial resolution. This made possible a new class of segmentation approaches, working directly in the 3D space. Region growing is the most popular one and consists of aggregating neighboring voxels to a pre-defined seed, according to similarity criteria. The neighborhood is defined with respect to the 3D connectivity used (6-connected, 18-connected or 26-connected, Fig. 16). The seed is selected either interactively[43] or is automatically set at the origin of the trachea.[44] Multiple seeds may be defined to increase the segmentation

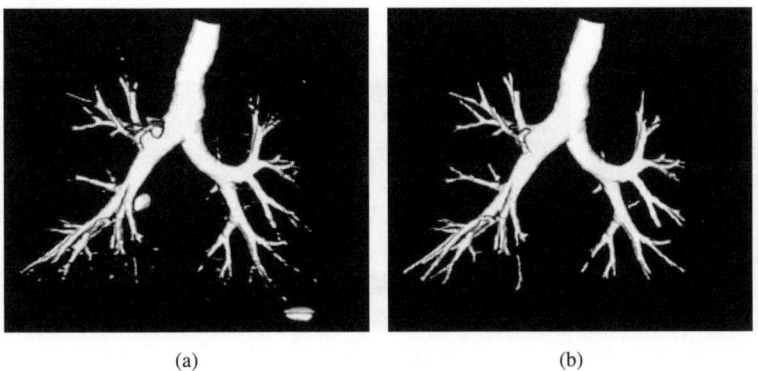

(a)   (b)

Fig. 15.   Example of a result produced by a 2D/3D segmentation approach[41] (a) 2D segmentation and 3D connectivity setup. (b) 3D reconstruction and filtering.

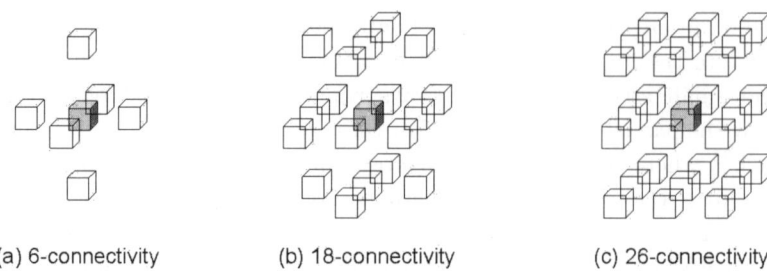

(a) 6-connectivity   (b) 18-connectivity   (c) 26-connectivity

Fig. 16.   Voxel neighborhood corresponding to a given 3D connectivity.

performance for distal bronchi or for bronchi affected by stenosis. The accuracy and robustness of the region growing techniques relies mainly on the definition of the similarity criteria. The most simple ones specify a threshold interval for accepting the aggregation of neighboring voxels to the growing set. While threshold-based techniques are effective for *in vitro* data,[43] they generally either produce an expansion of the growing set outside the airway lumen,[45] or stop the segmentation prematurely. Locally-adaptive thresholding[44,46] improves the result but do not eliminate the "leak" problem. Tschirren *et al.*[47] developed a method relying on multiseeded fuzzy connectivity which simultaneously grows two competing regions– the foreground and the background based on fuzzy-logic similarity criteria. The method prevents from significant overflow but the segmentation is generally limited to low-order subdivision bronchi. Figure 17 illustrates the two extreme cases wich may occur for region growing-based segmentation.

The concept of region growing is the basis of the 3D segmentation methods developed later on. Such methods aimed at improving the performances of the classic region growing approaches by working on two aspects: similarity criteria for overflow prevention, and seed initialization. Several authors proposed to combine 2D/3D and region growing approaches. The benefit of such a mixed technique is mutual: the 2D segmentation result is used to limit the region growing expansion

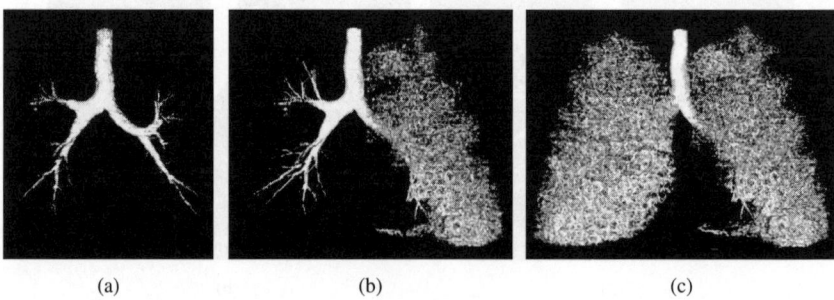

(a)   (b)   (c)

Fig. 17.   Airway segmentation using region growing. Depending on the similarity criterion used, the growing process may stop prematurely (a) or lead to overflow in the lung prenchyma (b), (c).

on one hand, and the region growing propagation is exploited to validate and restore the 2D segmented sections belonging to the airway tree, on the other hand. The resulting mixed approaches are mainly differentiated with respect to the 2D segmentation method implemented: succesive filtering based on anatomical knowledge,[48] fuzzy-logic approach,[49] detection using neural networks,[50] *a priori* knowledge,[51] morphological closing,[52] gray-level morphological reconstruction.[53]

Seed initialization plays also an essential role in the final 3D segmentation. When an interactive procedure is considered, the seed can be recursively updated at the level where propagation stoped. This is the current situation on the postprocessing sofware provided by the majority of CT scanner manufacturers. However, an automated seed setup is largely preferred. Generally, the seed (or a region) is automatically selected inside the trachea, which is easy to detect by using basic image processing tools. In Ref. 53, the seed is automatically updated when region growing stops and set up at the location of terminal bronchial segments previously detected.

Exploiting similar concepts, the work in Refs. 54 and 55 developed a fully-3D approach for airway segmentation. The seed here is a subset of the airway tree, segmented by means of advanced morphological filtering. A new morphological filter was introduced — the *sup-constrained connection cost* — which discriminates between aiway lumen and surrounding lung parenchyma. Such a filter exploits the image properties of the pulmonary tissues, namely the fact that airway lumen is associated with local minima. Defined on functions $f\colon X \subset \Re^n \to \Re$ of connected support $supp(f) = X$ and upper bounded, on any bounded subset of $supp(f)$, the sup-constrained connection cost $(\mathcal{RC}_f^m)$ affects the local minima of f according to connectivity and morphometric criteria. While a complete mathematical definition of $\mathcal{RC}_f^m$ can be found in Refs. 54 and 55, its intuitive interpretation will be given in the following. Let us imagine f as the surface of a relief. A point $x \in supp(f)$ is called *topographically connected* to a subset $Y \subset supp(f)$, if there is a descending path on f leading from x to Y. Computing $\mathcal{RC}_f^m(., Y)$ of f with respect to a non-empty subset $Y \subset supp(f)$ will result in "filling in", at constant level, all local minima of f topographically disconnected from Y. The "filling in" level is controlled by the size m of the structuring element (SE) associated with the $\mathcal{RC}_f^m$ operator. If such a SE is a n-D ball, the "filling in" depth of a "valley" is given by the level at which the "valley" width becomes larger than m (Fig. 18(a)).

By adjusting the m parameter, the $\mathcal{RC}_f^m$ can be implemented in a multi-resolution scheme, making it possible to segment a large subset of the airway lumen. The m value is chosen according to the trachea diameter T: $m_1 = T/2$, $m_2 = T$. The Y subset is defined outside the pulmonary field. Figure 18(b) illustrates the multiresolution principle by using a synthetic thoracic relief simulating the thorax cage, the lung parenchyma with noise and the trachea subdivision. When applying the first filter, $\mathcal{RC}_f^{T/2}$, the bronchi relief is not modified due to their topographical connection with the trachea. The second filtering, $\mathcal{RC}_f^T$, will select the airway network, without affecting the lung valleys.

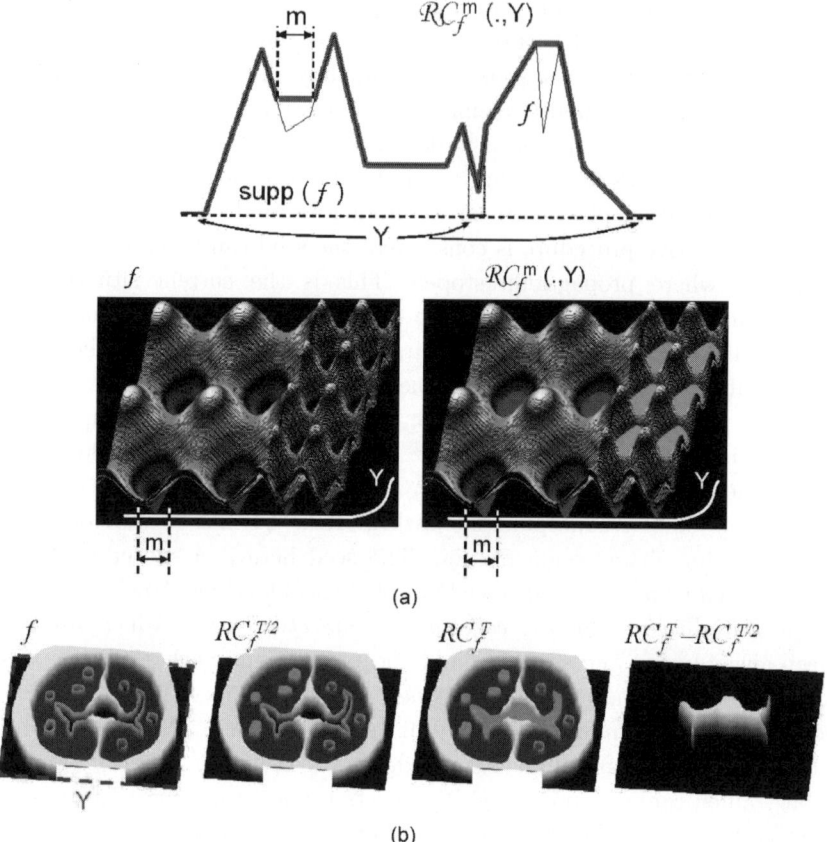

Fig. 18.   Principle of airway subset initialization[54]: (a) the $\mathcal{RC}_f^m(.,Y)$ operator illustrated in 1D and 2D case, (b) multiresolution segmentation scheme.

Figure 19(a) shows an example of low-order airways obtained from MDCT data with the described multiresolution filtering approach. High-order bronchi are then reconstructed by performing a region growing conditional to local constraints on gradient, topology and image intensity. The similarity criteria allowing the propagation at a point x on the boundary of low-order airway subset, in a given direction $\mathbf{d}$, is described by:

$$(\mathbf{d} \cdot \nabla f)(x) + \mathcal{T}(x, f, \mathbf{d}) - kf(x) > 0, \qquad (12)$$

where $\mathcal{T}$ characterizes the local directional topology with respect to f and $\mathbf{d}$, favoring the propagation inside small caliber bronchi,[54] and k is a normalizing parameter, set up according to the MDCT acquisition protocol.

Figure 19(b) shows the 3D segmentation result starting from the seed airway subset of Fig. 19(a). The tracheobronchial tree is here segmented up to the 6th

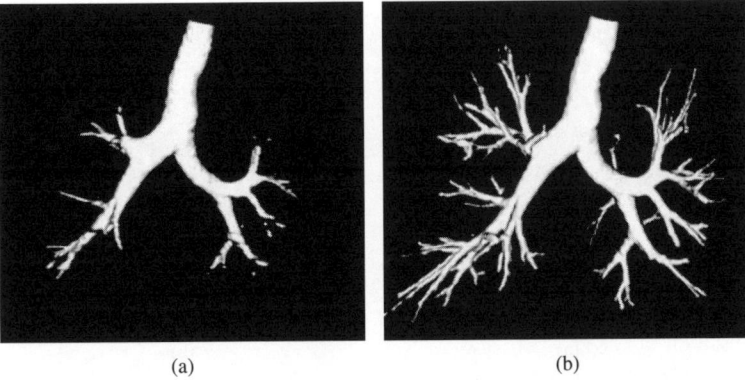

(a) (b)

Fig. 19. 3D segmentation of the tracheobronchial tree from MDCT using the[54] approach (same subject as in Figs. 15 and 17): (a) the seed airway subset computed by multiresolution filtering, (b) conditional region growing.

subdivision order. Note that the airway segmentation results illustrated further on in this paper were obtained with the latter 3D technique.[54]

5.1.1. *Global investigation of the bronchial tree*

The 3D segmentation of the airways provides the access to a global investigation of the bronchial morphology by using a volume rendering approach. The radiologist can navigate around the airway network and analyze the eventual morphological changes caused by disease. The inner airway wall surface can be displayed by using color/opacity transfer functions similar to those of Fig. 13.

An example of airway tree analysis of some subjects discussed in Sec. 4 is shown in Fig. 20 using volume rendering with shaded surface display. The morphological characteristics of bronchi are striking even for an unexperienced investigator.

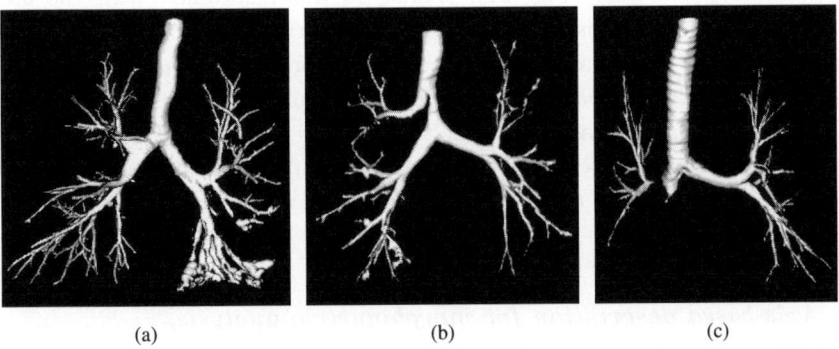

(a) (b) (c)

Fig. 20. 3D airway investigation using shaded volume rendering (subjects of Fig. 9): (a) cystic and varicose bronchiectasis in the LIL basilar bronchi, (b) congenital tracheal bronchus (RULB), (c) severe stenosis of RULB and occlusion of IB.

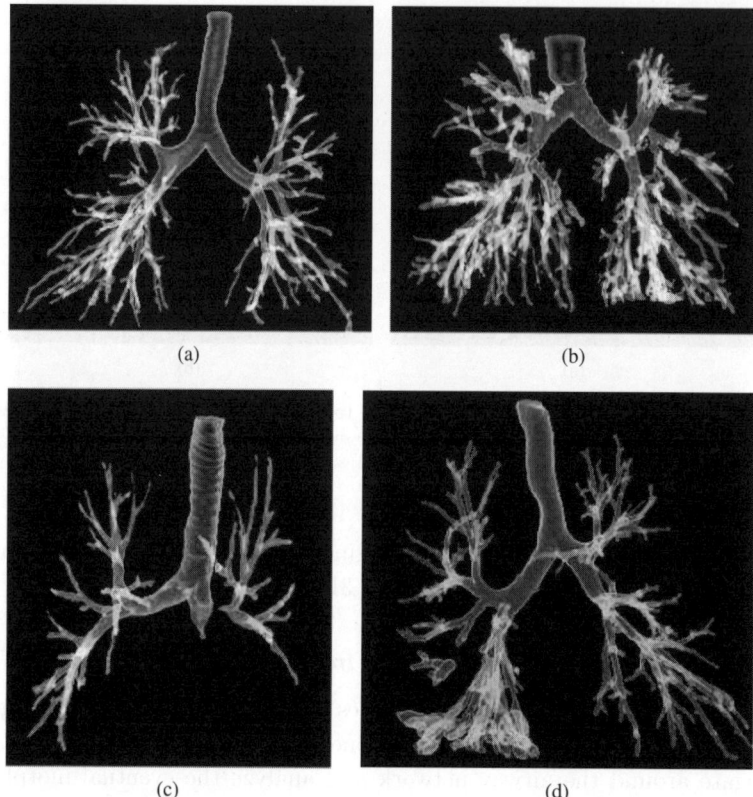

Fig. 21.   3D airway investigation using shaded volume rendering: (a) normal morphology, (b) cylindrical bronchiectasis, (c) severe stenosis of RULB and occlusion of IB (rear view), (d) cystic and varicose bronchiectasis in LIL basilar bronchi (rear view).

Another type of analysis consists in providing semi-transparent views of the segmented bronchial tree (Fig. 21), similar to those obtained with the ancient bronchography. They are useful for producing film-printed clichés for patient record. Such a modality is known as *virtual bronchography* or *CT bronchography*. As the 3D segmentation produces binary (two gray levels) volumetric images (255 is the object value, 0–the background value), specific transfer functions should be used to obtain the desired transparency effect (see Fig. 21(a)). Note also that a 3D smoothing using a Gaussian kernel is applied to the segmented data prior to rendering.

5.2. Axis-based description for morphometric analysis, interaction and navigation

Improving the airway analysis via local assessment requires to develop associated CAD tools for interaction, navigation and quantification. Such tools should rely on a compact representation of the bronchial tree morphology granting the access to specific locations for in-depth investigation.

By compact representation we understand a multi-valued hierarchical graph synthesizing the geometrical and topological information enclosed by the airway tree. A straightforward way for building up such a graph is to compute the axis of the segmented binary 3D airway structure, which will provide the subdivision geometry, and to complete it with topological and morphometric information. Computing the axis of a highly branching binary structure is however challenging and raises several constraints when an accurate result is expected:

- homotopy preservation (same number of simply-connected components),
- geometry preservation (branch length, subdivision angles, subdivision hierarchy),
- central position inside the airway structure,
- unitary dimension (set of curves in the 3D space, not surfaces),
- robustness with respect to noise.

Due to the discrete nature of the 3D segmented data, the airway axis will be built up as a collection of points governed by a connectivity relationship which establishes the topology of the tree structure and the subdivision hierarchy. In addition, each point of the airway axis may carry out information on its spatial position, lumen diameter, local tangent, subdivision order, access to its neighborhood, and so on. The following section presents the main approaches developed in the literature for airway axis computation.

5.2.1. *Axis computation of the tracheobronchial tree*

Three methodological classes for axis computation can be distinguished: thinning-based, using the Voronoi diagram, and relying on distance functions. The methods based on thinning consist of an iterative removal from the segmented airway structure of voxels belonging to the external layer, the suppression of which do not affect the object topology.[56] Such voxels are called *simple points*. Among them, certain points should however be preserved in order to maintain the geometry of the initial structure (*terminal points*). While such an approach applies effectively in two dimensions, the detection of simple and terminal points reveals to be more difficult in 3D and remains the key point of the developed algorithms. In addition, thinning of a 3D object generally produces a surface and subsequent processing is required for extracting an unitary axis. The presence of noise at the surface of the 3D object may induce fake segments in the computed axis (when noise and terminal points are mixed up) and thus, a pruning step is generally required. Different solutions have been proposed to ensure the preservation of both geometry and topology but, to our knowledge, a robust approach for the general case of high-order subdivision trees has not been found yet — for more details on this subject the reader could report to Refs. 57–64.

The axis computation methods based on the Voronoi diagram apply rather to sampled data object represented as a 3D polygonal mesh. The principle exploit a Kirkpatrick's remark[65] according to which the axis of a polygon is a subset of its Voronoi diagram.[66] Recall that the Voronoi diagram of a finite point set $E \subset \Re^n$ is defined as the contours of the Voronoi cells $\mathcal{V}$ given by:

$$\forall p \in E, \quad \mathcal{V}(p) = \{m \in \Re^n, d(m,p) \leq d(m,E)\}, \tag{13}$$

where $d(.,.)$ denotes the Euclidean distance function. The existing methods share a general procedure which consists of surface object sampling, computation of the Voronoi diagram and selection of a subset corresponding to the best approximation of the object axis. According to the latter point, several techniques were proposed: extracting the subset of the Voronoi diagram included in the object,[67-69] consider the intersection between the Voronoi graph and the object,[70] or compute the dual of the Delaunay triangulation of the polygonal approximation of the object. Note that all these techniques present a common drawback — the high sensitivity to the noise on the object surface — which imposes to develop additional simplification procedures.[71-73] In the case of complex 3D objects such as the bronchial tree, there is no warranty that the simplification step will preserve the correct geometry of their axis.

The last class of approaches, based on distance functions, includes the methods using an Euclidean distance map computed with respect to the object border (background).[74] The points of the axis are selected as a subset of the local maxima of the distance function. The key issue is the way that such a selection is performed. Several methods try to detect singularity points on the distance function, and link them together to reconstruct the object axis.[75-78] Other approaches use the distance function as a complementary information for a more robust detection of the simple points during a thinning procedure.[79-81] Numerically-interesting methods introduce a geodesic distance function computed with respect to a root point situated at the top of the trachea. Such geodesic distance map allows to extract the minimal path connecting end points (terminal or subdivision points, either manually defined[82] or automatically detected[83,84]) to the root point. The Euclidean distance map computed with respect to the background serves to constrain the minimal path to remain centered in the airway structure.[84-86]

Similar methods use an approximation of the geodesic distance map by performing a front propagation starting from the root point.[87,88] At each step, the new front is constituted by the current front's neighboring voxels. All voxels within a propagation front are considered to have the same geodesic distance with respect to the root point. The airway axis is progressively built up by including from each propagation front the point corresponding to the local maximum of the Euclidean distance map. The key issue is to accurately estimate the position of the subdivision points and the subdivision hierarchy (in order to preserve the geometry and topology, respectively) of the airway axis. The subdivision detection criterion relies generally on front splitting during propagation (Fig. 22(a)). In order to prevent geometry errors, either a backward propagation is performed (from the terminal points up to the root point) and the spatial position of the subdivision points is corrected,[87,88] or the subdivision detection criterion includes the Euclidean distance map information.[55,89] In the latter situation, a subdivision is also reported when several local maxima of the distance map are detected in the same propagation front (Fig. 22(b)). These methods are not sufficient to ensure the preservation of the subdivision hierarchy in general, as shown in Fig. 22(c).

A solution is proposed in Refs. 55 and 89. It consists in validating the subdivision topology each time a subdivision point is detected. The basic idea is that, for a quasi-tubular branching structure, a specific space partitioning procedure initiated at a hypothetical subdivion point in the tree is able to accurately decide if a subdivision occurs (Fig. 23). The space partitioning first defines the maximum sphere inscribed in the airway set, centered at the hypothetical subdivision point. Then, the points located on the sphere surface propagate toward lower values of the Euclidian

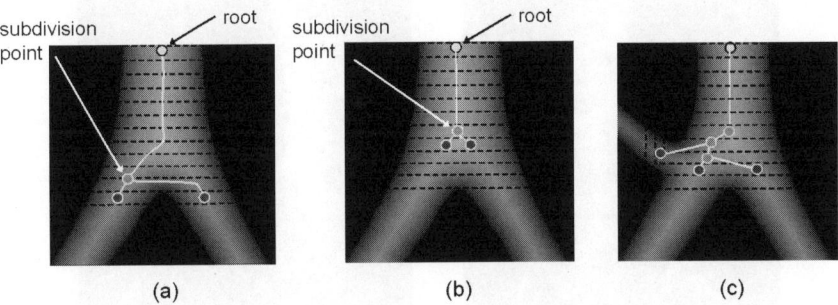

Fig. 22. Subdivision detection criteria: (a) front splitting — geometry errors, (b) follow-up of local maxima of the Euclidean distance map–geometry — preservation, (c) previous methods fail in preserving the geometry/subdivision hierarchy in the general situation.

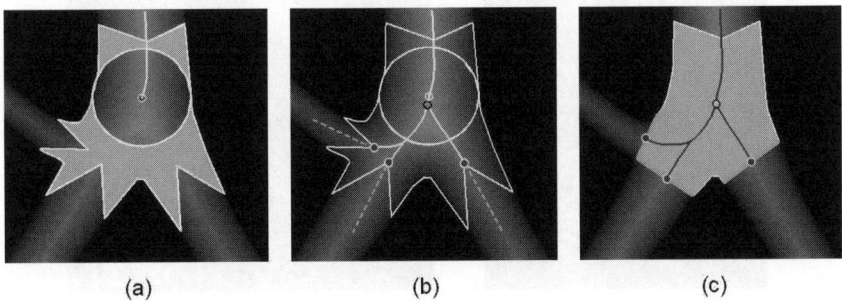

Fig. 23. Subdivision detection criterion preserving both the geometry and the subdivision hierarchy: (a) space partitioning starting at a hypothetical subdivision point, (b) airway axis reconstruction at the subdivision level, (c) partitioning in sub-trees and recursive procedure resumption.

distance map. This will give birth to a cone-shaped structure associated with each segment of the subdivision, irrespective to the degree of the subdivision (bifurcation, trifurcation, ...; Fig. 23(a)). The geometry of the airway axis at the subdivision level is then reconstructed by connecting the vertex of each cone-shaped structure to the subdivision point, following the maximum value path on the distance map (Fig. 23(b)). A subdivision in sub-trees is then performed (Fig. 23(c)) and the procedure is recursively applied to each sub-tree.

The airway axis computation approaches using Euclidean distance function and geodesic front propagation have the advantage to be less computationally expensive and more robust with respect to object surface irregularities/noise than thinning or Voronoi-based methods. Nevertheless, any technique cand be implemented in a computer-aided diagnosis system if it complies with the robustness, the accuracy and the interactivity degrees required by the application. Figure 24

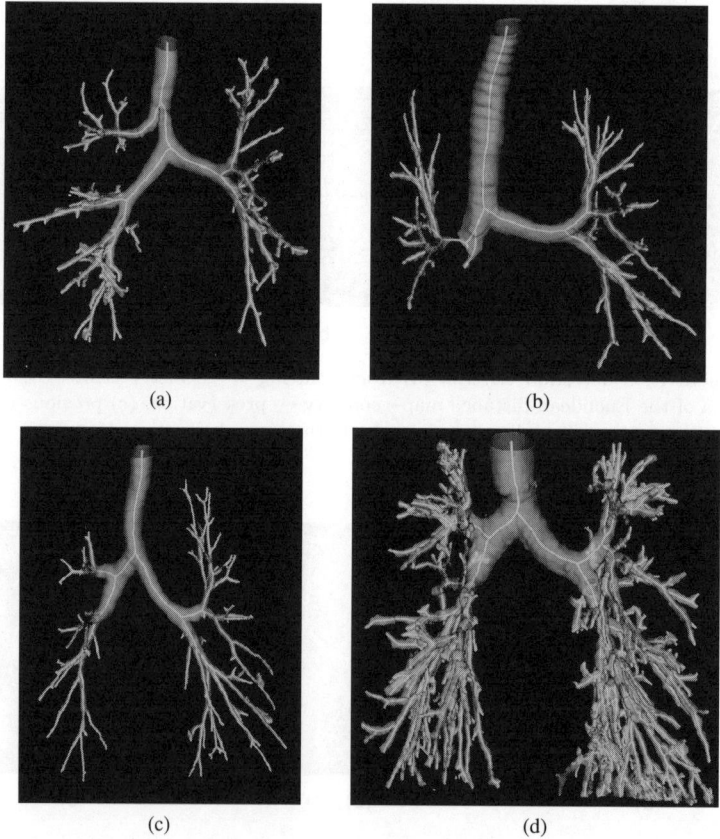

(a)   (b)

(c)   (d)

Fig. 24. Airway axis computed for different airway morphologies[55]: (a) congenital tracheal bronchus (RULB), (b) severe stenosis of RULB and occlusion of IB, (c) peribronchovascular thickening inducing airway lumen narrowing and occlusion, (d) cylindrical bronchiectasis.

illustrates some results of airway axis computation obtained by using the latter approach,[55,89] showing robustness with respect to various physiological and pathological morphologies of the airway tree.

The airway axis is built up as a discrete, hierarchic and multi-valued tree structure. Each point of the axis carries out data related to:

- the geometry (3D spatial coordinates, tangent vector),
- the topology (local neighborhood, node type: root, terminal, subdivision or regular),
- the subdivision order of the current bronchus segment,
- the approximate caliber of the bronchus (estimated from the Euclidean distance function),

which allows interactive or automated applications for medical investigation.

5.2.2. *Morphometric analysis*

By exploiting the airway axis structure, morphometric measurements of bronchi become straightforward. Such measurements include bifurcation angles, bronchi lengths, cross-section caliber estimation (Fig. 25(a)), longitudinal extent of pathologies (stenosis, bronchiectasis; Fig. 25(b)). Apart from being of clinical interest in pre/post-surgery analysis, the bronchi investigation based on the airway axis description may automatically provide useful morphometric informations at different subdivision levels. Average models concerning a target population may thus be built up and the effect of different perturbation factors studied with respect to these models.

By combining 3D segmentation and airway axis description, an indexation of the bronchial segments with respect to the subdivision order is achieved,[55] Fig. 25(c). Such an indexation differs from the one of the airway axis and provides the correct

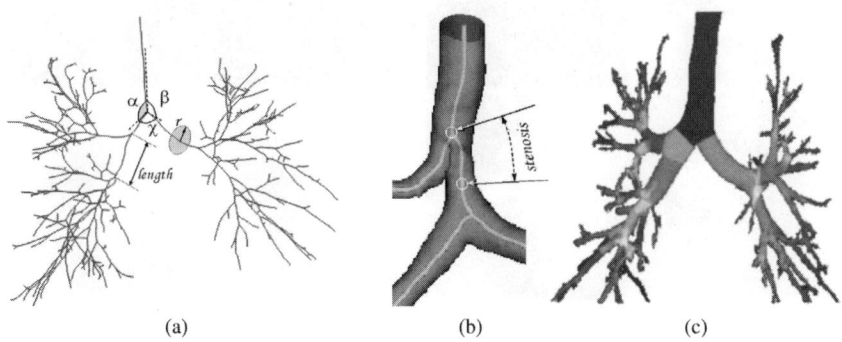

Fig. 25. Morphometric analysis based on airway axis information: (a) subdivision angles, segment lengths, cross-section caliber, (b) quantification of a stenosis, probably due to the aortic arch printing, (c) bronchus indexation.

labeling of the bronchial segments (*cf.* Fig 4). This is both useful to enrich the average models and to build up interactive anatomical atlases for medical learning.

5.2.3. *Interaction and navigation facilities*

The hierarchic tree structure of the airway axis makes it possible to develop associated tools for interacting with and navigating within the airway network. A straightforward example is the virtual endoscopy application.

By selecting two points on the axis, the endoluminal trajectory is automatically computed and the virtual camera guided along the axis. The virtual camera is centered in the bronchus segment and provides the optimal view during the navigation. The endoluminal images are obtained with shaded volume rendering techniques applied on the negative segmented binary data, and using color/opacity transfer functions similar to those in Figs. 13 and 14.

Performing virtual bronchoscopy investigation along the segmented airway tree instead of using native MDCT data (*cf.* Sec. 4.2) has two major advantages. First, it provides a higher robustness to the partial volume effects (Fig. 26(a)). Second, it allows a more distal investigation as the gray level values of the lumen wall are constant with respect to the subdivision order, which is not the case with native data. Indeed, in native MDCT data, the gray level associated with the bronchus wall decreases with the subdivision order because of the partial volume effect and the reduction of the wall thickness. Consequently, the opacity associated with the airway wall via the transfer functions decreases and the wall surface "fades out" while anatomical structures beyond it become visible (Fig. 26(b)–(d)).

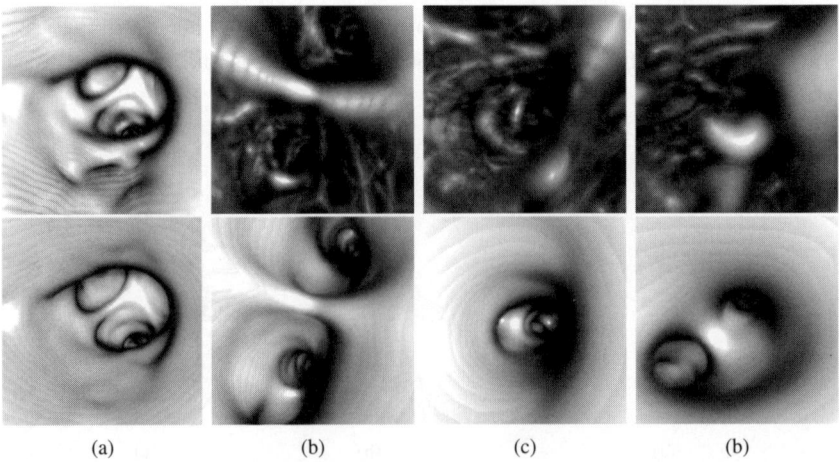

(a)   (b)   (c)   (b)

Fig. 26.   Virtual bronchoscopy using native (top) and segmented (bottom) data (same subject as in Fig. 13): (a) sensitivity to partial volume effects (RULB), (b) 4th order subdivision bronchus (subsegmental), (c) 5th order subdivision bronchus, (d) 6th order subdivision bronchus.

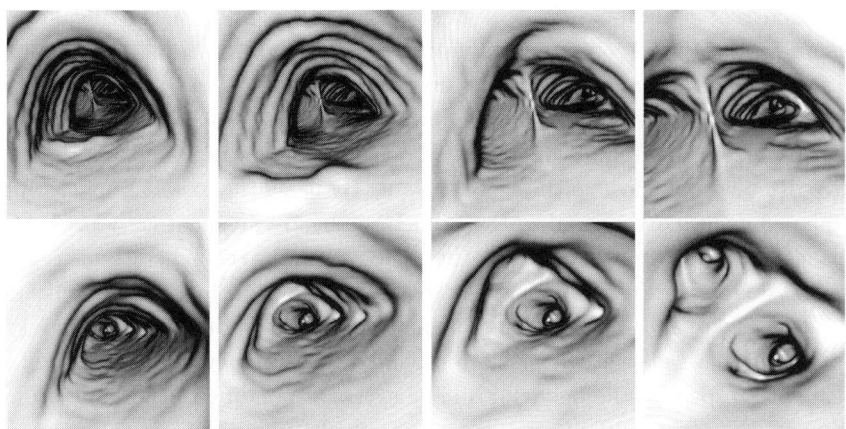

Fig. 27. Virtual bronchoscopy of airways affected by tracheobronchomalacia using the 3D segmentation and axis description (same viewpoints as in Fig. 14). From left to right and top to bottom, endoscopic views from trachea through the LMB, up to the subdivision into LULB and LILB.

Figure 27 illustrates a virtual bronchoscopy investigation by using the previous 3D segmentation and airway axis navigation facilities. The analysis concerns the same patient as in the endoscopic investigation based on native MDCT data, *cf.* Fig. 14. For comparison purposes, the same viewpoints were selected in both endoscopic investigations.

Another interaction facility provided by the airway axis description is the definition of the cutting planes for multiplanar image reformation (Sec. 4.1). Of a particular interest for quantification purposes are the MPR images reconstructed in the bronchus cross-section plane, at selected location points. As the tangent to the bronchus axis is one of the parameters enclosed by each node of the airway axis, the cross-section image reconstruction is fully-automatic and reproducible. Such essential properties are exploited for airway lumen/wall area quantification in the framework of bronchial reactivity and wall remodeling assessment.

5.2.4. *Assessment of airway reactivity and bronchial wall remodeling*

Pathologies such as asthma and COPD induce airway remodeling which can be noticed on clinical MDCT investigations as bronchial wall thickening and lumen narrowing. Such a remodeling occurs in the affected subjects in response to various external stimuli. The challenge is to provide accurate quantification tools in order to evaluate the degree of obstruction and its associated risks. Patient follow-up consequently to an administered medication also requires the ability to assess changes in airway remodeling prior and after therapy. In this framework, MDCT imaging may play the role of biomarker when associated with accurate CAD facilities.

The current techniques for assessing the airway lumen narrowing and wall thickening with MDCT consist in evaluating the bronchus lumen/wall areas or their variation in longitudinal studies.[b] The first requirement for an accurate estimation is to perform the measurements in the bronchus cross-section plane, otherwise the estimation errors may climb up to +40% when investigating small airways, even slightly tilted with respect to the section plane. By using the axis-based description, multiplanar images orthogonal to the bronchus axis are automatically provided for quantification at locations selected by the radiologist. The second key issue is related to the 2D quantification technique used to assess the bronchial parameters, which has to be accurate and reproducible. Such a requirement should be considered from two points of view: (1) with respect to repeated measurements on the same image and (2) with respect to the behavior on images corresponding to the same bronchus location in the same patient, but coming from distinct MDCT acquisitions (for example, in the case of pre/post-treatment analysis).

Several (semi-)automatic approaches for airway wall quantification have been proposed in the literature. We can mention here "full-width at half maximum" (FWHM), pattern-based and shape-independent approaches. Well-known and largely used in the medical community, FWHM methods[90,91] estimate the locations of the inner/outer wall contours of a bronchus from gray-level profiles computed along rays cast from its center. However, it has been shown[92] that measures using FWHM are biased for small or thin-wall airways. Pattern-based approaches[93-95] use the assumption that airway cross-sections have circular or elliptical shapes. Such an assumption applies well to images of excised animal lungs but holds no longer for in-vivo CT data, thus making estimation errors possible. Shape-independent techniques gather various approaches for inner/outer wall contour detection such as gradient-based,[96] mathematical morphology,[97] knowledge-based,[94] etc. A recent technique,[98] especially designed for airway remodeling quantification in asthma, exploits the benefits provided by the airway axis descriptive structure and by a fully-automated 2D segmentation approach. Due to the diffuse nature of the disease, quantifying a theraphy effect on the airway wall remodeling requires to simultaneously assess several bronchi throughout the lung. In this respect, an experienced radiologist identifies and selects the bronchi where quantification should be performed by clicking on the corresponding landmarks on the airway axis (Fig. 28(a)). A series of cross-section images are automatically generated at different sampling locations on each selected bronchus axis (Fig. 28(b)). The 2D quantification of lumen/wall areas is then automatically performed on each cross-section image (Fig. 28(c)) by using a dedicated deformable contours approach. The quantification results are reported both individually and averaged by bronchus segment, and comparisons between data before/after treatment are performed.[99]

---

[b]Studies reproduced at different time intervals.

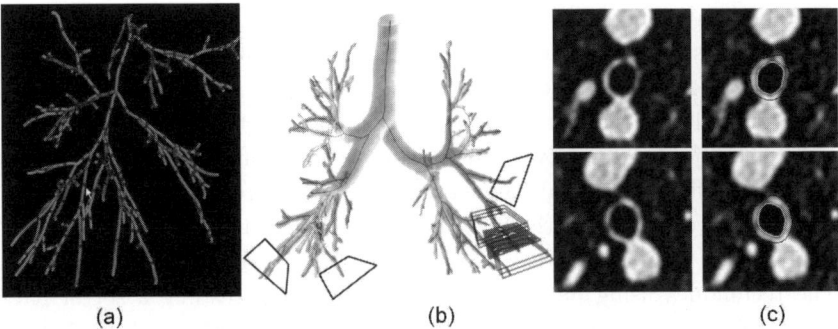

Fig. 28. Quantification of airway reactivity and bronchus wall remodeling:[98,99] (a) selection of bronchi under evaluation, (b) cross-section image reformation, (c) airway lumen/wall quantification.

Considering the impact that such quantitative studies on airway reactivity and bronchus wall remodeling may have on the healthcare policy, new questions arised regarding the effectiveness of the cross-section assessment procedures, and new methodological trends appeared to tackle them. These issues will be discussed later in this paper.

5.3. *Patient-specific model synthesis for data exchange and functional investigation*

Data exchange, virtual surgery, high-speed rendering, numerical functional simulation, are some of the applications which require the elaboration of patient-specific models combining both low bitrate coding and high representation accuracy. Mesh surface modeling offers such desired attributes together with interaction facilities with the object surface.

5.3.1. *3D mesh modeling of the tracheobronchial tree*

Generating an accurate surface mesh of the 3D binary data issued from the bronchial tree segmentation raises several difficulties related to the high branching complexity and to the caliber variability of the airway structure. The existing algorithms performing the extraction of an object 3D surface from volumetric data can be grouped into the following categories: planar contour based methods, deformable models, particle systems and *Marching Cubes*.

Planar contour based methods consist in generating on equally-spaced 2D planes (usually the axial image plane) the set of intersection contours between the object and the plane. Then, the 2D contours are spatially aligned in 3D and a triangulation is performed between adjacent contours.[100,101] Such methods are not adapted to represent complex morphologies implying random subdivisions.

The deformable models[102] obey the following principle in building up an object surface mesh. A specific mesh model is initialized inside the object then the model is progressively deformed under elastic constraints, until the object surface is reached. The main difficulty consists in adapting the topology of the initial model to the one of the target object. Interactive[103] or dynamical adaptation,[104-106] together with the use of specific (cylindrical) models[107,108] may improve the final mesh of the airway tree. However, due to the high morphological variability of the (segmented) bronchial tree, it is difficult to provide a generic deformable model for initialization.

The techniques using particle systems consist in spreading a set of particles along the object surface according to a diffusion equation.[109,110] When the equilibrium is reached, the particles are connected by means of a Delauney triangulation approach. The main inconvenient of these techniques is the convergence slowness. Several methods have been proposed to speed up the convergence[111-113] while preserving the object topology. Another approaches to be mentioned here are those relying on implicit surface sampling by means of point insertion.[114-116] They use the concept of restricted Delauney triangulation which guarantees the preservation of the surface geometry and topology. Paradoxically, due to their accuracy in reproducing surface irregularities, such techniques are less adapted to binary volumetric discrete data. The reason is that they will not interpret the voxel 3D connectivity in the same manner as in 3D discrete geometry, namely, they will not provide a tubular geometry from a row of 26-connected voxels as one would expect.[55]

Widely used in medical imaging[117] for its low computational cost, Marching Cubes[118,119] is an approach conceived to extract *isosurface* meshes from 3D discrete data. Its principle consists in subdividing the data volume in logical cubes of vertices formed by adjacent voxels and classify each cube vertex as being inside/outside the surface. Such classification is performed according to the vertex data value with respect to a selected *isovalue* characterizing the object surface. The precise locations of the intersections between the cubes edges and the isosurface are computed using linear interpolation between the isovalue and the values of the adjacent vertices. A look-up table describing all possible intersection configurations for a cube allows to greatly increase the computational speed.

Applying Marching Cubes to extract the surface of the binary 3D segmented airway tree reveals strong irregularities corresponding to the voxel contours, as well as some discontinuities in the small caliber segments.[89] In order to prevent such effects, the commonly used approach consists in smoothing the binary data by means of a Gaussian filtering prior to applying the Marching Cubes.[117] The surface smoothness directly depends on the considered filter size. In the case of segmented airways, a large filter size induces geometrical distortions (segment shortening, diameter increasing and branch discontinuities) at the level of small caliber segments, while a small filter size preserves the surface irregularities for large caliber bronchi. In addition, data smoothing also requires a tune-up of the isovalue parameter in order to preserve the original caliber of the bronchi in the reconstructed mesh. The smoothing kernel and the isovalue should thus be adaptiveley selected according to the bronchial caliber. Such an adaptive approach is developed in Refs. 55 and 89 where, instead of changing the isovalue according to the bronchus caliber (which might result in holes on the mesh surface), the smoothed data values are shifted accordingly, while the isovalue is kept constant. The adaptation of the kernel size and the shift value is based on a look-up table built up according to the bronchial segment indexation (*cf.* Fig. 25). Figure 29 illustrates the results obtained using the latter approach, showing smooth meshes and caliber preservation for small, large and stenosed airways.

Surface mesh modeling of airways offers several facilities in clinical investigation. First, it enables effective data compression for exchange or telemedicine purposes. For example, an initial MDCT exam including 550 axial images reconstructed on a 768 × 768 matrix requires 618 MB for storage. The binary volume including the segmented airway tree will request 35 MB, while the airway mesh model will only need 9 MB.

Second, mesh modeling allows real time display and interaction using surface rendering approaches,[29] for which hardware graphics accelerators are widely developed. Global analysis or endoluminal investigation are performed in the same way as using volume rendering techniques, *cf.* Secs. 5.1.1 and 5.2 (Fig. 30).

Third, such patient-specific models make it possible to simulate and analyze the functional behavior of normal and pathologic airway morphologies via computational fluid dynamics techniques. Finally, surface models of the airway lumen represent an essential morphological knowledge to be exploited in segmenting

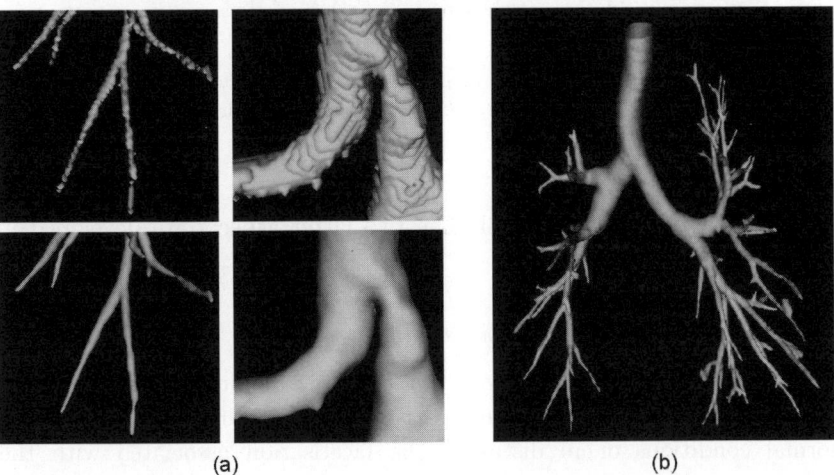

(a) (b)

Fig. 29. Adaptive mesh modeling of airway surface illustrated with shaded surface rendering: (a) comparison between adaptive (bottom) and classic (top) Marching Cubes approaches showing caliber preservation and surface smoothness, (b) surface mesh of an airway tree showing lumen narrowing and occlusions.

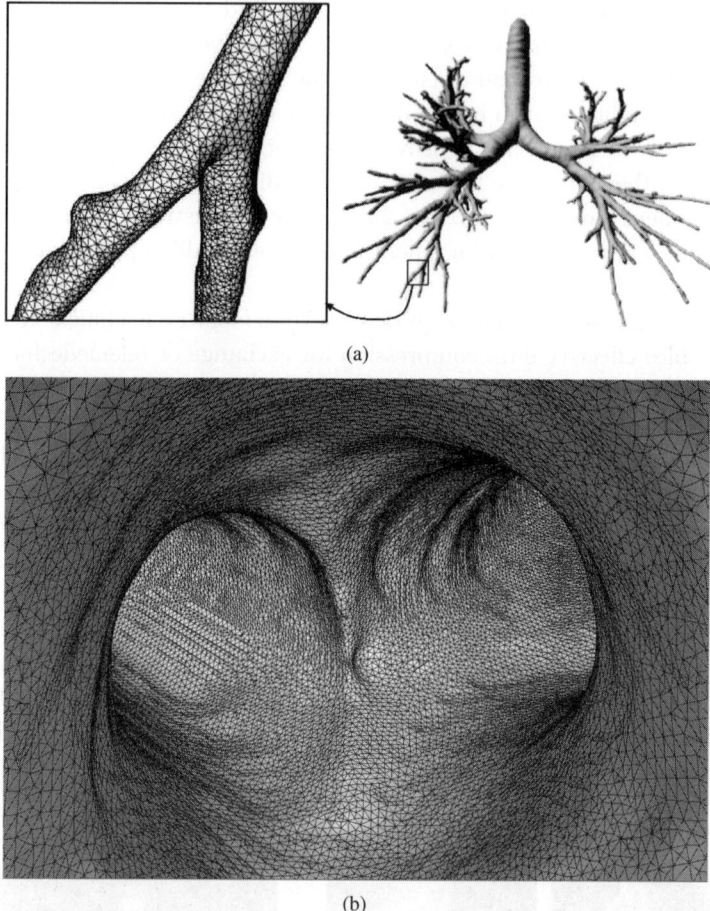

(a)

(b)

Fig. 30. Surface rendering of airway mesh models (same patient as in Fig. 13): (a) Global investigation with a zoom-in on a bronchus segment, (b) Virtual endoscopy (wireframe superimposed on the shaded surface).

and quantifying the bronchial wall. The two latter aspects are developed in the following sections.

5.3.2. Airflow simulation in proximal airways

Computational models of oscillatory laminar flow of air can be carried out in image-based domains of the proximal part of human tracheobronchial trees, either in normal conditions or in diseases. The facetisation associated with the 3D segmentation of the tracheobronchial tree is improved to get a computation-adapted surface triangulation, which leads to a volumic mesh composed of tetrahedra. The tracheobronchial models are composed of the trachea and the proximal generations, down to generation five, six, and sometimes seven, according to the image quality and the airway bore. A given bronchus, indeed, generates two, sometimes three, branches of unequal size (asymmetric branching).

The surface meshes must match strong requirements related both to the accuracy of the surface approximation and to the element shape and size quality for the computations. In a first step, redundant elements are removed but the accuracy of the geometric approximation of the underlying surface is preserved. The simplification procedure is based on the Hausdorff distance. The required smoothing is based on a bi-laplacian operator.[120] Whereas the surface triangulation is coarsened in the regions where the local curvatures are sufficiently large, maintaining the main local curvatures, the mesh is enriched in sharp regions with possible flow complex behaviour. Besides, the boundary conditions must be set at cross sections sufficiently far from the exploration volume in order to avoid pressure cross gradient and boundary-dependent flow disturbances, and to keep both upstream and downstream 3D effects of the pipe geometry.[121] Finally, element shapes and sizes must be controlled as they usually impact the accuracy of the numerical results. Therefore, an anisotropic geometric metric map based on the local principal directions and radii of curvatures is constructed in the tangent planes related to the mesh vertices. This metric map prescribes element sizes proportional to the local curvature of the surface.[122] The conforming surface triangulation must be topologically accurate to generate a volumic tetrahedral mesh.

The air inhaled and exhaled during quiet breathing is supposed to be homogeneous, incompressible (according to the values of the Mach and Helmholtz numbers) and Newtonian. The inhaled air is heated, being at the body temperature. Moreover, it is saturated with water vapor. Consequently, the physical properties of the air in the respiratory tract are the following: the air density $\rho = 19.04\,10^{-6}\,\mathrm{kg.m^{-3}}$, the dynamic viscosity $\mu = 1.068\,Pl$, and the kinematic viscosity $\nu = 17.8\,10^{-6}\,\mathrm{m^2.s^{-1}}$. The governing equations of an airway flow are derived from the mass and momentum conservations, the so-called Navier–Stokes equations. The values of the peak tracheal Reynolds numbers based on the peak cross-sectional average velocity and on the tracheal radius at the end cross section ranges from 700 to 900. The Stokes numbers based on the radius at the cross section of the tracheal end varies between four and five.

The boundary of the fluid domain is partitioned into a surface set: the cross section of the tracheal end, at which a Dirichlet boundary condition is applied, the cross sections of the bronchial ends, over which normal constraint is equal to zero, and the airway wall, which is assumed to be rigid during quiet breathing. The wall of the explored bronchus generations are reinforced by cartilaginous (complete or not) rings, which are assumed to be not flexible during rest ventilation. The classical no-slip condition is then applied to the airway wall. A time-dependent uniform injection velocity is prescribed at the inlet which can be associated with a sharp constriction in order to mimic the laryngeal lumen narrowing. It provides a zero-mean sinusoidal flow.

The Navier–Stokes equations associated with the classical boundary conditions and different values of the flow dimensionless parameters are solved using the finite element method. The computational method is suitable to unsteady flow. The finite element type is P_1-P_1 bubble element.[123] The pressure is defined at the four vertices of the tetrahedron and the velocity at both the vertices and the barycenter. The order of the method in the L^2 norm is $\mathcal{O}(\xi^2)$ for the velocity and $\mathcal{O}(\xi)$ for the pressure, ξ being the characteristic size of the tetrahedron. The convective term is approximated by the method of characteristics.[124] The solution is obtained via a generalized Uzawa-preconditioned-conjugate gradient method.[125] The initial condition is given by a Stokes problem with the same boundary condition as the unsteady one (period of 1 s).

After investigating the cycle reproducibility and mesh size effects on the numerical results, the flow distribution among the set of bronchi (the parameter of interest for the physician) is computed during the respiratory cycle. The flow distribution can be calculated for the five lobes of the two lungs. Six phases have been selected to depict the numerical results: mid acceleration phase, peak, and mid deceleration phase of inspiration and expiration.

The relative flow contribution is given at the selected phases of the respiratory cycle (Table 1). However, the flow distribution is estimated, rather than properly quantified, due to the crude boundary conditions used in the present numerical simulations, since the impedance of the small bronchi is unknown.

Moreover, the heterogeneous deformation of the lungs, which is usually assumed to be caused by gravity and interactions between the lungs and the chest wall, has not been taken into account, due to unknowns. The regional distribution of prestresses is, indeed, determined not only by the hydrostatic pressure in the pleural space but also by the shape of the lung with respect to the thoracic cage. Under normal conditions, the lung weight is only a minor determinant of the topographic distribution of parenchymal stress and strain. Helpful qualitative data are provided rather than accurate quantitative results in the context of multimodeling, from image acquisition to numerical simulations.

Table 1. Between-lobe flow distribution in the lung lobes of a normal tracheobronchial tree (R: right, L: left, U: upper, M: middle, I: inferior) at selected phases of the respiratory cycle (MAI: mid acceleration phase of inspiration, PI: peak inspiration, MDI: mid deceleration phase of inspiration, MAE: mid acceleration phase of expiration, PE: peak expiration, MDE: mid deceleration phase of expiration, q_R: flow in the right part of the tracheobronchial tree, q_t: tracheal flow rate).

Phase	$\frac{q_L}{q_t}$	$\frac{q_R}{q_t}$	RUL	RML	RIL	LUL	LIL
MAI	40	60	15	8	37	16	24
IP	39	61	13	8	39	15	24
MDI	40	60	14	8	37	16	24
MAE	36	64	18	9	37	15	21
EP	34	66	19	9	39	13	20
MDE	31	69	17	10	42	11	20

5.3.3. *New trends in airway wall quantification: a volumetric approach*

As mentioned in Sec. 5.2.4, non-invasive airway wall quantification based on MDCT imaging plays a key role in evaluating the efficiency of a treatment prescribed to reverse the airway remodeling induced by asthma or COPD. The discussed cross-section quantification methodologies allow detecting clinically significant variations of lumen diameter and wall thickness between successive CT acquisitions prior and after medication,[126] provided a set of conditions is met:

- First, the follow-up MDCT acquisitions have to be performed at the same inspiratory volume to avoid differences in wall thickness due to different bronchus elongations. Note however that, despite using pneumotachographycally-controlled acquisitions, the total lung capacity of a patient may vary after medication (due to the overall effect of the treatment on the inflammatory condition) and so does the length of the bronchi. Remains to determine how this variation will affect the quantification result.
- Second, to be relevant, cross-section analysis can be performed only in the locations outside of a subdivision zone (Fig. 31(a)). In addition, some cross-section configurations of bronchus-vessel pairs should be avoided for a confident quantification result (Fig. 31(b)).[127] In this respect, a confidence index (CI) was defined in Ref. 127 for accepting or rejecting a measure. Such CI condition should be observed for a number of consecutive sections along the bronchus axis.[126] Consequently, bronchus wall thickness variations within subdivision areas or within zones of low CI cannot be monitored with cross-section quantification techniques.
- Third, the quantification result is strongly conditioned by the correct estimation of the airway axis. While sometimes the notion of central axis is locally questionable, problems may occur even for unambiguous situations. For example, irregular lumen walls may induce irregular airway axis which will result in

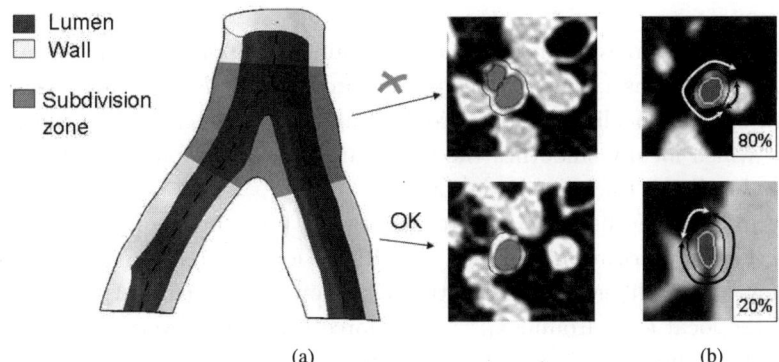

(a)   (b)

Fig. 31.   Measure validation with cross-section quantification methods: (a) exclusion of the bronchus subdivision zone, (b) acceptance/rejection based on the confidence index value.

asymmetric and tilted sampling of wall regions, leading to wall cross-section area overestimation.

In the highly challenging context of therapy follow-up, a novel automated approach for volumetric quantification of the bronchial wall has been proposed in.[128] Its objective was to increase the detection sensitivity with respect to the cross-section techniques and to eliminate the dependency on the airway axis geometry. The developed approach exploits the knowledge of the inner bronchus wall shape provided by the airway mesh modeling described at the begining of Sec. 5.3. This knowledge is incorporated into a deformable mesh model in the form of initial conditions, shape constraints, and orientation of the deformation. The algorithm carries out the evolution of the mesh model relative to image data and shape regularity constraints guaranteeing a fast and robust segmentation of the outer bronchial wall.

The behavior of the model is governed by an adapted and discretized formulation of a Lagrangian equation of a snake. The Newtonian law of motion is applied at each vertex allowing it to move in a force field governed by internal and external forces:

$$m_i \ddot{\mathbf{x}}_\mathbf{i} + \gamma_i \dot{\mathbf{x}}_\mathbf{i} = F_{ext}\left(\mathbf{x}_\mathbf{i}\right) + F_{int}\left(\mathbf{x}_\mathbf{i}\right), \qquad (14)$$

where $\ddot{\mathbf{x}}_\mathbf{i}$ and $\dot{\mathbf{x}}_\mathbf{i}$ are the acceleration and velocity of vertex i, m_i the mass, γ_i a damping factor, F_{int} the internal forces and F_{ext} the external forces. In pratice, m_i is set to 0 in order to constrain the deformation process to be constant. Equation (14) is integrated forward through time using an explicit first-order Euler method. This method approximates the temporal derivatives with forward finite differences. It updates the positions of the model vertex from time t to $t + \Delta_t$ according to the formula:

$$\mathbf{x}_\mathbf{i}^{\mathbf{t}+\boldsymbol{\Delta}\mathbf{t}} = \mathbf{x}_\mathbf{i}^\mathbf{t} + \frac{\Delta_t}{\gamma_i}\left(F_{ext}\left(\mathbf{x}_\mathbf{i}^\mathbf{t}\right) + F_{int}\left(\mathbf{x}_\mathbf{i}^\mathbf{t}\right)\right). \qquad (15)$$

The internal forces are intented to maintain the topology of the initial model. F_{int} will be defined as a composition of three forces, $F_{int} = F_t + F_\delta + F_r$, a tensile force F_t which spreads localized deformations along the whole surface, a regularization force F_r which locally smoothes the shape and an elastic force F_δ which linearly penalizes local wall thickness variations.

The internal tensile force acts to maintain a uniform spacing between model vertices. The regularization term, F_r, exploits the local normal curvature, computed according to the differential geometry definition: $F_r = (-\nabla(A)/2A)$, where A denotes the local area around $\mathbf{x}_\mathbf{i}$.[129] This force brings back vertices to their local tangent plane and minimizes surface curvature.

The elastic force is defined as the distance from the vertex $\mathbf{x}_\mathbf{i}$ to the inner wall surface mesh, weighted by the mean distance computed over the vertices situated in a cross-section slab orthogonal to the bronchus axis and including x_i: F_δ enhances F_{int} to prevent the propagation to penetrate within the contact zone between the bronchus and the vessel. The shape of the external surface of the bronchus at the level of vessel-bronchus contact zone is mainly constrained by the elastic component to follow the inner wall contour shape.

The model deformation toward the outer surface of the bronchus wall is guided by the external forces acting at each vertex x_i, $F_{ext} = F_I + F_\nabla$. They represent the influence of the image on the embedded surface. The force F_I guides the surface toward the image high intensity values while the force F_∇ drives the surface to regions of strong gradient. Both forces are normalized by the invariant maximum gray-level value $\hat{I}$. External forces are computed from the raw data by transforming the discrete volumetric image I into a continuous scalar field using tri-linear interpolation. The force F_I acts as a balloon force[130] and aims to inflate the model locally at high intensity regions.

As gray-level values decrease when approaching the outer surface of the bronchial wall, F_{ext} is strengthened by a force which drives the surface along the local gradient of the image. The gradient value is averaged over the local neighborhood of x_i improving the robustness against noise. The model is attracted to strong contours of the wall guided by the force F_∇, thus allowing to match bronchus wall irregularities.

In the context of medical data, the resolution of the triangulated deformable surface model must match the resolution of the volume image. The size of each surface mesh element (e.g. each triangle) should be close to the voxel size of the image volume. However, as a result of vertex displacement, the inter-vertices distance will change, leading either to skip important image features in the case of a too large distance, or to increase computational cost when too dense vertex distributions occur. In order to maintain adequate surface mesh resolution and high computational efficiency, the edge length is constrained during the deformation process, according to $\xi \leq d_E(u,v) \leq \lambda\xi$, where $d_E(u,v)$ denotes the Euclidean distance between two u, v vertices, ξ determines the global resolution of the surface, and λ the admissible length ratio between the longest and the shortest edges. Edges not holding these constraints are removed or subdivided by methods used in progressive meshing.[131] The vertex displacement step between two iterations, k, as well as mesh density ξ, are set according to the highest CT data spatial resolution. The deformable model is initialized with a coarse resolution and deformed toward its energy minimum. Then the mesh is globally refined and the process is repeated. The step and the density parameters are iteratively decreased in order to reach the optimal mesh resolution at the convergence until all the mesh triangles have the same dimension as image voxels. The finest image structures can subsequently be detected and the costs of the first deformations are significantly reduced. Mesh deformation may also lead to surface self-intersections, especially in the case of bronchus subdivision. To prevent this problem, auto-collision is checked for each vertex.[132]

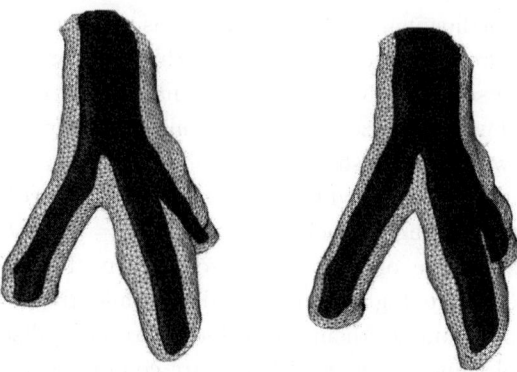

Fig. 32.   3D segmentation applied on clinical data. Before (left) and after (right) treatment.

Figure 32 illustrates the 3D segmentation of the airway wall achieved for a bronchus subdivision, before and after medication, by using the described approach. The visual analysis of the result clearly indicates the enlargement of the airway lumen and the wall thinning after the treatment. However, an accurate quantification of the variations between these examinations will require to accurately delimit the same bronchial extent in both cases.

6. Conclusion

In the context of the emerging paradigm in the medical community — "imaging as a biomarker" — the role of medical imaging is progressively evolving from a qualitative analysis toward quantitative assessment. Such an evolution is mainly imposed by the needs expressed in the patient follow-up and in new therapy design and evaluation in clinical trials.

This paper oriented its topics toward such a transition in the development of computer-assisted diagnosis tools, within the framework of bronchial systems analysis. The presented panorama covered multiple aspects, starting with simple visualization techniques and progressively adding new facilities to end up with a quantitative assessment. The contribution of each new developed data analysis methodology was stressed with respect the CAD tools that it makes possible to implement. The evolution of these clinical tools for bronchial systems investigation was thus guided by the aspects related to 3D segmentation, axis-based description and mesh surface modeling, for which both a general overview and specific solutions were presented. Hot topic issues on functional modeling via computational fluid dynamics simulation and on therapy assessment in asthma in clinical trials were also addressed, and current solutions as well as new trends were discussed.

Acknowledgment

Authors would like to thank Dr. Diane Perchet and Dr. Pierre-Yves Brillet for the enriching discussions we had on the topic of bronchial systems analysis, which largely influenced the orientation of this presentation.

References

1. A. Jain, Image reconstruction from projections, in *Fundamentals of Digital Image Processing.* (Englewood Cliffs Ed., Prentice Hall, NJ, 1989).
2. J. Beutel, H. Kundel and R. Van Metter, Tomographic imaging, in *Handbook of Medical Imaging. Volume 1: Physics and Psychophysics*, (2000), pp. 511–554.
3. M. W. Vannier and G. Wang, Principles of spiral CT, in *Spiral CT of the Chest*, eds. M. Rémy-Jardin and J. R. Ed., (Springer, Berlin, 1996), pp. 1–32.
4. G. Ferreti, I. Bricault and M. Coulomb, Virtual tools for imaging of the thorax, *Eur. Respir. J.* **18** (2001) 381–392.
5. K. Hopper, T. Iyriboz, R. Mahraj, S. Wise, C. Kasales, T. TenHave, R. Wilson and J. Weaver, CT bronchoscopy: optimization of imaging parameters, *Radiology* **209** (1998) 872–877.
6. C. Shaeffer-Prokop and M. Prokop, Spiral CT of the trachea and main bronchi, in *Medical Radiology Spiral CT of the Chest*, eds. M. Rémy-Jardin and J. R. Ed., (1996), pp. 161–183.
7. P. Grenier, C. Beigelman-Aubry, C. Fetita and Y. Martin-Bouyer, Multidetector-row CT of the airways, *Sem. Roentgenol.* **38**(2) (2003) 146–157.
8. D. Naidich, N. L. Müller, E. A. Zerhouni and G. McGuinness, Airways, in *Computed Tomography and Magnetic Resonance of the Thorax, Third Edition.* (Lippincott-Raven Ed., Philadelphia, 1999).
9. J. O. Shepard, The bronchi, in *Thoracic Radiology: The Requisites.* (Theresa C McLoud, Mosby Inc., St. Louis, 1998).
10. J. Westcott and J. Volpe, Peripheral bronchopleural fistula: CT evaluation in 20 patients with pneumonia, empyema, or postoperative air leak, *Radiol.* **196** (1995) 175–181.
11. J. Semenkovich, H. Glazer, D. Anderson, J. J. Arcidi, J. Cooper and G. Patterson, Bronchial dehiscence in lung transplantation: CT evaluation, *Radiol.* **194** (1995) 205–208.
12. C. Beigelman, N. Howarth, C. Chartrand-Lefebvre and P. Grenier, Congenital anomalies of tracheobronchial branching patterns: spiral CT aspects in adults, *Eur. Radiol.* **8** (1998) 79–85.
13. G. McGuinness, D. Naidich, S. Garay, A. Davis, A. Boyd and H. Mizrachi, Accessory cardiac bronchus: CT features and clinical significance, *Eur. Radiol.* **189** (1993) 563–566.
14. J. Kim, N. Muller, C. Park, P. Grenier and C. Herold, Cylindrical bronchiectasis: diagnostic findings on thin-section CT, *AJR Am. J. Roentgenol.* **168** (1997) 751–754.
15. G. McGuinness, D. Naidich, B. Leitman and D. McCauley, Bronchiectasis: CT evaluation, *AJR Am. J. Roentgenol.* **160** (1993) 253–259.
16. J. Tagasuki and J. Godwin, Radiology of chronic obstructive pulmonary disease, *Radiol. Clin. North Am.* **36** (1998) 29–55.

17. P. Stark and A. Norbash, Imaging of the trachea and upper airways in patients with chronic obstructive airway disease, *Radiol. Clin. North Am.* **36** (1998) 91–105.
18. E. Stern, C. Graham, W. Webb and G. Gamsu, Normal Trachea during forced expiration: dynamic CT measurements, *Radiol.* **187** (1993) 27–31.
19. R. Gilkeson, L. Ciancibello, R. Ilejal, H. Montenegro and P. Lange, Tracheobroncho-malacia: dynamic airway evaluation with multidetector CT, *Am. J. Roentgenol.* **176** (2001) 36–42.
20. P. Grenier, I. Mourey-Gerosa, K. Benali, M. Brauner, A. Leung, S. Lenoir, M. Cordeau and B. Mazoyer, Abnormalities of the airways and lung parenchyma in asthmatics: CT observations in 50 patients and inter- and intraobserver variability, *R. Eur. Radiol.* **6** (1996) 199–206.
21. D. Lynch, J. Newell, B. Tschomper, T. Cink, L. Newman and R. Bethel, Uncomplicated asthma in adults: comparison of CT appearance of the lungs in asthmatic and healthy subjects, *Radiol.* **188** (1993) 829–833.
22. F. Paganin, V. Trussard, E. Seneterre, P. Chanez, J. Giron, P. Godard, J. Senac, F. Michel and J. Bousquet, Chest radiography and high resolution computed tomography of the lungs in asthma, *Am. Rev. Respir. Dis.* **146** (1992) 1084–1087.
23. C. Park, N. Muller, S. Worthy, J. Kim and M. Awadh, N. and 0 Fitzgerald, Airway obstruction in asthmatic and healthy individuals: inspiratory and expiratory thin-section CT findings, *Radiol.* **203** (1997) 361–367.
24. P. Grenier, C. Beigelman-Aubry, C. Fetita, F. Prêteux, M. Brauner and S. Lenoir, New frontiers in CT imaging of airway disease, *Eur. Radiol.* **12** (2002) 1022–1044.
25. L. Quint, R. Whyte, E. Kazerooni, F. Martinez, P. Cascade, J. Lynch, M. Orringer, L. Brunsting and G. Deeb, Stenosis of the central airways: evaluation by using helical CT with multiplanar reconstructions, *Radiology* **194** (1995) 871–877.
26. J. Rémy, M. Rémy-Jardin, D. Artaud and M. Fribourg, Multiplanar and three-dimensional reconstruction techniques in CT: impact on chest diseases, *Eur. Radiol.* **8** (1998) 335–351.
27. B. Cabral, N. Cam and J. Foran, Accelerated volume rendering and tomographic reconstruction using texture mapping hardware. in *VVS '94: Proceedings of the 1994 Symposium on Volume Visualization*, (ACM Press, 1994), pp. 91–98.
28. R. Drebin, L. Carpenter and P. Harrahan, Volume Rendering, *SIGGRAPH'88.* (1988), pp. 665–674.
29. K. Hohne, M. Bomans, A. Pommert, U. Tiede and G. Weibeck, Rendering tomographic volume data: Adequacy of methods for different modalities and organs, in *3D Imaging in Medicine*, eds. K. Hohne, H. Fuchs and e. S.M. Pizer, (1990), pp. 197–215.
30. M. Levoy, Display of surfaces from volume data, *IEEE Comput. Graph. Appl.* **8** (1988) 29–37.
31. R. Robb and C. Barillot, Interactive display and analysis of 3-D medical images, *IEEE Trans. Med. Imaging* **8** (1989) 17–226.
32. R. Robb, *Three-Dimensional Biomedical Imaging: Principles and Practice.* (VCH Publishers, New York, 1994).
33. G. Rubin, Techniques of reconstruction, in *Medical Radiology Spiral CT of the Chest*, eds. M. Rémy-Jardin and J. R. Ed., (1996), pp. 101–107.
34. P. Grenier, C. Beigelman-Aubry, C. Fetita and F. Prêteux, in Large airways at CT: Bronchiectasis, Asthma and COPD, *Functional Imaging of the Chest*, (Springer-Verlag, Berlin, Germany, 2004), pp. 39–54.
35. W. Krueger. The application of transport theory to visualization of 3D scalar data fields. in *VIS '90: Proc. 1st Conf. Visualization '90* (IEEE Comput. Soc. Press, 1990), pp. 273–280.

36. H. McAdams, S. Palmer, J. Erasmus, E. Patz, J. Connolly, P. Goodman, D. Delong and V. Tapson, Bronchial anastomotic complications in lung transplant recipients: virtual bronchoscopy for noninvasive assessment, *Radiology* **209** (1998) 689–695.

37. M. Rémy-Jardin, J. Rémy, F. Deschildre, D. Artaud, P. Ramon and J. Edme, Obstructive lesions of the central airways: evaluation by using spiral CT with multiplanar and three-dimensional reformations, *Eur. Radiol.* **6** (1996) 807–816.

38. H. Kitaoka and T. Yumoto, Three-dimensional CT of the bronchial tree. A trial using an inflated fixed lung specimen, *Invest. Radiol.* **25** (1990) 813–817.

39. T. Mitsa, J. Qian and J. Galvin, 3-D modeling of lung morphogenesis using fractals, *Proc. SPIE.* **1898** (1993) 540–548.

40. T. Tozaki, Y. Kawata, N. Niki, H. Ohmatsu, K. Eguchi and N. Moriyama, Three-dimensional analysis of lung areas using thin-slice CT images, *Proc. IEEE 13th Int. Conf. Pattern Recogn.* **3** (1996) 548–552.

41. C. Fetita, F. Prêteux and P. Grenier, Three-dimensional reconstruction of the bronchial tree in volumetric computerized tomography: application to CT bronchography, *J. Electron. Imaging* **15**(2) (2006) 23004-1–17.

42. F. Prêteux, On a distance function approach for gray-level mathematical morphology, in mathematical morphology in image processing, ed. E. Dougherty (Marcel Dekker, New York, 1992).

43. S. A. Wood, J. D. Hoford, E. A. Hoffman, E. Zerhouni and W. A. Mitzner, Quantitative 3-D reconstruction of airway and pulmonary vascular tree using HRCT, *Proc. SPIE.* **1905** (1993) 316–323.

44. K. Mori, J. Hasegawa, J. Toriwaki, H. Anno and K. Katada, Recognition of bronchus in three-dimensional X-ray images with applications to virtualized bronchoscopy system, *Proc. 13th Int. Conf. Pattern Recogn.* **3** (1996) 328–332.

45. M. Lacrosse, J.-P. Trigaux, B. Van Beers and P. Weynants, 3D spiral CT of the tracheobronchial tree, *J. Comput. Assisted Tomography* **3** (1995) 341–347.

46. T. Schlatholter, C. Lorenz, I. Carlsen, S. Renisch and T. Deschamps, Simultaenous segmentation and tree reconstruction of the airways for virtual bronchoscopy, *Proc. SPIE.* **4684** (2002) 103–113.

47. J. Tschirren, E. Hoffman, G. McLennan and M. Sonka, Intrathoracic airway trees: segmentation and airway morphology analysis from low-dose ct scans, *IEEE Trans. Med. Imaging* **24**(12) (2005) 1529–1539.

48. M. Sonka, W. Park and E. A. Hoffman, Rule-based detection of intrathoraic airway trees, *IEEE Trans. Med. Imaging* **15**(3) (1996) 314–326.

49. W. Park, E. A. Hoffman and M. Sonka, Fuzzy logic approach to extraction of intrathoracic airway trees from three-dimensional CT images, *Proc. SPIE.* **2710** (1996) 210–219.

50. J. S. Kim and M. Sonka, Neural network-based method for intrathoracic airway detection from three-dimensional CT images, *Proc. SPIE.* **2433** (1995) 191–202.

51. R. Chiplunkar, J. M. Reinhardt and E. A. Hoffman, Segmentation and quantification of the primary human airway tree, *Proc. SPIE.* **3033** (1997) 403–414.

52. A. Kiraly, W. Higgins, G. McLennan, E. Hoffman and J. Reinhardt, Three dimensional human airway segmentation methods for clinical virtual bronchoscopy, *Acad. Radiol.* **9** (10), 1153–1168, (2002).

53. D. Aykac, E. A. Hoffman, G. McLennan and J. M. Reinhardt, Segmentation and analysis of the human airway tree from three-dimensional X-ray CT images, *IEEE Trans. Med. Imaging* **22**(8) (2003) 940–950.

54. C. Fetita, F. Prêteux, C. Beigelman-Aubry and P. Grenier, Pulmonary airways: 3D reconstruction from multi-slice CT and clinical investigation, *IEEE Trans. Med. Imaging* **23**(11) (2004) 1353–1364.

55. D. Perchet, *Modélisation in-silico des voies aériennes: reconstruction morphologique et simulation fonctionnelle*. PhD thesis (Université RenDescartes-Paris V, 2005).
56. L. Lam, S.-W. Lee and C. Y. Suen, Thinning methodologies — a comprehensive survey, *IEEE Trans. Pattern Anal. Machine Intell.* **14**(9) (1992) 869–885.
57. S. Lobregt, P. Verbeek and F. Groen, Three-dimensional skeletonization: principle and algorithm, *IEEE Trans. Pattern Anal. Machine Intell.* **2** (1980) 75–77.
58. C. Ma and M. Sonka, A fully parallel 3D thinning algorithm and its applications, *Comput. Vision Image Understanding* **64**(3) (1996) 420–433.
59. P. Saha, B. Chaudhuri and D. Dutta Majumder, A new shape preserving parallel thinning algorithm for 3D digital images, *Pattern Recogn.* **30**(12) (1997) 1939–1955.
60. K. Palágyi and A. Kuba, A 3D 6-subiteration thinning algorithm for extracting medial lines, *Pattern Recogn. Lett.* **19** (1998) 613–627.
61. C.-M. Ma, S.-Y. Wan and H.-K. Chang, Extracting medial curves on 3D images, *Pattern Recogn. Lett.* **23** (2002) 895–904.
62. W. Xie, R. P. Thompson and R. Perucchio, A topology-preserving parallel 3D thinning algorithm for extracting the curve skeleton, *Pattern Recogn.* **36** (2003) 1529–1544.
63. D. Paik. *Computer Aided Interpretation of Medical Images*. PhD thesis (Stanford, 2002).
64. E. Sorantin, C. Halmai, B. Herdhelyi, K. Palagyi, G. Nyul, K. Olle, B. Geiger, F. lindbichler, G. Friedriche and K. Kiesler, Spiral-CT-based assessment of tracheal stenoses using 3D-skeletonisation, *IEEE Trans. Med. Imaging* **21**(3) (2002) 263–273.
65. D. Kirkpatrick. Efficient computation of continuous skeletons, in *IEEE 20th Ann. Symp. Foundations Comput. Sci.* (1979) 18–27.
66. J. Brandt and R. Algazi, Continuous skeleton computation by Voronoi diagram, *CVGIP: Image Understanding* **55**(3) (1992) 329–338.
67. J. Brandt, Convergence and continuity criteria for discrete approximation of the continuous planar skeletons, *CVGIP: Image Understanding* **59**(1) (1994) 116–124.
68. D. Attali, P. Bertolino and A. Montanvert, Using polyballs to approximate shapes and skeletons, in *12th Int. Conf. Pattern Recogn.* (1994) 626–628.
69. N. Amenta, S. Choi and R. Kolluri, The power crust, unions of balls and the medial axis transform, *Int. J. Comp. Geometry Appl.* **19**(2–3) (2001) 127–153.
70. R. Ogniewicz and M. Ilg. Vorono skeletons: Theory and applications, in *Proc. IEEE Conf. Comput. Vision Pattern Recogn.* (Champagne, Illinois, 1992), pp. 63–69.
71. D. Attali and A. Montanvert, Computing and simplifying 2D and 3D continuous skeletons, *Comput. Vision Image Understanding* **67**(3) (1997) 261–273.
72. R. Ogniewicz and O. Kübler, Hierarchic Voronoi Skeletons, *Pattern Recogn.* **28**(3) (1995) 343–359.
73. M. Näf, G. Székely, R. Kikinis, M. Shenton and O. Kübler, 3D Voronoi skeletons and their usage for the characterization and recognition of 3D organ shape, *CVIU* **66**(2) (1997) 147–161.
74. C. Arcelli and G. Sanniti di Baja, Finding local maxima in a pseudo-euclidian distance transform, *Comput. Vision Graph. Image Processing* **43** (1988) 361–367.
75. G. Malandain and S. Fernández-Vidal, Euclidian skeletons, *Image Vision Comput.* **16**(5) (1998) 317–327.
76. J. A. Sethian, *Level Set Methods and Fast Marching Methods* 2nd edition (Cambridge University Press, 1999).
77. R. Kimmel, D. Shaked, N. Kiryati and A. Bruckstein, Skeletonization via distance maps and level sets, *Comput. Vision Image Understanding* **62**(3) (1995) 382–391.

78. K. Siddiqi, S. Bouix, A. Tannenbaum and S. Zucker. The Hamilton-Jacobi skeleton, in *Int. Conf. Comput. Vision ICCV '99* (1999) 828–834.
79. C. Pudney, Distance-ordered homotopic thinning: a skeletonization algorithm for 3D digital images, *Comput. Vision Image Understanding* **72**(3) (1998) 404–413.
80. G. Borgefors, I. Nyström and G. Sanniti di Baja, Computing skeletons in three dimensions, *Pattern Recogn.* **32**(7) (1999) 1225–1236.
81. S. Svensson, I. Nyström and G. Borgefors, Fully reversible skeletonization for volume images based on anchor-points from the D26 distance transform, in *Proc. 11th SCIA* (Kangerlussuaq, Greenland, 1999), pp. 601–608.
82. A. Kanitsar, R. Wegenlittl, P. Felkel, D. Fleischmann, D. Sandner and E. Groller, Computed tomography angiography: a case study of periferal vessel investigation, *Visualization'01* (2001) 477–480.
83. S. He, B. Ai, R. Dand Lu, C. Cao, H. Bai and B. Jing, Medial Axis Reformation: a new visualization method for CT angiography, *Acad. Radiol.* **8**(8) (2001) 726–733.
84. Y. Zhou and A. Toga, Efficient skeletonization of volumetric objects, *IEEE Trans. Visualization Comput. Graph.* **5**(3) (2001) 196–209.
85. D. Chen, B. Li, Z. Liang, M. Wan, A. Kaufman and M. Wax, A tree-branch searching multiresolution approach to skeletonization for virtual endoscopy, *Proc. SPIE Med. Imaging* (2000) 726–734.
86. I. Bitter, A. Kaufman and M. Sato, Penelized distance volumetric skeleton algorithm, *IEEE Trans. Visualization Comput. Graph.* **7**(3) (2001) 195–206.
87. F. Queck and C. Kirbas, Vessel extraction in medical images by wave-propagation and traceback, in *IEEE Trans. Med. Imaging* **20** (2001) 117–131.
88. C. Pisupati, L. Wolff, W. Mitzner and E. Zerhouni, A central axis algorithm for 3D bronchial tree structures, *Proc. IEEE Int. Symp. Comput. Vision* (1995) 259–264.
89. D. Perchet, C. Fetita, L. Vial, F. Prêteux, G. Caillibotte, G. Sbirlea-Apiou and M. Thiriet, Virtual investigation of pulmonary airways in volumetric computed tomography, *Comput. Anim. Virtual Worlds* **15**(3-4) (2004) 361–376.
90. B. Baxter and J. Sorenson, Factors affecting the measurement of size and CT number in computed tomography, *Invest. Radiol.* (1981) 337–341.
91. O. Saba, E. Hoffman and J. Reinhardt, Maximizing quantitative accuracy of lung airway lumen and wall measures obtained from X-ray CT imaging, *J. Appl. Physiol.* **95** (2003) 1063–1075.
92. E. Hoffman, J. Reinhardt and M. Sonka, Characterization of the intersistal lung diseases via density based and texture-based analysis of computed tomography images of lung structure and function, *Acad. Radiol.* **10** (2003) 1104–1118.
93. F. Chabat, X. Hu, D. Hansell and G. Yang, ERS transform for the automated detection of bronchial abnormalities on CT of the lungs, *IEEE Trans. Med. Imaging* **20** (2001) 942–952.
94. G. King, N. Muller, K. Whittall, Q. Xiang and P. Pare, An analysis algorithm for measuring airway Lumen and Wall areas from high-resolution computed tomographic data, *Am. J. R. Cr. Care Med.* **161** (2000) 574–580.
95. R. Wiemker, T. Blaffert, T. Blow, S. Renisch and C. Lorenz, Automated assessment of bronchial lumen, wall thickness and bronchial tree using high-resolution CT, *International Cong Ser.* **1268** (2004) 967–972.
96. P. Berger, V. Perot, P. Desbarats, J. M. Tunon-de Lara, R. Marthan and F. Laurent, Airway wall thickness in cigarette smokers: quantitative thin-section CT assessment, *Radiol.* **235** (2005) 1055–1064.

97. F. Prêteux, C. Fetita, P. Grenier and A. Capderou, Modeling, segmentation and caliber estimation of bronchi in high-resolution computerized tomography, *J. Electron. Imaging* **8** (1999) 36–45.

98. A. Saragaglia, C. Fetita, F. Prêteux, P. Brillet and P. Grenier, Accurate 3D quantification of bronchial parameters in MDCT, *Proc. SPIE Conf. Math. Methods Pattern Image Anal.* **5916** (2005) 323–334.

99. P. Brillet, M. Becquemin, C. Beigelman-Aubry, C. Fetita, A. Capderou, V. Attali, T. Similowski, P. Grenier and M. Zelter, Assessment by multidetector CT (MDCT) of bronchi dimensions in mild to moderate asthmatics follo wing 12 weeks treatment by salmeterol/fluticasone 50/250 Diskus bd (SFC), in *Proc. Am. Thoracic Soc. (ATS'2006)* (San Diego, CA, 2006).

100. J. Boissonnat, Shape reconstruction from planar cross sections, *Comput. Vision, Graph. Image Process.* **44**(1) (1988) 1–29.

101. G. Kwon, S. Chae and L. Lee, Automatic generation of tetrahedral meshes from medical images, *Computers and Structures* **81** (2003) 765–775.

102. T. McInerney and D. Terzopoulos, Deformable models in medical image analysis: a survey, *Med. Image Anal.* **1**(2) (1996) 91–108.

103. H. Delingette, Simplex meshes: a general representation for 3D shape reconstruction, *Proc. Int. Conf. Comput. Vision Pattern Recogn.* (1994) 856–857.

104. F. Leitner and P. Cinquin. Complex topology 3D objects segmentation, in *Model-Based Vision Develop Tools*, vol. 1609, *SPIE Proc.*, (SPIE, 1991) 16–26.

105. J.-O. Lachaud and A. Montanvert, Deformable meshes with automated topology changes for coarse-to-fine three-dimensional surface extraction, *Med. Image Anal.* **3**(2) (1998) 197–207.

106. J.-Y. Park, T. McInerney, D. Terzopoulos and M.-H. Kim, A non self-intersecting adaptive deformable surface for complex boundary extraction from volumetric images, *Comput. Graph.* **25** (2001) 421–440.

107. A. Frangi, W. J. Niessen and R. Hoogeveen, Model-based quantification of 3-D magnetic resonance angiographic images, *IEEE Trans. Med. Images* **18** (1999) 946–956.

108. P. Yim, J. J. Cebral, R. Mullick, H. Marcos and P. Choyke, Vessel surface reconstruction with a tubular deformable model, *IEEE Trans. Med. Images* **20**(12) (2001) 1411–1421.

109. L. de Figueiredo, J. de Miranda Gomes, D. Terzopoulos and L. Velho, Physically-based methods for polygonization of implicit surfaces, *Graph. Interface'92.* (1992) 250–257.

110. G. Turk, Generating textures for arbitrary surfaces using reaction-diffusion, *Comput. Graph. (Proc. SIGGRAPH'91).* **25** (1991) 289–298.

111. A. Witkin and P. Heckbert, Using particules to sample and control implicit surfaces, *Comput. Graph. (Proc. SIGGRAPH'94).* (1994) 269–278.

112. M. Desbrun, N. Tsigos and M.-P. Gascuel, Adaptive sampling of implicit surfaces for modeling and interaction, *Proc. Implicit Surfaces* (1995) 171–185.

113. J. Hart and B. Stander, Guaranteeing the topology of an implicit surface polygonization for interactive modeling, *Proc. SIGGRAPH'97.* (1997) 279–286.

114. L. Chew, Guaranteed-quality mesh generation for curved surfaces, *Proc. 9th Annu. ACM Symp. Comput. Geom.* (1993) 274–280.

115. J.-D. Boissonnat and S. Oudot, Provably good surface sampling and approximation, *Eurograph. Symp. Geomet. Processing* (2003).

116. J.-D. Boissonnat and S. Oudot, An effective condition for sampling surfaces with guarantees, *ACM Symp. Solid Modeling Appl.* (2004), pp. 101–112.

117. R. Summers and J. Cebral. Tracheal and central bronchial aerodynamics using virtual bronchoscopy, in *Physiology and Function from Multidimensional Images, C.-T. Chen and, A. V. Clough, eds., Proc. SPIE*, vol. 4321, (2001), pp. 22–31.

118. W. Lorensen and H. Cline, Marching Cubes: a high resolution 3D surface construction algorithm, *Comput. Graph.* **21** (1987) 163–169.

119. Z. Wood, P. Schroder, D. Breen and M. Desbrun, Semi-regular mesh extraction from volumes, *IEEE Visualization* (2000), pp. 275–282.

120. G. Taubin, Curve and surface smoothing without shrinkage, *5th Int. Conf. Comput. Vision Proc.* (1995) 852–857.

121. M. Thiriet, R. Issa and J. Graham, A pulsatile developing flow in a bend, *J. Phys. III.* **3** (1992) 995–1013.

122. P. Frey and H. Borouchaki, Surface meshing using a geometric error estimate, *Int. J. Num. Methods Eng.* **58** (2003) 227–245.

123. D. Arnold, F. Brezzi and M. Fortin, A stable finite element for the Stokes equations, *Calcolo.* **21** (1984) 337–344.

124. O. Pironneau, On the transport-diffusion algorithm and its application to the Navier-Stokes Equations, *Num. Math.* **38** (1982) 309–332.

125. R. Glowinski, Numerical methods for nonlinear variational problems (Springer Series in Computational Physics, 1984).

126. P. Brillet, C. Fetita, C. Beigelman-Aubry, A. Saragaglia, D. Perchet, F. Prteux and P. Grenier, 3D quantitative assessment of bronchial reactivity and wall thickening in asthmatics at MDCT, in *Proc. First World Cong. Thoracic Imaging (WCTI'2005)*, (Florence, Italy, 2005), p. 160.

127. P. Brillet, C. Fetita, C. Beigelman-Aubry, D. Perchet, F. Prêteux and P. Grenier, Automatic segmentation of airway wall area for quantitative assessment at MDCT: preliminary results in asthmatics, *Eur. Cong. Radiol.* (2005).

128. A. Saragaglia, C. Fetita, F. Prêteux and P. Grenier, Assessment of airway remodeling in asthma: volumetric versus surface quantification approaches, *MICCAI.* Vol. 4191, R. Larsen, M. Nielsen and J. Sporring, eds. (Springer-Verlag, 2006), pp. 413-420.

129. M. Desbrun, M. Meyer and P. Alliez, Intrinsic parameterizations of surface meshes, *Comput. Graph. Forum* **21** (2002) 209–218.

130. L. Cohen, On active contour models and ballons, *Computer Vision, Graphics and Image Processing: Image Understanding* **53**(2) (1991) 211–218.

131. H. Hoppe, T. DeRose, T. Duchamp, J. McDonald and W. Stuetzle, mesh optimization, *Comput. Graph. SIGGRAPH 93 Proc.* (1993) 19–26.

132. J.-O. Lachaud and B. Taton. Deformable model with adaptive mesh and automated topology changes, in *IEEE Proc. 4th Int. Conf. 3D Digital Imaging Modeling*, (2003) 12–19.

CHAPTER 5

COMPUTATIONAL APPROACH TO LEFT VENTRICULAR FLOW FOR DEVELOPING CLINICAL APPLICATIONS

MASANORI NAKAMURA

The Center for Advanced Medical Engineering and
Informatics, Osaka University
1-3 Machikaneyama, Toyonaka 560-8531, Japan
masanori@me.es.osaka-u.ac.jp

SHIGEO WADA

Department of Mechanical Science & Bioengineering
Graduate School of Engineering Science, Osaka University
1-3 Machikaneyama, Toyonaka 560-8531, Japan

TAKAMI YAMAGUCHI

Department of Bioengineering and Robotics
Graduate School of Engineering, Tohoku University
Aoba 6-6-1, Sendai 980-8579, Japan

It is now possible to simulate flow in various organs in detail, due to the rapid advances in computational technology. Our ultimate goal is to build a system that can assist clinicians in diagnosis, treatment planning, and as patients differ in terms of anatomical configuration and disease condition, a wide variety of patient data must be accumulated, not only for statistical analysis but also to improve the processing system. While the computer simulation of a phenomenon plays a key role in this success, it is still necessary to elucidate the mechanism that elicits a phenomenon inside the patient's body. This paper gives brief descriptions of heart anatomy and physiology, reviews the past *in vivo*, *in vitro* and numerical studies on the left ventricular flow and introduces the recent attempts on computational fluid modeling of the left ventricular flow and its clinical applications. The studies demonstrate that computational modeling of intraventricular flow has great potential to advance clinical diagnosis of the left ventricular function.

Keywords: Computational fluid dynamics; left ventricle; mitral valve; blood flow; color M-mode Doppler echocardiogram.

1. Introduction

The great advances in computer technology during the past decade have enabled us to analyze various biological and physiological phenomena that were previously impossible to study numerically. One of the most successful applications is the study of blood flow. This paper introduces the recent work on computational fluid modeling of the left ventricular flow and its clinical applications. In this context, this chapter briefly describes the anatomy and physiology of the heart in Sec. 2, explains left ventricular diastolic function and its clinical assessment using echocardiography in Sec. 3, and reviews the history of the study of blood flow in the heart in Sec. 4. In Sec. 5, we describe our philosophy for performing computational biomechanics from the perspective of its application to clinical diagnosis. Section 6 introduces two case studies modeling left ventricular flow aimed at developing clinical applications. Finally, we provide conclusions in Sec. 7.

2. Anatomy and Physiology of the Heart

The heart is a muscular organ enclosed in a fibrous sac located slightly to the left of the middle of the thorax, underneath the sternum. It is slightly larger than a human fist and weighs 250–350 g in adults. The heart must beat continuously over person's lifetime. Beating 80,000–100,000 times and pumping approximately 7,000 l a day, the heart will beat 2–3 billion times and pump 200–300 million liters of blood over a 70–90 year life span. The wall of the heart is made of specialized muscle cells capable of sustaining continuous beating without fatigue.

The anatomy of the heart is illustrated in Fig. 1. In mammals and birds, the heart consists of four chambers: the upper chambers are called the left and right atria and the lower chambers are the left and right ventricles. The atria collect blood as it enters the heart. The ventricles pump blood out of the heart to the lungs or other parts of the body. From the perspective of circulation, the heart is divided into the right and left sides, which are separated by a septum. The right side of the heart pumps blood to the lungs for gas exchange (the pulmonary circulation). Then, oxygen-rich blood returns from the lungs to the left side of the heart, which pumps it to the body (the systemic circulation). As the right ventricle needs to pump blood only to the pulmonary circulation (15–20 mm Hg), its wall is not very

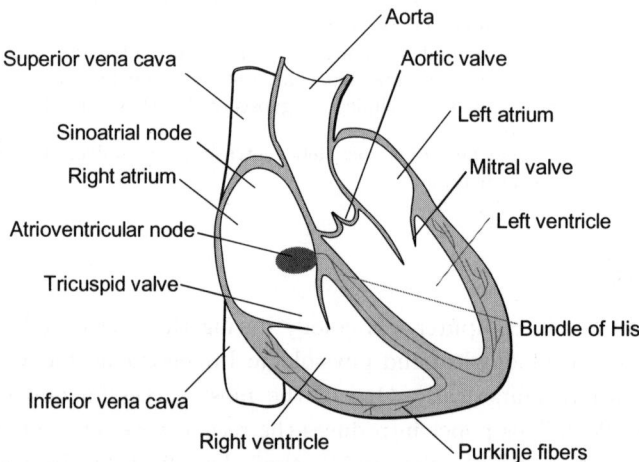

Fig. 1.   Anatomy and conducting-system of the heart. The pulmonary artery and vale are not illustrated in this cross-section.

thick (0.3–0.5 cm). It is more triangular in shape when viewed anteriorly and curves over the left ventricle. In contrast, the left ventricle is nearly conical in shape. In cross section, its cavity appears circular. The wall of the left ventricle is much more muscular (1.3–1.5 cm thick) as it has to pump blood around the entire body, which involves exerting a considerable force to overcome the high resistance at vascular pressures (80–120 mm Hg).

There are four valves in the heart (Fig. 2). Located between the atrium and ventricle on each side are the atrioventricular (AV) valves, which allow blood to flow from the atrium to the ventricle. The right AV valve is called the tricuspid valve, and the left is called the mitral valve (bicuspid valve). The mitral valve is the only heart valve that has two cusps, as it must cope with much strain and pressure. These AV valves are tethered to the wall of the ventricle by chordae tendinae to prevent the valve from prolapsing into the atria when it closes. The chordae tendinae are attached to papillary muscles that produce tension to hold the valve. The papillary muscles and chordae tendinae are now considered to have no effect on the opening and closing of the valves. The semilunar valves are present between the arteries and the ventricles. They prevent blood from flowing back from the arteries into the ventricles. The pulmonary valve is between the right ventricle and the pulmonary artery, while the aortic valve is between the left ventricle and the aorta. The aortic and pulmonary valves are similar anatomically, each consisting of three symmetrical valve cusps. Opening and closing of the heart valves are caused entirely by the pressure gradient across the valves.

The contraction of the heart is triggered by depolarization in a small group of conducting-system cells, the sinoatrial (SA) node, located in the right atrium near the entrance of the superior vena cava (Fig. 1). The SA node is the normal pacemaker for the entire heart and the heart rate is determined by the frequency of depolarization of the SA node. The action potential generated in the SA node spreads rapidly throughout the right atrium first and then throughout the left atrium to induce the contraction of the two atria. The spread of the action potential from the atria to the ventricles is via the conducting system called

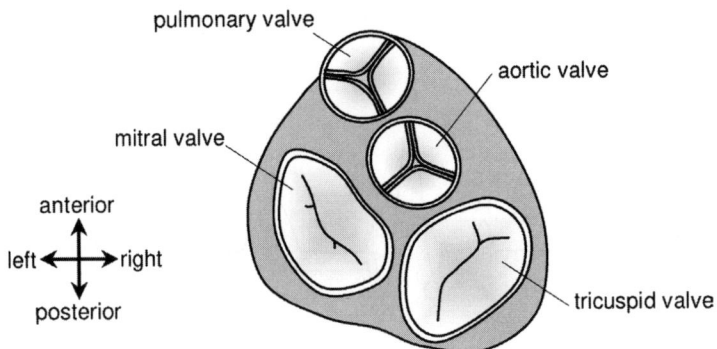

Fig. 2.   Anatomy of heart valves. The heart is looked down from the atrium side.

the atrioventricular (AV) node, which is located at the base of the right atrium. The propagation of the action potential through the AV node is relatively slow (taking approximately 0.1 s), allowing the atrial contraction to be completed before ventricular contraction begins. After leaving the AV node, the action potential enters the interventricular septum via conducting fibers called the bundle of His. Within the interventricular septum, the bundle of His divides into left and right branches, which leave the septum and enter the walls of the left and right ventricles, respectively. The branches are in turn connected to Purkinje fibers, which rapidly distribute the action potential throughout the ventricles. Depolarization and contraction of the ventricles begin slightly earlier in the apex of the ventricle and spread upward to squeeze blood into the arteries.

The electrocardiogram (ECG) is a device that records these electrical activities of the heart. Figure 3 illustrates a typical normal ECG. The first deflection is called the P wave and it is the electrical signature of atrial contraction. The second deflection, the PQR complex, which occurs approximately 1.5 s later, corresponds to the current that causes ventricular contraction. The final deflection is the T wave, the result of ventricular repolarization. Atrial repolarization is usually not evident on the ECG because it occurs at the same time as the QRS complex, which is much larger.

The orderly process of the electrical events in the heart triggers a recurring cycle of atrial and ventricular contraction and relaxation (Fig. 4). The cycle is divided into two major phases: the period of ventricular relaxation and blood filling or diastole, which is followed by the period of ventricular contraction and blood ejection, or systole. The explanation of the cycle begins with the end of systole. After the ventricles finish ejection, they begin to relax, and the aortic and pulmonary valves close. At this time, all valves are closed, allowing no blood to enter or leave the ventricles. This period is called isovolumetric relaxation. During the isovolumetric relaxation, the blood pressure in the ventricles decreases. When the blood pressure in the ventricles falls below that in the atria, the AV valves open and blood flows into the ventricles to fill them. This phase is called early diastole or the ventricular filling phase. Normally, approximately 80% of ventricular filling takes place during this phase. Near the end of diastole, the atrium depolarizes on excitation of the SA

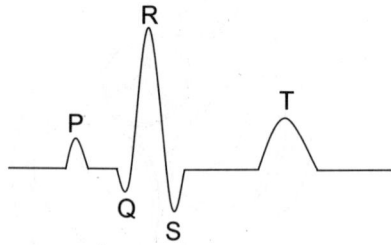

Fig. 3. Typical electrocardiogram. P, atrial depolarization; QRS, ventricular depolarization; T, ventricular repolarization.

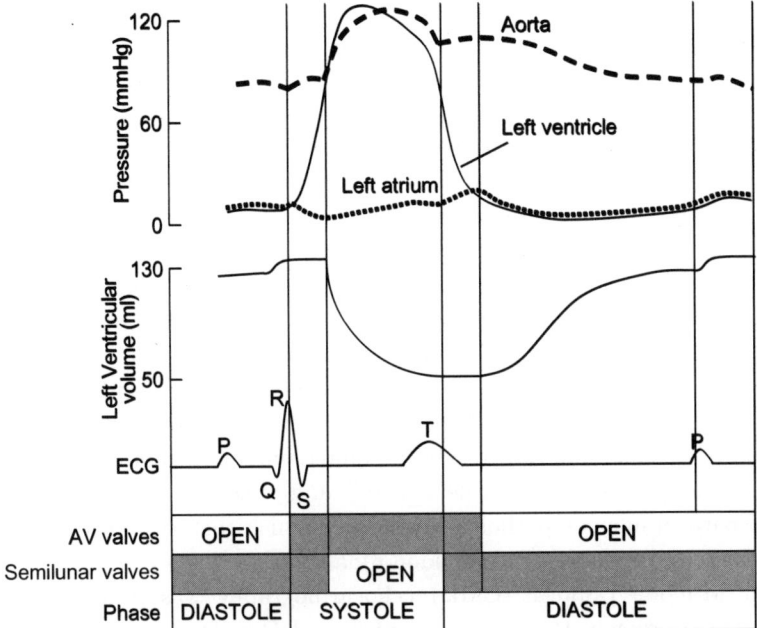

Fig. 4. Summary of events in the heart during a cardiac cycle.

node and atrial contraction occurs to give rise to additional filling of the ventricles. The propagation of the action potential from the AV node induces ventricular contraction. This rapidly elevates the blood pressure in the ventricles, which closes the AV valves. Since the semilunar valves are still closed and there has been no change in volume, this phase is referred to as the isovolumetric contraction. Once the blood pressure in the ventricles exceeds that in the arteries, the semilunar valves open and ventricular ejection occurs. Systole ends when the ventricular pressure falls below the arterial pressure.

3. Left Ventricular Diastolic Function and its Clinical Assessment Using Color M-mode Doppler Echocardiography

Cardiac disorders are the leading cause of death worldwide. The ability of the heart to distribute blood to the periphery of the vascular system is often evaluated from the perspective of the contractility of the left ventricle. However, it has been pointed out that diastolic function of the left ventricle, defined as the function of drawing blood from the left atrium at a normal intraventricular pressure, is also a key determinant of cardiac pump function.[1,2] For example, impaired expansibility of the left ventricle due to dilated cardiomyopathy leads to a reduction of blood storage in the left ventricle during diastole, resulting in deterioration of cardiac function.[3] In fact, it is reported that one-third of patients with cardiac dysfunctions have only diastolic dysfunction of the heart, while their systolic function is normal. Therefore, it is necessary to assess left ventricular diastolic function in clinical practice.

A number of diagnostic techniques, both invasive and noninvasive, are currently in use to detect abnormal cardiac function. While some successes have been achieved in detecting abnormalities in patients with advanced disease, relatively poor results have been obtained in patients with early disease. Therefore, there is impetus to develop a new method to assess ventricle function with sufficient sensitivity to detect latent cardiac disease.

Pulsed Doppler echocardiography has been widely used clinically to assess the diastolic function of the human left ventricle, as it is a convenient, noninvasive method. Cardiologists have attempted to evaluate the diastolic function of the left ventricle based on the ratio of the magnitudes of the E and A waves of the transmitral flow velocity profile recorded using this method (Fig. 5).[4-8] However, limitations of this method have also been pointed out;[9] for example, the transmitral velocity is readily affected by the heart rate[10] and preload.[11] Moreover, it can show a normal pattern in some pathological cases in which the atrioventricular pressure gradient increases; this is called pseudonormalization.[12]

Color M-mode Doppler (CMD) echocardiography was proposed as a new method that overcomes the drawbacks of pulsed Doppler echocardiography. This method measures the distribution of blood velocity along the wave direction of an ultrasound beam transmitted from a probe as a function of time, and presents the measured velocity distribution as a spatiotemporal map in which the magnitude of the blood velocity is expressed by the color and brightness (Fig. 6). Using this method, Jacobs et al.[13] recorded the velocity distribution of ventricular filling flow along the long axis of the left ventricle, from the ventricular apex to the center of the mitral orifice, and measured the times at which the peak velocity of the filling flow appeared at different levels from the mitral valve to the apex. The results showed that propagation of the peak velocity of the ventricular filling flow was delayed in

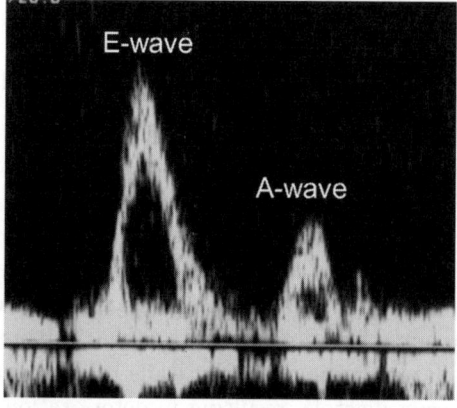

Fig. 5.   Transmitral flow wave: E-wave and A-wave.

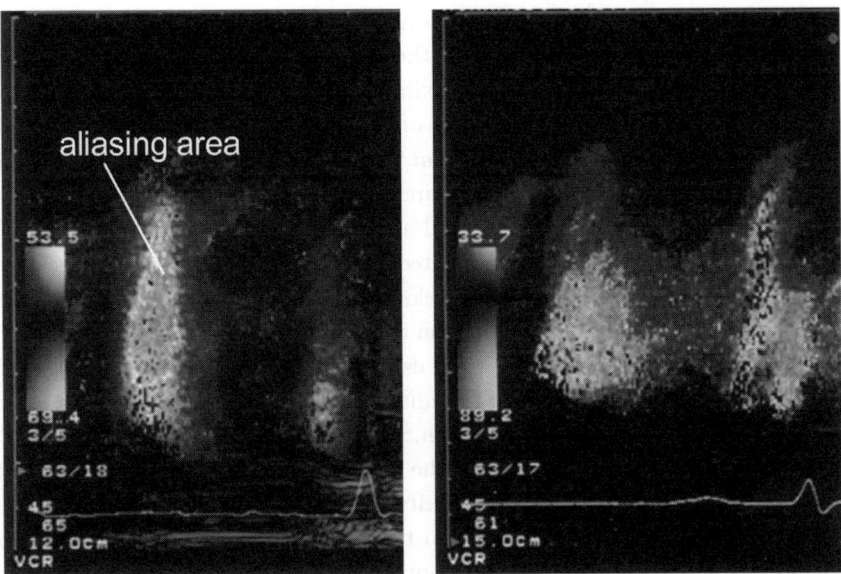

Fig. 6.   Color M-mode Doppler echocardiogram. Normal (left) and diastolic dysfunction (right).

the left ventricle with dilated cardiomyopathy. The validity of using the propagation rate of the peak velocity of the ventricular filling flow as an indicator of the diastolic function was confirmed by comparing it with invasively measured parameters, such as a time constant of the pressure decay of the left ventricle during isovolumetric relaxation.[14] Subsequently, CMD echocardiography has attracted the attention of cardiologists as a new method to evaluate diastolic function of the left ventricle.

The flow propagation velocity is a quantitative index describing the topology of a CMD echocardiogram of the flow in the left ventricle. Currently, five different approaches are used to quantify the topology of a CMD echocardiogram.[15] Since De Mey et al.[15] recapitulated these algorithms with clear schematic representations of CMD echocardiographic images, we provide brief descriptions here. Brun et al.[14] was the first to introduce the concept of flow propagation velocity. They defined it as the slope of the line drawn at the black-to-color boundary of a straight upward column of the early filling wave, called Phase I.[16] However, as the black-to-color boundary, as defined by Brun et al.[14] is not always clear, Duval-Moulin et al.[17] and Garcia et al.[18,19] modified this method by changing the aliasing limit of the velocity and creating clearly visible iso-velocity contours. The flow propagation velocity is then calculated by taking a slope of its leading edge. Stugaard et al.[20,21] measured the occurrence of the maximum velocities at several positions on the long-axis of the ventricle during diastole. The flow propagation velocity is calculated as the ratio of the spatial distance between the tips of the mitral leaflet and the middle of the long axis to the time difference between the occurrence of the maximum velocity at those locations. Thomas et al.[22] used eigenvector analysis of the CMD echocardiographic image to determine the flow propagation velocity. In their algorithm, a selected region of the iso-velocity contour of the ventricular filling flow in the M-mode image is approximated as an ellipse. The flow propagation velocity is then obtained from the angle of rotation of the long axis of the ellipse. In the method proposed by Takatsuji et al.[23] the aliasing limit of the color Doppler signals is changed to 70% of the spatiotemporal maximum velocity during diastole to create a blue aliasing area within the red area in the CMD echocardiogram. Then, the flow propagation velocity is calculated as the slope of a line connecting the point of the spatiotemporal maximum velocity to the point nearest the ventricular apex on the aliasing boundary. In addition to the propagation velocity, the traveling distance of the maximum velocity point, estimated as the distance from the mitral valve opening point to the center of the aliasing area, has also been proposed as an index of left ventricular diastolic function.[24]

Clinically, the diastolic function of the left ventricle is evaluated using the flow propagation velocity. Due to the complexity in the pattern of blood flow in the left ventricle, however, it is difficult to grasp the pattern of intraventricular flow as a whole and the wall motions of the left ventricle only from a CMD echocardiogram, which provides information only along its scan line. Therefore, the theoretical bases of the relationship between the topology of a CMD echocardiogram and the diastolic function of the left ventricle are not well understood. In order to advance the diagnosis of the diastolic function of the left ventricle using CMD echocardiography, it is necessary to analyze the relationship between intraventricular flow and the wall motion of the left ventricle during diastole, and to clarify how this relationship is reflected in the topology of a CMD echocardiogram.

4. Fluid Mechanics of Intraventricular Blood Flow

Blood flow within the left ventricle exhibits a complex structure that quickly changes in a three-dimensional spatial domain as a function of time with movement of the ventricular wall. To date, numerous approaches have been used to gain fluid mechanical insights into the full three-dimensional, temporal variation in the blood velocity within the ventricle over the cardiac cycle. However, none of them successfully reproduce the complete flow because of the highly complex nature of intraventricular flow.

To our knowledge, Bellhouse and Bellhouse[25] made the first *in vitro* model of the left ventricular flow in 1969. They used a transparent diaphragm to fabricate a left ventricle model and hypothesized that the ventricular vortex generated during diastole was a crucial factor for closure of the mitral valve. Later, Bellhouse[26] examined the flow field in an enlarged left ventricle and reported that enlargement of the left ventricle eliminated the vortex and resulted in a delay in mitral valve closure. However, since ventricular contraction was not started before the flow had come to a standstill, the strong deceleration in mitral flow that is now considered to be the mechanism of valve closure was missed.[27] Flow visualization studies in mock left ventricles have shown that a vortex, which sometimes has a ring structure, is a key feature of intraventricular diastolic flow. Studies have revealed that the vortex deforms rapidly, depending on the ventricular size[28] and the radius of the mitral orifice.[29] While past studies relied on video systems to visualize flow, recently introduced particle image velocimetry (PIV) enables a more precise analysis of the flow, particularly in eddies and turbulence downstream from artificial valves.[30,31]

Flow has also been measured *in vivo* using Doppler ultrasound and magnetic resonance imaging (MRI). Although Doppler ultrasound cannot measure more than one component of velocity and requires translation and rotation of the ultrasound transducer, the development of dynamic three-dimensional Doppler echocardiography has enabled the visualization of blood flow in three dimensions. Unfortunately, the resolution is low, which remains a problem.[32,33] MRI produces clear pictures of flow patterns in terms of spatial resolution, although it has limited temporal resolution. MRI studies[34−36] have confirmed the formation of the ventricular diastolic vortex predicted by *in vitro* studies. An attempt was also made to reconstruct the pressure field from the obtained velocity field within the ventricle.[37]

Computational fluid dynamics (CFD) have also been used to investigate intraventricular flow.[38−45] In the past, researchers have focused mainly on aspects of systolic function that are linked directly to the function of pumping blood. Georgiadis *et al.*[46] investigated the spatial distribution of intraventricular pressure during systole using an axisymmetric model of the left ventricle, assuming a potential flow. Later, Schoephoerster *et al.*[47] proved the importance of the viscous effects of blood, casting doubt on the use of potential flow models to study left ventricular fluid dynamics. They also constructed a human heart model based on successive cine-angiographic images to describe an asymmetric flow pattern. In 1994, they simulated the systolic flow dynamics in a left ventricle with abnormal wall motions,[48] which was later extended to a three-dimensional flow simulation.[49] Yoganathan *et al.*[50] modeled the left ventricle as a thin-walled cavity with contracting fibers, and studied systolic ejection using the immersed boundary method.[38−42] Taylor *et al.*[51] adopted a finite volume method to solve a full set of Navier–Stokes equations, and carried out a computer simulation of blood flow ejected from an axisymmetric model of the left ventricle. They modified the left ventricle model by constructing an anatomically realistic model of the left ventricle from a resin-molded canine heart and studied the three-dimensional structure of blood flow during a ventricular contraction.[52,53] Using the same geometric model of the left ventricle, they extended their study to examine the effect of partial cardiac infarction on intraventricular systolic flow.[54] In contrast, relatively few attempts have been made to model flow in the left ventricle during diastole numerically, although there have been a few recent attempts. Lemmon *et al.*[55,56] studied the change in the intraventricular flow field and pressure due to deterioration in left ventricular diastolic function. Saber *et al.*[45,57] constructed an anatomically realistic model of a human left ventricle using MRI and simulated the flow evolution during a cardiac cycle. Baccani et al.[58] simulated the diastolic flow in a left ventricle with dilated cardiomyopathy. The results were presented in an M-mode style to allow physical interpretation of the pattern detected in clinical measurements. They also examined the influence of mitral valve opening on the ventricular filling flow, focusing on the traveling speed of the vortices.[59] Domenichini et al.[60] introduced a direct numerical simulation to clarify the vortex structure within in the ventricle. They examined the process of vortex development in early diastole, although the results seem to be limited by the assumption of a quiescent flow at the onset of diastole. Although these studies have provided fluid mechanics insight into intraventricular flow dynamics, there has been little discussion on how the simulated flow is captured with current medical devices, such as Doppler echocardiography, and observed by clinicians. Consequently, despite computational studies providing a large amount of information to elucidate physiological phenomena, they are not helpful for clinicians and therefore have not contributed very much to advances in clinical diagnosis.

5. Advancing Clinical Diagnosis Using Computational Biomechanics

Measurement is the first step in clinical diagnosis. Based on information obtained from measurements, a medical doctor analyzes the phenomena occurring in a patient to grasp his/her physical condition to make a diagnosis. Until now, engineering resources have mainly been poured into developing measurement devices and technologies. This has increased the amount of information available for diagnosis, and consequently the accuracy of clinical diagnosis has improved markedly.

Now, medical doctors are required to analyze more complex physiological phenomena. Accordingly, they require more detailed and sophisticated information from the measurements, and tend to rely on the development of measurement technologies. Engineers have tackled such problems by modifying and inventing measurement devices to increase the amount of information available for diagnosis. In fact, the evolution of measurement devices has contributed to the advancement of clinical diagnosis; for example, it has made it possible to grasp complex phenomena that could not be previously captured. However, with this evolution, medical devices have become much larger and more complex, which has led to social issues, such as the growth of medical expenses and the reduction in the number of medical institutions in which a patient can receive a specific type of medical care. In addition, when the phenomenon to be diagnosed becomes more complicated, it is difficult for a medical doctor to construct a picture of the phenomenon based solely on information obtained by measurement. Therefore, we have to be aware of the limits and effectiveness of advances in diagnosis that depend solely on the development of measurements.

Currently, medical doctors analyze the information obtained from measurements based on experience and knowledge. By utilizing the power of computational biomechanics to analyze phenomena, we expect advances in the analysis of information. While the computer simulation of a phenomenon plays a key role in this success, in order to advance clinical diagnosis, it is still necessary to elucidate the mechanism that elicits a phenomenon occurring inside the patient's body. It is also important to understand how that phenomenon is seen or captured using measurement devices. By meeting these requirements, it should be possible to analyze complex phenomena from information obtained by measurement, thereby advancing clinical diagnosis.

The success in simulating a phenomenon using computational biomechanics demonstrates the potential to advance medical measuring devices. In the process of making a measurement, because of the limited resolution of measuring devices, some information, which is sometimes essential to grasp the physical condition of the patient, cannot be obtained. However, if a physiological phenomenon occurring inside the patient's body can be reproduced on a computer screen using computer simulation, it is possible to perform complementary procedures to determine the missing information. The combined use of computer simulations with measuring devices will upgrade low-technology medical devices so that they are equivalent to high-technology medical devices in terms of the quality of information.

By using computational biomechanics in conjunction with measurement, it should be possible to break out of the current situation in which the collection of information is dependent solely on advances in measurement technology, and to establish new diagnosis systems that place the emphasis on the analysis of a phenomenon.

6. Toward Clinically Applying the Computational Modeling of Intraventricular Flow

The computational modeling of intraventricular flow has great potential to advance clinical diagnosis. In Sec. 6.1, we briefly summarize computational modeling of left ventricular flow dynamics, with the intent to advance the clinical diagnosis of diastolic function in the left ventricle. In the next two sections, we introduce two case studies involving the clinical application of the computational modeling of intraventricular flow. In Sec. 6.2, we discuss how a change in left ventricular diastolic function is reflected in the blood flow in the left ventricle, the pattern of the CMD echocardiogram, and Doppler-derived clinical indices from a fluid mechanics perspective. In Sec. 6.3, we discuss the influence of the opening mode of the mitral valve orifice on intraventricular flow, focusing on the intraventricular vortex.

6.1. *Modeling left ventricular flow*

6.1.1. *Modeling the left ventricle*

The geometry of the left ventricular cavity at the end of diastole was defined using medical images so that it approximated the general anatomy of a human

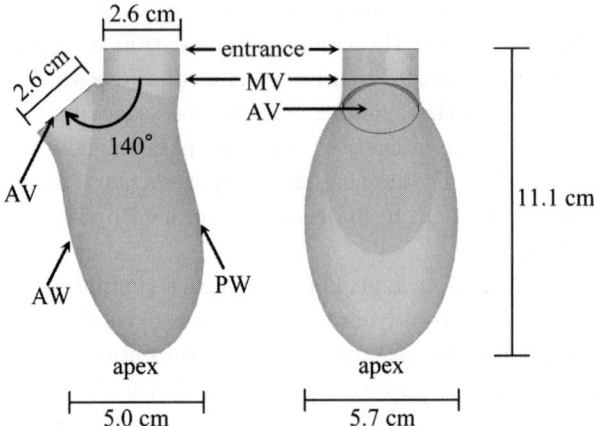

Fig. 7.   The geometry of the left ventricle model at its maximum expansion that was constructed based on the anatomical data. AV: aortic valve orifice, MV: mitral valve orifice, AW: anterior wall, PW: posterior wall. From Nakamura et al.[61] Reproduced by permission.

left ventricle. The ventricular volume was set to $120\,cm^3$ for a normal left ventricle and $180\,cm^3$ for an enlarged left ventricle, which represents dilated cardiomyopathy. The geometry of the normal left ventricle model in this design is shown in Fig. 7. For simplicity, the left ventricle was assumed to be symmetric with respect to the plane bisecting the mitral and aortic valves. We regarded the left ventricle as a U-shaped tube with the mitral valve at one end and the aortic valve at the other. We defined Ψ as the cross section of the left ventricle obtained by cutting it with a plane radiating from the line of intersection of the planes containing the two valve orifices. In designing the fully expanded left ventricle model, all Ψ cross sections were assumed to be elliptical.[61] A global Cartesian coordinate system, with coordinates (x, y, z), was defined at the origin, O, which was located at the point where the two planes containing the mitral and aortic orifices intersected the symmetric plane of the left ventricle. The x-axis lies along the intersection of the plane containing the mitral orifice and the symmetric plane, and the y-axis lies along the intersection of the two planes containing the mitral and aortic orifices.

It is generally thought that deformation of the left ventricle is caused by spontaneous relaxation and contraction of myocardium. Clinical data on the magnitude of intraventricular blood pressure suggest that the blood pressure during diastole is not high enough to significantly deform the left ventricular wall.[62] Thus, we assumed that the movement of the ventricular wall was not affected by intraventricular flow dynamics. In addition, twisting and untwisting were neglected since their effects on intraventricular flow are relatively small.[63]

For modeling of the ventricular wall motion, we assumed that a point on the wall moves in the direction of a line connecting the point to the centroid of cross section Ψ. The velocity of the ventricular wall at the apex was determined to satisfy

$$V'(t) = \iint\limits_{S} v_a(t)W(x, y, z)\,\mathbf{e} \cdot \mathbf{n}dS,\tag{1}$$

where $V'(t)(= dV(t)/dt)$ is the time derivative of $V(t)$, $v_a(t)$ is the velocity of the ventricular apex, $W(x, y, z)$ is a weighting function of the moving velocity of the wall, $\mathbf{n}$ is a unit vector normal to the ventricular surface, and $\mathbf{e}$ is a unit vector parallel to the direction of wall movement. For the derivation of this equation, refer to Nakamura *et al.*[61,64] If $V'(t)$ and $W(x, y, z)$ are provided, $v_a(t)$ is calculated from Eq. (1) . Then, the velocity at any point on the wall is simply obtained from $v_a(t)$ and the weighting function $W(x, y, z)$. In this study, the weighting function $W(x, y, z)$ was set such that the wall at the base including the two valve orifices did not move, while the velocity of the wall increased going toward the apex.

6.1.2. *Modeling the mitral and aortic valve orifices*

The gradual opening of the mitral valve orifice is important for the formation of an intraventricular vortex.[65] Therefore, the mitral valve was modeled as a planar, circular object with a core allowing blood to flow into the left ventricle. Hereafter, the core is referred to as the mitral valve orifice. Four different opening mode types of the mitral valve orifice were modeled: axisymmetric, anteroposterior, bilateral opening, and instantaneous, as illustrated in Fig. 8. The temporal change in the size of the orifice was kept the same for all modes and expressed as a function of the rate of volume change of the left ventricle.

6.1.3. *Analysis of blood flow*

Blood was treated as an incompressible Newtonian fluid with a density of $\rho = 1.05 \times 10^3\,\mathrm{kg/m^3}$ and a viscosity of $\nu = 3.5 \times 10^{-3}\,\mathrm{Pa \cdot s}$. Computations were performed using the CFD program ANSYS ver. 7.1 (Cybernet, Tokyo, Japan), which adopts

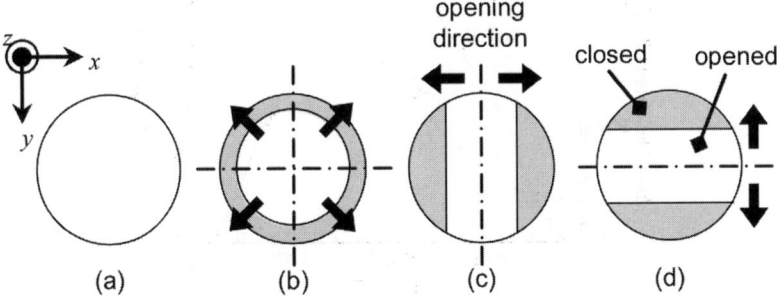

Fig. 8.   Schematic drawings of the modes of valve opening as seen from the top of the left ventricle: (a) instantaneous opening, (b) axisymmetric opening, (c) anteroposterior opening (parallel to the x-axis) and (d) bilateral opening (parallel to the y-axis).

a finite element method to solve the laminar flow model described by the Navier–Stokes and continuity equations:

$$\frac{\partial \mathbf{U}}{\partial t} + (\mathbf{U} \cdot \nabla)\mathbf{U} = -\frac{1}{\rho}\nabla P + \nu \nabla^2 \mathbf{U} \qquad (2)$$

$$(\nabla \cdot \mathbf{U}) = 0, \qquad (3)$$

where $\mathbf{U}$ is the three-dimensional velocity vector and P is the pressure. As boundary conditions, zero pressure and zero velocity were given to the opened and closed parts of the valve, respectively, and the velocity of the wall was applied to the ventricular wall based on a non-slip condition.

6.2. Analysis of left ventricular diastolic flow and its relation to the pattern of a CMD echocardiogram

To understand the intraventricular flow during diastole and to elucidate the mechanism linking the left ventricular diastolic function with the CMD echocardiogram and its derived indices, blood flow in the left ventricle was analyzed numerically. The volume change during diastole was determined from clinical data. The times from the beginning of diastole ($t = 0$) to the peak dV/dt and to the end of diastole were set to 0.12 s and 0.24 s, respectively. The maximum of dV/dt in diastole was set so that a net change in the volume within the framework of early diastole, equivalent to the left ventricular diastolic function, was 20–70 cm^3 with an interval of 5 cm.^{3} The volume change for the normal left ventricle with a net change of 60 cm^3 is shown in Fig. 9. The axisymmetric opening mode was chosen for the mitral valve as it produced a flow pattern similar to the one observed *in vivo*.[65]

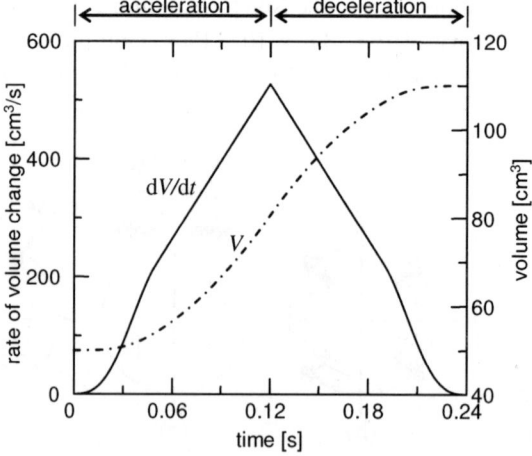

Fig. 9.   Temporal change of the left ventricular volume V (dot-dashed) and its rate of the change dV/dt (solid) during diastole. Diastole was divided into the acceleration phase and the deceleration phase according to dV/dt. From Nakamura et al.[66] Reproduced by permission.

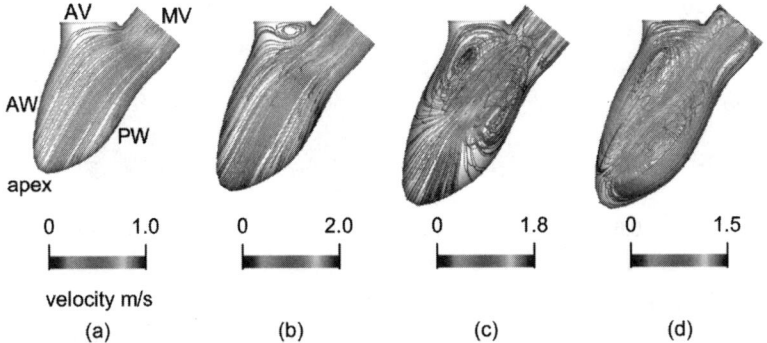

Fig. 10. Streamlines of blood flow for the left ventricle with a normal diastolic function. (A) $t = 0.06\,$s, (B) $t = 0.12\,$s, (C) $t = 0.18\,$s, (D) $t = 0.24\,$s. MV: mitral valve, AV: aortic valve, AW: anterior wall, PW: posterior wall. From Nakamura *et al.*[66] Reproduced by permission.

The simulation results showed the formation of an annular vortex under the aortic valve that was asymmetrically enlarged regardless of diastolic function. Figure 10 shows the flow patterns in the left ventricle with a net volume change of $60\,$cm.[3] From the onset of diastole, blood flowed into the cavity through the mitral valve orifice to fill the ventricular cavity. The main flow headed toward the apex, while the other flows gradually diverged and headed toward the wall. Immediately after the peak of early diastole ($t = 0.12\,$s), the fluid elements under the aortic valve were induced to coil, forming a vortex. With further expansion, the vortex not only grew in size, but also extended in a circumferential direction, developing into an annular vortex that surrounded the blood inflow along the left ventricular long axis, as shown in Fig. 11, where the annular vortex was observed from the top of the ventricle. At the mid-late stage of early diastole ($t = 0.18\,$s), another small vortex appeared in the space between the main flow heading straight toward the apex and the posterior wall. At this time, two asymmetric vortices were seen in the bisector plane. Toward the end of diastole, the annular vortex was amplified greatly.

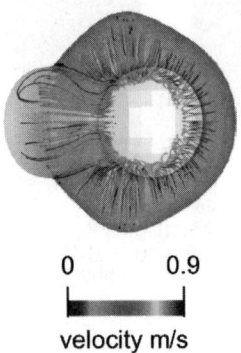

Fig. 11. Development of the annular vortex in the left ventricle at $t = 0.18\,$s during diastole.

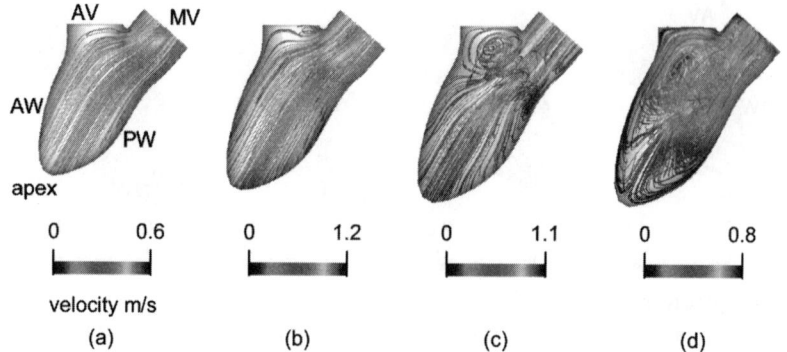

Fig. 12.   Streamlines of blood flow for the left ventricle with a deteriorated diastolic function.
(A) $t = 0.06$ s, (B) $t = 0.12$ s, (C) $t = 0.18$ s, (D) $t = 0.24$ s. MV: mitral valve, AV: aortic valve,
AW: anterior wall, PW: posterior wall. From Nakamura et al.[66] Reproduced by permission.

After the annular vortex was formed, the position of the fluid elements with a high
velocity (the maximum velocity point) shifted toward the apex along the long axis,
past the middle of the cavity.

The development of the vortex was retarded as the left ventricular diastolic
function deteriorated, as seen in Fig. 12. In this case, the annular vortex did not
grow much larger, compared to the one observed in the normal left ventricle. The
position of the maximum velocity point on the long axis did not shift toward the
apex as much.

The difference in left ventricular diastolic function was clearly reflected in the
pattern of the CMD echocardiograms of the inflow velocity along the left ventricular
long axis, as illustrated in Fig. 13. Here, the horizontal and vertical axes show the

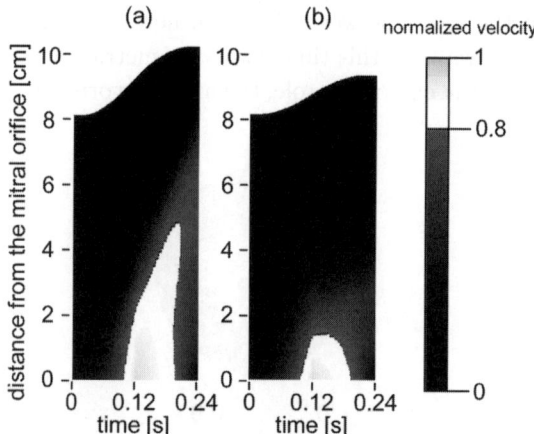

Fig. 13.   Color M-mode Doppler (CMD) echocardiogram of a ventricular filling flow along the
left ventricular long axis. The magnitude of the velocity is normalized by the spatiotemporal
maximum velocity. (a) volume change $= 60$ cm^3. (b) volume change $= 40$ cm^3. From Nakamura et
al.[66] Reproduced by permission.

time that as elapsed from the onset of the diastolic phase and the distance from the entrance of the left ventricle, respectively. The magnitude of the velocity at each point is expressed as a color according to the scale of the color bar shown on the right-hand side. The area that appears in white in the middle of the abscissa indicates the region where the velocity of fluid elements exceeded 80% of the maximum velocity in the early diastolic phase and is called the aliasing area. More quantitatively, the relationship between the left ventricular diastolic function and the traveling distance of the maximum velocity point is plotted in Fig. 14. The traveling distance of the maximum velocity point was evaluated as the distance from the mitral valve orifice to the tip of the aliasing area in the CMD echocardiogram.[24] Figure 15 plots the relationship between the left ventricular diastolic function and the propagation velocity.[23] The flow propagation velocity increased linearly as the left ventricular diastolic function improved.

The fluidic mechanism required to bring about a change in the pattern of the CMD echocardiogram in accordance with the left ventricular diastolic function is controversial. Sugawara *et al.*[67] insisted that this was due to a difference in the propagation of blood pressure in the ventricle. Kawano *et al.*[24] attributed it to a difference in the magnitude of the pressure gradient. In fact, a pressure gradient was formed from the base to the apex and the pressure propagated toward the apex. However, it occurred before the peak of early diastole, whereas the aliasing area elongated after the peak of early diastole. A detailed description of the intraventricular flow provided an opportunity to discuss the fluid mechanics factors that determine the shape of the aliasing area. At the beginning of diastole, the blood inflow through the mitral orifice diverged and its velocity decreased as it entered the main body of the left ventricle. This was due to the enlargement of the flow channel from the mitral orifice. As the annular vortex developed around

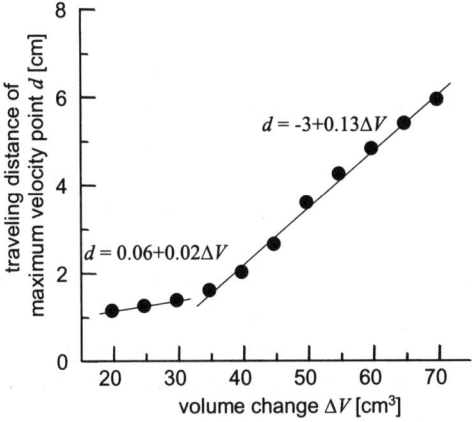

Fig. 14.   Relationship between the volume change of the left ventricle and traveling distance of the maximum velocity point during diastole. From Nakamura *et al.*[66] Reproduced by permission.

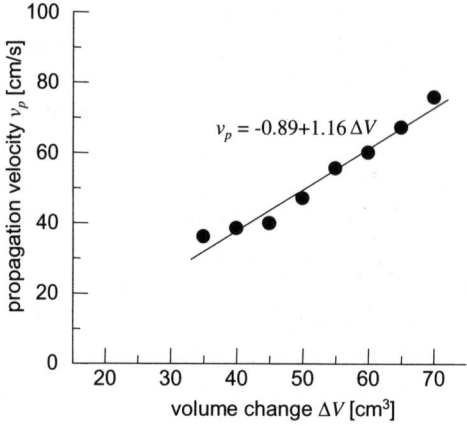

Fig. 15.   Relationship between the volume change of the left ventricle and the propagation velocity obtained on the basis of Takatsuji's method.[23] From Nakamura et al.[66] Reproduced by permission.

the blood inflow along the left ventricular long axis, it narrowed the passage of the blood inflow. Consequently, the fluid elements surrounded by the annular vortex increased their velocities locally via the vena contracta effect, inducing the maximum velocity point at the same depth as the center of the annular vortex. Furthermore, since the center of the annular vortex moved toward the apex of the left ventricle as the vortex grew in size and increased in intensity, the maximum flow velocity propagated toward the apex. Therefore, the elongation of the aliasing area in the CMD echocardiogram is associated with the growth of the annular vortex toward the apex. Such an idea on the relationship between the intraventricular vortex and the CMD echocardiogram was consistent with the conclusion obtained from the axisymmetric model studies.[68−70] We confirmed that their interpretation could be extended to a non-axisymmetric model of the left ventricle where an asymmetric vortex formed.

In general, the volume change during early diastole decreases as the left ventricular diastolic function deteriorates. The data in Takatsuji et al.[23] suggest that the volume change of a left ventricle with low function during early diastole decreases by approximately 30% compared to one with normal diastolic function. If we assume that the net volume change for the normal left ventricle during early diastole is $60 \, \text{cm}^3$, the left ventricle with the deteriorated diastolic function has a volume of $42 \, \text{cm}^3$. According to this simulation, the respective traveling distance of the maximum velocity point and the flow propagation velocity for these cases are 4.8 cm and 60.7 cm/s for the normal left ventricle, and 2.5 cm and 39.8 cm/s for the deteriorated left ventricle. In other words, these indices decrease by 50% and 33%, respectively, in the deteriorated left ventricle. These results suggest that it is possible to detect a change in left ventricular diastolic function based on the CMD echocardiogram.

Computational fluid dynamics of the intraventricular flow during early diastole were used to investigate the relationship between left ventricular diastolic function and the pattern of the CMD echocardiogram. The findings suggest that a CMD echocardiogram, which expresses the spatiotemporal distribution of velocity along the long axis of the left ventricle, reflected the growth of an intraventricular annular vortex toward the ventricular apex during diastole, and the clinical evaluation of diastolic function of the left ventricle with this method indirectly captured the development of the intraventricular vortex.

6.3. *Influence of the mitral valve orifice opening mode on intraventricular diastolic flow*

The mitral valve plays an important role in regulating a flow direction in the heart. If the valve is too damaged to permit repair, it must be replaced with an artificial valve. A wide variety of the artificial valves have been devised.[71] The performance of an artificial mitral valve has been evaluated in terms of biology, including thrombosis and hemolysis,[72,73] and engineering, including noise,[74] energy loss,[75,76] and regurgitation.[77] These parameters are mainly concerned with the blood flow dynamics near the valve. In contrast, little attention has been paid to the intraventricular flow dynamics downstream from the valve.

Here, we address the importance of the opening mode of the mitral valve orifice for intraventricular blood flow, to investigate designs of the mitral valve opening mode favored by fluid mechanics.[78] Four different opening modes were examined: gradually axisymmetric, gradually anteroposterior (anatomical), gradually bilateral (anti-anatomical), or instantaneous opening and closing as already shown in Fig. 8. In all of these models, the mitral valve orifice had the same shape when fully open.

The framework of the velocity profile of transmitral flow was built during the phase of mitral valve opening, which was characterized by the mode of valve opening, as seen in Fig. 16, which shows the velocity profile of the transmitral flow immediately after the mitral valve has fully opened. After the mitral valve opened completely, the transmitral velocity profile developed, while maintaining its topological features created during the opening phase, as illustrated in Fig. 17, which plots the transmitral flow at $t = 0.35$ s just before the mitral valve started to close toward the end of early diastole. These results suggest that the opening

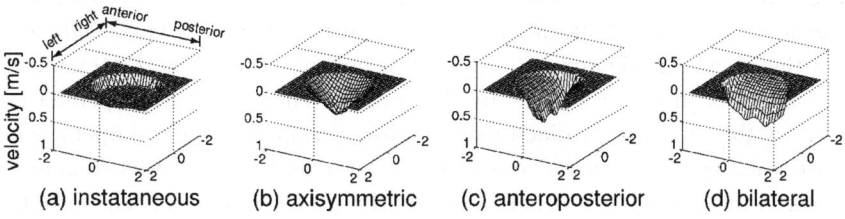

Fig. 16. Velocity profiles of the transmitral flow just after the valve has finished opening for cases (b)–(d). From Nakamura *et al.*[78] Reproduced by permission.

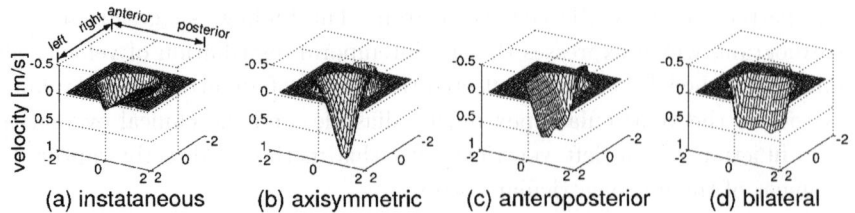

Fig. 17.   Velocity profiles of the transmitral flow just before the valve started to close for cases (b)–(d). From Nakamura et al.[78] Reproduced by permission.

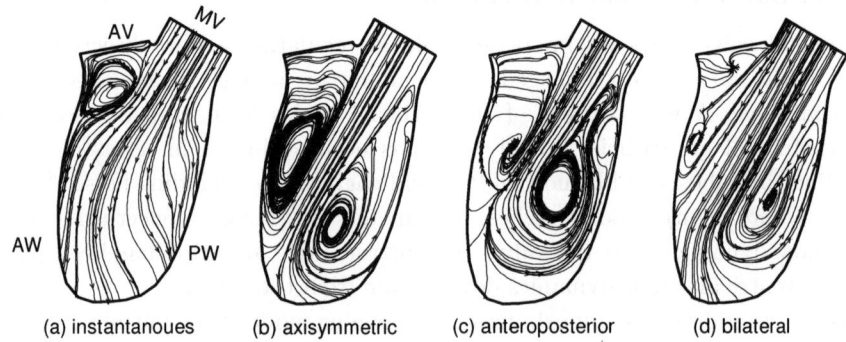

Fig. 18.   Flow patterns at the end of early diastole.

mode of the mitral valve influenced the transmitral velocity profile, not only during opening, but also throughout diastole.

The difference in the transmitral velocity profiles gave rise to differences in the intraventricular flow dynamics. Instantaneous streamlines on the long axis plane of the left ventricle at the end of diastole are plotted in Fig. 18 to gain overall insight into the flow patterns. A remarkable difference was observed in the vortex structure, in addition to the velocity field. Great variation persisted in the flow field between the different opening modes, as depicted in Fig. 19.

It has been postulated that the vortex under the aortic valve helps redirect blood preferentially toward the aorta without a loss of flow momentum, thereby accommodating ventricular flow ejection.[36] Moreover, the vortex contributes to the mixing of blood to prevent it from coagulating. Consequently, a larger vortex under the aortic valve seems desirable in terms of cardiac function. This study showed that in the axisymmetric and anteroposterior opening modes, the vortex under the aortic valve was sufficiently large during diastole. Therefore, these opening modes might favorably increase cardiac function. However, in the bilateral opening mode, the vortex under the aortic valve was not as large and the flow was stagnant near the apex, which could potentially lead to thrombus formation. The problem of thrombogenesis is much greater in patients with mechanical heart valves, suggesting that the bilateral opening mode is not a promising design. To confirm these

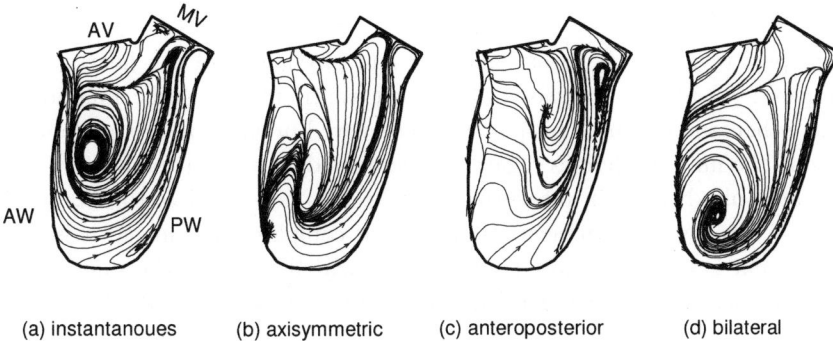

(a) instantanoues   (b) axisymmetric   (c) anteroposterior   (d) bilateral

Fig. 19.   Flow patterns at the end of systole.

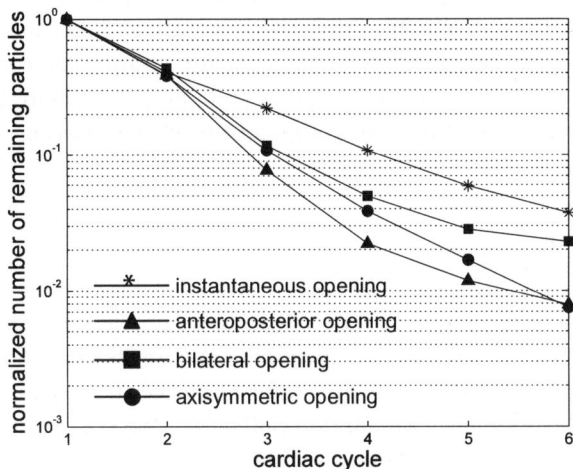

Fig. 20.   Logarithmic plot of the number of particles at the end of each cardiac cycle. Note that the number of particles is normalized using the value in the first cardiac cycle. From Nakamura *et al.*[78] Reproduced by permission.

speculations, we performed particle tracking in the resulting flow field. Figure 20 plots the number of particles remaining at the end of systole in each cardiac cycle. After the third cardiac cycle, there was a difference in the number of particles that had not been ejected. The graph shows that the efficiency of ventricular ejection was worst with instantaneous opening mode. In the bilateral opening mode, the particles were not ejected as efficiently as in the anteroposterior and axisymmetric opening modes.

The results demonstrated that even if the shape of the valve orifice is the same when it opens fully, the vortex pattern in the ventricle might change if the orifice shape differs during the process of valve opening. Therefore, we suggest that the opening mode of the valve orifice should also be emphasized in the design of artificial valves.

7. Conclusions

This chapter reviewed the basic anatomy and physiology of the heart and some techniques used for the diagnosis of the left ventricular diastolic function using Doppler echocardiography. This paper also reviewed *in vitro*, *in vivo*, and numerical studies on the fluid mechanics regarding the hemodynamics in the heart.

Because of advances in measuring devices, it is now possible to obtain a huge amount of data by measurement. However, for complex phenomena, it is difficult to grasp what is occurring based solely on measured data. At the same time, the evolution of measuring devices has led to larger medical systems and inflated medical costs. We believe that these problems could be solved by introducing computational analyses to measurements. Information obtained in computer simulations plays an important role in analyzing the data obtained from clinical measurements and linking them to clinical diagnosis. The results shown in this paper demonstrate the potential of supplying such missing information using computational fluid dynamics. It complements the measurement by CMD echocardiography and consequently helps to reveal concealed phenomena. With aid of computational analysis, the diagnosis of left ventricular diastolic function will be advanced even further.

Acknowledgment

The authors acknowledge Prof. Takeshi Karino for his comments from a fluid mechanical point of view and Prof. Taisei Mikami for providing medical images. This work was supported by a Research Fellowship from JSPS for Young Scientists No. 06787. It was also funded by Grant-in-Aid for Scientific Research No. 15086204 and No. 17300138 "Revolutionary Simulation Software (RSS21)" project supported by next-generation IT program of Ministry of Education, Culture, Sports, Science and Technology (MEXT), Grants in Aid for Scientific Research by the MEXT and JSPS Scientific Research in Priority Areas (768) "Biomechanics at Micro- and Nanoscale Levels" and Scientific Research(A) No.16200031 "Mechanism of the formation, destruction, and movement of thrombi responsible for ischemia of vital organs".

References

1. W. Grossman and W. H. Barry, *Fed. Proc.* **39** (1980) 148.
2. H. Pouleur, C. Hanet, O. Gurne and M. F. Rousseau, *Br. J. Clin. Pharmacol.* **28** (1989) 41S.
3. S. Fujimoto, K. H. Parker, H. B. Xiao, K. S. Inge and D. G. Gibson, *Br. Heart J.* **74** (1995) 419.
4. A. Kitabatake, M. Inoue, M. Asao, J. Tanouchi, T. Masuyama, H. Abe, H. Morita, S. Senda and H. Matsuo, *Jpn. Circ. J.* **46** (1982) 92.
5. B. J. Delemarre, H. Bot, A. S. Pearlman, C. A. Visser and A. J. Dunning, *J. Clin. Ultrasound* **15** (1987) 115.
6. M. Bessen and M. Gardin, *Cardiol. Clin.* **8** (1990) 315.

7. M. F. Stoddard, A. J. Labovitz, and A. C. Pearson, *Echocardiogr.* **9** (1992) 387.
8. S. Fujimoto, T. Kagoshima, T. Nakajima and K. Dohi, *Cardiol.* **83** (1993) 217.
9. M. Takeuchi, H. Monnaka, T. Tsukamoto, T. Hayashi, S. Tomimoto, M. Odake, Y. Yokota and H. Fukuzaki, *J. Cardiol.* **21** (1991) 679.
10. C. P. Appleton, *J. Am. Coll. Cardiol.* **17** (1991) 227.
11. C. Y. Choong, H. C. Herrmann, A. E. Weyman and M. A. Fifer, *J. Am. Coll. Cardiol.* **10** (1987) 800.
12. C. P. Appleton, L. K. Hatle and R. L. Popp, *J. Am. Coll. Cardiol.* **12** (1988) 426.
13. L. E. Jacobs, M. N. Kotler and W. R. Parry, *J. Am. Soc. Echocardiogr.* **3** (1990) 294.
14. P. Brun, C. Tribouilloy, A. M. Duval-Moulin, L. Iserin, A. Meguira, G. Pelle and J. L. Dubois-Rande, *J. Am. Coll. Cardiol.* **20** (1992) 420.
15. S. De Mey, J. De Sutter, J. Vierendeels and P. Verdonck, *Eur. J. Echocardiogr.* **2** (2001) 219.
16. T. Steen and S. Steen, *Cardiovasc. Res.* **28** (1994) 1821.
17. A. M. Duval-Moulin, P. Dupouy, P. Brun, F. Zhuang, G. Pelle, Y. Perez, E. Teiger, A. Castaigne, P. Gueret and J. L. Dubois-Rande, *J. Am. Coll. Cardiol.* **29** (1997) 1246.
18. M. J. Garcia, M. A. Ares, C. Asher, L. Rodriguez, P. Vandervoort and J. D. Thomas, *J. Am. Coll. Cardiol.* **29** (1997) 448.
19. M. J. Garcia, J. D. Thomas and A. L. Klein, *J. Am. Coll. Cardiol.* **32** (1998) 865.
20. M. Stugaard, O. A. Smiseth, C. Risoe and H. Ihlen, *Circulation* **88** (1993) 2705.
21. M. Stugaard, U. Brodahl, H. Torp and H. Ihlen, *Eur. Heart J.* **15** (1994) 318.
22. J. D. Thomas, M. J. Garcia and N. L. Greenberg, *Heart Vessels* **12** (1997) 135.
23. H. Takatsuji, T. Mikami, K. Urasawa, J. Teranishi, H. Onozuka, C. Takagi, Y. Makita, H. Matsuo, H. Kusuoka and A. Kitabatake, *J. Am. Coll. Cardiol.* **27** (1996) 365.
24. Y. Kawano, K. Ohmori, Y. Wada, I. Kondo, K. Mizushige, S. Senda, S. Nozaki and M. Kohno, *Heart Vessels* **15** (2000) 205.
25. B. J. Bellhouse and F. H. Bellhouse, *Nature* **224** (1969) 615.
26. B. J. Bellhouse, *Cardiovasc. Res.* **6** (1972) 199.
27. H. Reul, N. Talukder and E. W. Muller, *J. Biomech.* **14** (1981) 361.
28. A. P. Shortland, R. A. Black, J. C. Jarvis, F. S. Henry, F. Iudicello, M. W. Collins and S. Salmons, *J. Biomech.* **29** (1996) 503.
29. H. Bot, J. Verburg, B. J. Delemarre and J. Strackee, *J. Biomech.* **23** (1990) 607.
30. V. Gariety, T. Gandelheid, J. Fusezi, R. Pelissier and R. Rieu. *Int. J. Artif. Organs* **18** (1995) 380.
31. O. Pierrakos, P. P. Vlachos and D. P. Telionis, *ASME J. Biomech. Eng.* **126** (2004) 714.
32. A. Delabays, L. Sugeng, N. G. Pandian, T. L. Hsu, S. J. Ho, C. H. Chen, G. Marx, S. L. Schwartz and Q. L. Cao, *Am. J.Cardiol.* **76** (1995) 1053.
33. F. J. Pinto, F. Veiga, M. G. Lopes and F. de Padua, *Rev. Port. Cardiol.* **16** (1997) 787.
34. W. Y. Kim, P. G. Walker, E. M. Pedersen, J. K. Poulsen, S. Oyre, K. Houlind and A. P. Yoganathan, *J. Am. Coll. Cardiol.* **26** (1995) 224.
35. P. G. Walker, G. B. Cranney, R. Y. Grimes, J. Delatore, J. Rectenwald, G. M. Pohost and A. P. Yoganathan, *Ann. Biomed. Eng.* **24** (1996) 139.
36. P. J. Kilner, G. Z. Yang, A. J. Wilkes, R. H. Mohiaddin, D. N. Firmin and M. H. Yacoub, *Nature* **404** (2000) 759.
37. T. Ebbers, L. Wigstrom, A. F. Bolger, B. Wranne and M. Karlsson, *ASME J. Biomed. Eng.* **124** (2002) 288.
38. C. S. Peskin, *J. Comp. Phys.* **25** (1977) 220.

39. C. S. Peskin and D. M. McQueen, *J. Comp. Phys.* **81** (1989) 372.
40. C. S. Peskin and D. M. McQueen, *J. Comp. Phys.* **82** (1989) 289.
41. C. S. Peskin and D. M. McQueen, *Crit. Rev. Biomed. Eng.* **20** (1992) 451.
42. C. S. Peskin and D. M. McQueen, *Symp. Soc. Exp. Biol.* **49**(1995) 265.
43. E. L. Yellin, S. Nikolic and R. W. Frater, *Prog. Cardiovasc. Dis.* **32** (1990) 247.
44. T. N. Jones and D. N. Metaxas, *Proc. MICCAI'98*, (1998) Springer LNCS.
45. N. R. Saber, A. D. Gosman, N. B. Wood, P. J. Kilner, C. L. Charrier and D. N. Firmin, *Ann. Biomed. Eng.* **29** (2001) 275.
46. J. G. Georgiadis, M. Wang and A. Pasipoularides, *Ann. Biomed. Eng.* **20** (1992) 81.
47. R. T. Schoephoerster, C. L. Silva and G. Ray, *J. Eng. Mech.* **119** (1993) 733.
48. R. T. Schoephoerster, C. L. Silva and G. Ray, *J. Biomech.* **27** (1994) 125.
49. E. Gonzalez and R. T. Schoephoerster, *Ann. Biomed. Eng.* **24** (1996) 48.
50. A. P. Yoganathan, J. D. Jr. Lemmon, Y. H. Kim, P. G. Walker, R. A. Levine and C. C. Vesier, *ASME J. Biomed. Eng.* **116** (1994) 307.
51. T. W. Taylor, H. Okino and T. Yamaguchi, *ASME J. Biomed. Eng.* **116** (1994) 127.
52. T. W. Taylor and T. Yamaguchi, *Biorheology* **32** (1995) 61.
53. T. W. Taylor and T. Yamaguchi, *Med. Eng. Phys.* **17** (1995) 602.
54. T. W. Taylor, H. Suga, Y. Goto, H. Okino and T. Yamaguchi, *ASME J. Biomed. Eng.* **118** (1996) 106.
55. J. D. Lemmon and A. P. Yoganathan, *ASME J. Biomed. Eng.* **122** (2000) 109.
56. J. D. Lemmon and A. P. Yoganathan, *ASME J. Biomed. Eng.* **122** (2000) 297.
57. N. R. Saber, N. B. Wood, A. D. Gosman, R. D. Merrifield, G. Z. Yang, C. L. Charrier, P. D. Gatehouse and D. N. Firmin, *Ann. Biomed. Eng.* **31** (2003) 42.
58. B. Baccani, F. Domenichini, G. Pedrizzetti and G. Tonti, *J. Biomech.* **35** (2002) 665.
59. B. Baccani, F. Domenichini and G. Pedrizzetti, *J. Biomech.* **36** (2003) 355.
60. F. Domenichini, G. Pedrizzetti and B. Baccani, *J. Fluid Mech.* **539** (2005) 179.
61. M. Nakamura, S. Wada, T. Mikami, A. Kitabatake and T. Karino, *Biomech Model. Mechanobiol.* **2** (2003) 59.
62. H. N. Sabbah and P. D. Stein, *Circ. Res.* **48** (1981) 357.
63. M. Nakamura, S. Wada, A. Kitabatake, T. Karino and T. Yamaguchi, *Technol. Health Care* **13** (2005) 269.
64. M. Nakamura, S. Wada, T. Mikami, A. Kitabatake, T. Karino and T. Yamaguchi, *Med. Biol. Eng. Comp.* **42** (2004) 509.
65. M. Nakamura, S. Wada, T. Mikami, A. Kitabatake and T. Karino, *JSME Int. J. Ser. C* **45** (2002) 913.
66. M. Nakamura, S. Wada, T. Mikami and T. Yamaguchi, *Trans. JSME* **70** (2004) 1254 (in Japanese).
67. M. Sugawara and S. Maeda, *Blood Rheology and Flow* (Corona Publishing Co. Ltd., Tokyo, 2003), pp. 108–109 and pp. 122–123 (in Japanese).
68. M. Nakamura, S. Wada, T. Mikami, A. Kitabatake and T. Karino, *JSME Int. J. Ser. C* **44** (2001) 1013.
69. J. A. Vierendeels, K. Riemslagh, E. Dick and P. R. Verdonck. *ASME J. Biomed. Eng.* **122** (2000) 667.
70. J. A. Vierendeels, E. Dick and P. R. Verdonck. *J. Am. Soc. Echocardiogr.* **15** (2000) 219.
71. M. Aazami and H. J. Schafers. *J. Interv. Cardiol.* **16** (2003) 535.
72. J. T. Ellis, T. M. Wick and A. P. Yoganathan, *J. Heart Valve Dis.* **7** (1998) 376.
73. R. Paul, O. Marseille, E. Hintze, L. Huber, H. Schima, H. Reul and G. Rau. *Int. J. Artif. Organs* **21** (1998) 548.

74. A. Sezai, M. Shiono, Y. Orime, H. Hata, S. Yagi, N. Negishi and Y. Sezai. *Ann. Thorac. Surg.* **69** (2000) 507.
75. M. Butterfield, D. J. Wheatley, D. F. Williams and J. Fisher. *J. Heart Valve Dis.* **10** (2001) 105.
76. D. K. Walker, A. M. Brendzel and L. N. Scotten. *J. Heart Valve Dis.* **8** (1999) 687.
77. K. B. Manning, V. Kini, A. A. Fontaine, S. Deutsch and J. M. Tarbell. *Artif. Organs* **27** (2003) 840.
78. M. Nakamura, S. Wada and T. Yamaguchi, *Ann. Biomed. Eng.* **34** (2006) 927–935.

CHAPTER 6

THE BIOMEDICAL APPLICATIONS OF COMPUTED TOMOGRAPHY

HO SAEY TUAN

Division of Bioengineering, Faculty of Engineering
National University of Singapore
10 Kent Ridge Crescent, Singapore 119280, Singapore
g0201956@nus.edu.sg

DIETMAR W. HUTMACHER

Division of Bioengineering, Faculty of Engineering
Department of Orthopaedic Surgery, Yang Loo Lin School of Medicine
National University of Singapore, Engineering Drive 1
Singapore 119260
Tel: 65-6516-1036/3100; Fax: 65-6516-3069
biedwh@nus.edu.sg

Computed Tomography (CT) imaging is playing an increasingly important role in the biomedical sciences of today as clinicians and scientists begin to recognize its potential in health care and research. Clinical CT facilitates the early diagnosis of diseases thus allowing the selection of appropriate therapies which improves the patient's overcome. Pre-surgical imaging aids operation planning while real time scans assist complicated high risk surgeries. One of the primary concerns in clinical CT procedures would be the adverse radiation side effects thus only low dosages are allowed. The resolution of clinical imaging is insufficient for research, hence the micro CT set up has to be used. The advent of micro CT imaging has ushered in the possibility of non destructive quantitative analysis for trabeculae architectures, scaffolds, soft tissues and biological constructs. This paper highlights the inherent potential and emerging biomedical applications of CT.

1. Introduction

Recently, non-destructive analysis is gaining popularity and one particular technique which has witnessed tremendous development is the X-ray computed tomography (CT). CT is a relatively new innovation and the surge of interest can be attributed to various factors. First, it is a non-destructive evaluation method, hence fragile and rare specimens can be studied. Priceless fossils,[1] ancient Egyptian mummies[2] and antique statues[2] were examined via CT imaging. CT is capable of providing 2D and 3D visualization of the specimen, furthermore regions of interest within the sample can be digitally extracted out for close ups. This radiographic technique is appealing because visualizations can be accompanied by quantitative assessments. Moreover, CT results have been proven to be reliable and accurate by concurrent destructive studies.[3,4] The strategic potential of this radiographic technique has attracted specialists from several sectors, especially so from the biomedical field. The quality of imaging is largely determined by the resolution hence set ups are classified according to this feature. Initially, scanners could only operate at a resolution of 1 mm.[5] Higher resolution imaging became possible with stronger X-ray sources and precise instrumentations and some of these imagers found clinical applications but clinical resolution is inadequate for research.[6] However with the invention of the micro CT, high resolution imaging became feasible. In short, computed tomography can be divided into two broad categories. They are clinical CT ($>100\,\mu$m) and micro CT ($<100\,\mu$m). The following discussion will elaborate on the two setups and their applications.

2. Basics of CT

The fundamental principle in CT is data acquisition by X-ray projection. The main components of set up are the collimated X-ray source which is positioned on one side of the specimen and a detector that is located on the other side (Fig. 1). The collimated X-rays would penetrate through the exposed section of the sample while the detector array would capture the emitted radiation. A reduction in X-ray intensity occurs as energy is lost during the transit through the section. This energy absorption is known as attenuation and it is influenced by the material properties within the section.[1,7] Once the detector picks up the emitted X-rays, electronic signals are transmitted to the computer. Each X-ray path would generate a line integral[8] which would be used to calculate the attenuation coefficients encountered along the path within the sample section. Each section is irradiated at various angles and this creates a set of corresponding line integrals. This process is repeated for every section, and a series digital slices comprising of line integrals represents the specimen. Attenuation coefficients derived from the integrals are mapped onto pixels and the pixel map is reflective of the densities and spatial distributions of the materials within the section. An eventual integration of these 2D maps creates a 3D digital model and this process is known as tomography.[8] The 3D element associated with each pixel are known as voxel and each voxel bears a CT number which corresponds to the appropriate attenuation coefficient. The CT number is commonly expressed as grey values or Hounsfield units (HU).[9] For high resolution imaging, thinner slices are scanned but this generates a greater amount of data thus data storage and processing become a concern. This general data acquisition principle is found in both the clinical and micro CT.

3. Radiation Dosage

One of the major concerns in clinical CT imaging is the detrimental effects of X-rays. X-rays are ionizing and they can cause chromosomal aberrations thereby resulting in genetic mutations and cancers.[10–12] This is especially worrisome when the dosage per CT scan is approximately 50 times that of a plain film radiography.[13]

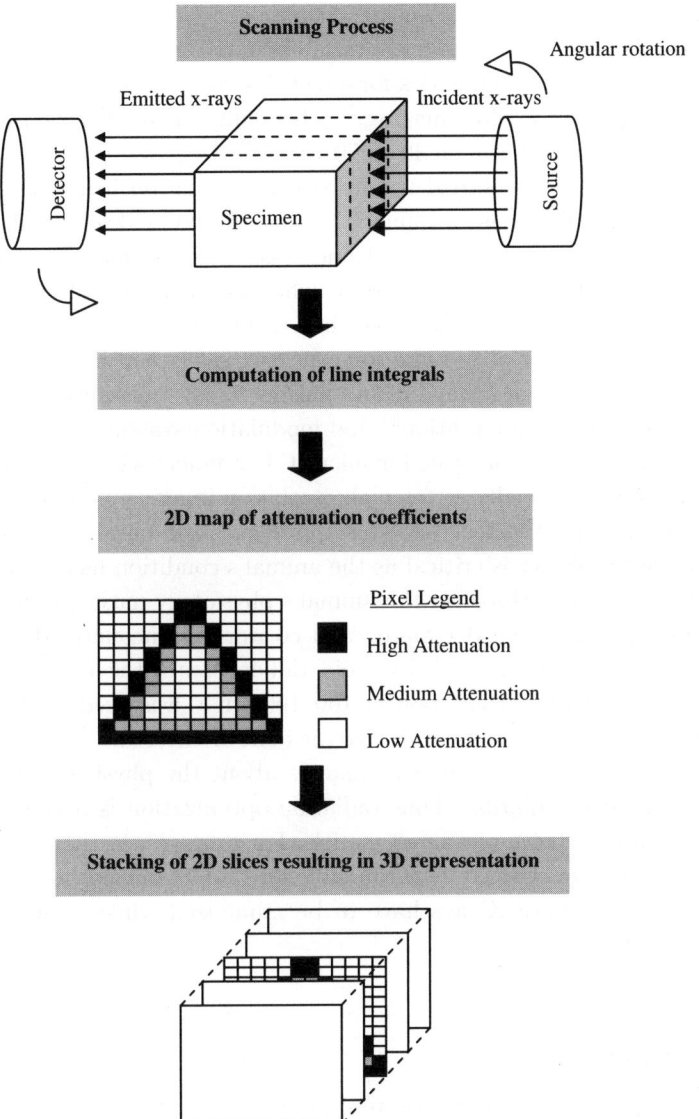

Fig. 1. Schematic representation of the basic stages in CT.

Appropriate exposures are used as drastic reduction in radiation dosage would lead to poor resolution and noise to signal ratios.[14,15] To manage the risks involved in clinical CT, deterministic and stochastic studies are conducted. The deterministic model assumes the occurrence of genetic mutation when a dose of 100 mGy is exceeded[11] and this assumption is supported by the atomic survivor data.[16,17] Stochastic modeling associates a measure of risk to low level exposures which are below the stipulated thresholds[11] and Prokop's population studies employ this model.[16] It should be noted that considerations such as age, gender, lifestyle, organs imaged and CT screening frequency are variables in risk assessments.[17] For example, Brenner *et al.* has shown a higher risk for lung CT screening (5.5% at 95% confidence level) when compared to colon imaging.[18] This danger is further aggravated if the patient is a female, aged between 40 to 70 years.[19,20]

Official guidelines are needed to address this radiation health concern. FDA stipulates a limit of 0.05 Gy as an annual individual radiation dosage and it allows for 15 head CT or five full body scans.[11,21] Unnecessary referrals for CT are discouraged and imaging is deemed only appropriate when the benefits offset the risks. In addition, Siegel stressed that extra care has to be exercized with regards to the pediatric population.[22] To allay radiation concerns, safety features are incorporated into clinical CT set ups and they include pulsing X-ray emissions, noise reduction filters,[23] automated dose adaptation[24] and modulation systems.[25–27]

Radiation safety is a non-issue for micro CT scanners when inanimate objects are imaged. This is especially so for high resolution imaging as long duration and intensive exposures are selected.[28,29] This approach is not suitable for *in vivo* micro CT imaging. Survivability is critical as the animal's condition has to be monitored at different time points. Moreover the animal's physiology must not be affected by the radiation exposure. Van der Sloten and co workers encountered this problem while working on Guinea pigs.[30] To avoid radionecrosis, the radiation dose was reduced from 3 to 1.7 Gy. Radiation of 100–1000 mGy was used by Kinney *et al.* and Waarsing *et al.* in the study of *in vivo* rat bone architecture.[29,31] Despite of the excellent results, Waarsing *et al.* was anxious about the physiological alterations induced by excessive radiation. Thus radiation optimization is necessary and this is dependent on the choice of animal models. For example, in the investigation of bone healing, a dosage of 15 Gy is permissible for rabbits but not for rats.[32,33] The undesirable side effects of X-rays have to be minimized while achieving scans of reasonable quality.

4. Contrast Reagents

Imaging contrast is as important as resolution because the region of interest on the scan should be easily discerned from the remaining features. This is often the problem when evaluating soft tissues as they attenuate X-rays poorly. Fortunately, this limitation can be resolved with high radiodensity chemicals. The initial usage of these agents can be traced back to the 18th century when doctors were attempting to examine cadavars via soft X-rays imaging.[34] Being highly attenuating, these radiopaque substances enhance the contrast of the occupied spaces. But one has to be mindful that the blatant clinical use of such reagents is not permitted as there are safety constraints. Concentration, osmolity, retention time and administered volumes have to be closely monitored.[35–38]

Barium sulfate and iodinated compounds are clinically accepted contrast agents. Barium sulfate is well characterized and there are established guidelines which govern its use in imaging ulcers, polyps and gastrointestinal tumors.[11,39] Iodinated agents are more frequently used than barium sulfate suspensions as they are less viscous. Imaging applications would include urography and visualization of vascular associated malignancies.[22,40,41] Iodinate compounds have a biological half life of 10–90 min, after which it is excreted via the liver and kidneys.[14] Despite of mainstream clinical acceptance, there are risks associated with the use of contrast agents. Bettmann has cautioned on the use of iodinate compounds as cases of adverse reactions such as heart complications, brain damage and even death were reported.[34] Delayed side effects were also observed.[42] Such occurrences may be rare but unpredictable. Therefore iodated compounds of appropriate osmolality and the formulations are chosen[34] while special attention is given to children, diabetic and asthmatic patients.[22]

Patient safety is not applicable in micro CT imaging but researchers have to grapple with other technical constraints when it comes to the usage of contrast agents. Guldberg and co-workers were dissatisfied with the use of barium sulfate in the study of vasculature growth.[43] They observed clumping and settling of barium sulfate which makes the perfusion of fine arterioles and veins difficult.[43–45] As a result, barium sulfate was replaced by a better contrast agent known as Microfill (Flow tech, Inc., Carver, Massachusetts). Microfill comprises of a homogeneous mix of silicone rubber and lead chromate[46] and it can be easily perfused into the fine vasculature. Some heavy metallic compounds are also suitable contrast enhancers. Examples include silver nitrate[47] and osmium tetroxide[48] which have been employed in the imaging of lung tissues. In the scanning of cartilage specimens, Wehmeyer *et al.* employed gadolinium to correct for the lack of imaging contrast.[49] Higher quality imaging with excellent contrast would facilitate evaluations and this is desired by both researchers and clinicians.

5. Clinical CT

In 1979, Sir Godfrey N. Hounsfield and Allan M. Cormack received the Nobel Prize in Medicine for their invention of the CT imager.[50] The first documented use of this technology was in head CT scans.[5] A larger set up which accommodates full body scans was developed later.[50,51] Such an innovation stirred up much excitement in the medical community as numerous clinical possibilities became apparent. The detailed anatomic imaging capabilities of the CT make it a much sought after imaging solution than plain film radiography. Soon a frenzy of research and development was observed in clinical CT and applications ranging from diagnosis to surgery were demonstrated.

5.1. *Clinical CT equipment*

The demand for non-invasive clinical imaging has accelerated the progress of CT technology such that four generations of clinical scanners had evolved within six years since its invention.[52] In the last three decades, Multidetector CT (MDCT), electron beam tomography and spiral scans were introduced and they became standard clinical imaging procedures.

Imaging is carried out in the first generation set up[52] by translating a single source-detector pair past the stationary patient as shown in Fig. 2(a). The translation step would be followed by an angular rotation[1] and the scan time per slice was approximately 5 min.[11] This primitive design was subsequently replaced by the second generation imager (Fig. 2(b)) that uses a fan shaped X-ray beam instead of a pencil beam.[11] Data acquisition was facilitated by a series of detectors thus shortening the imaging time to 30 s per slice.[1,53] Capitalizing on the strengths

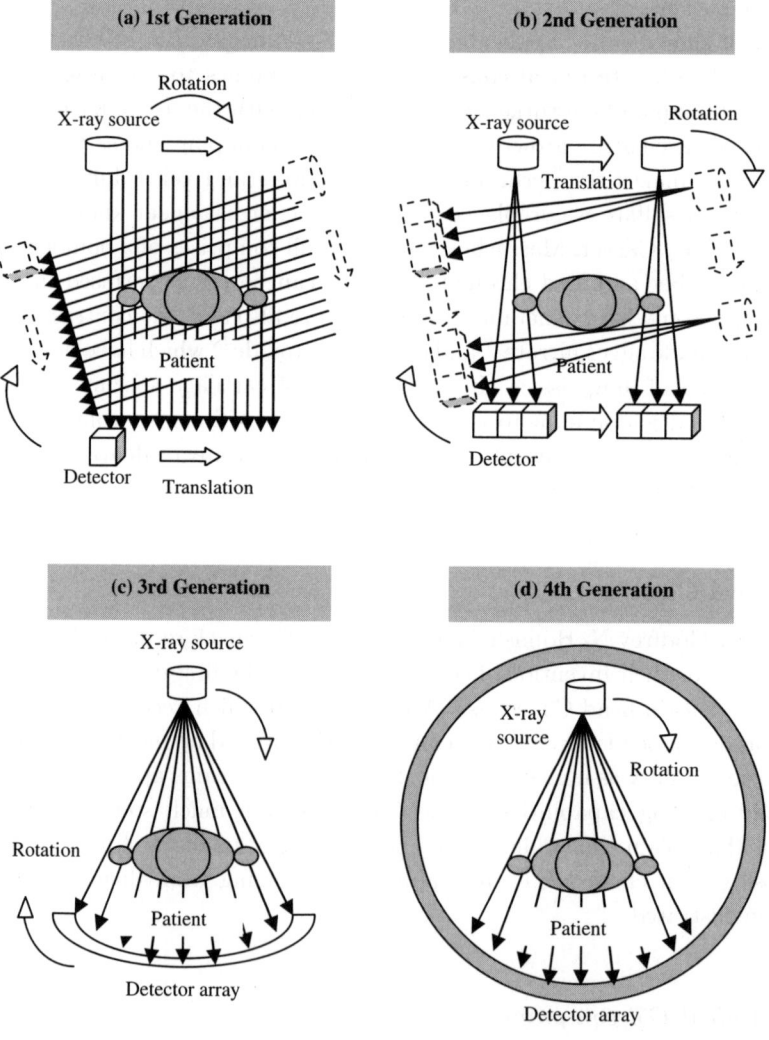

Fig. 2.   Various models of clinical the CT scanner.

of the improved scanner, engineers equipped third generation series (Fig. 2(c)) with a wider fan beam and a curvilinear detector array.[52] This upgraded imager is capable of 350 μm resolution at an imaging time of 1 s per slice, but ring artifacts are encountered and to solve this problem, the fourth generation imager is introduced. For this latest design, the X-ray source rotates within a circular detector array (Fig. 2(d)).[53] Besides upgrading the hardware aspect of the scanner, different scanning modes are also attempted. One example would be the use of spiral scan which reduces imaging time. In spiral scans, the patient is continuously translated into the scan region as the source-detector pair circles simultaneously as shown in Fig. 3.[9,11] This scanning mode shortens a full torso scan from 10 min to single breath holds. Moreover the single row of detector elements can be replaced by multiple rows in MDCT hence higher resolutions scans can be accomplished much quickly.[36] Since its introduction in 1989, the MDCT has become a standard imager for hospitals.[52]

The Electron Beam Computed Tomography (EBCT) is a unique set up based on a radically new design. It is equipped with an electron beam emitter instead of an X-ray source. The EBCT possesses a circular gantry which consists of two halves (Fig. 4). A curved tungsten target forms the lower half while the other upper half is a detector array.[11] An electron beam is focused onto the curved target and upon collision an X-ray beam is generated. The scanning time is a mere 50 ms per slice and this makes the EBCT the fastest clinical CT scanner in the world.[52,54] This set up is commonly used in cardiac imaging.[53,55]

5.2. *Clinical imaging: circulatory system*

Patients with vasculature and cardiac maladies are usually screened with CT techniques. One of these methods is dynamic MDCT angiography.[55] In this method, a dose of contrast agents is administered intravenously to the patient. Time serial imaging follows and the contrast enhanced circulatory network is

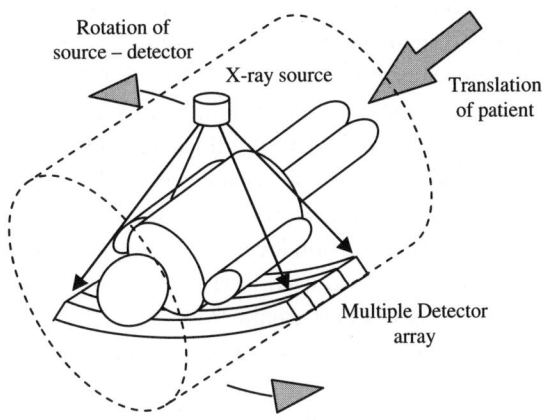

Fig. 3.   Multidetector spiral CT.

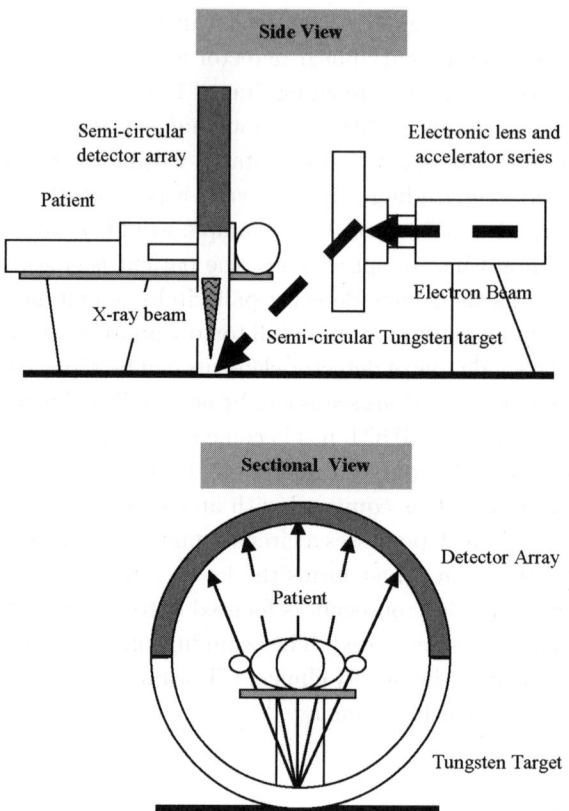

Fig. 4.   Electron Beam CT (EBCT) imager.

unraveled. This method works well for peripheral[27] and pulmonary[37] arteries but not for the pulsing heart.[56] However, with gating techniques and EBCT,[55] heart imaging is made feasible and images of high resolutions are obtainable even for neonates with congenital heart conditions.[22] This technical advantage enabled Kopp *et al.* and Masuda *et al.* to conduct full cardiac cycle scans and they were able to measure myocardial perfusion, ventricular end-diastolic and end-systolic volumes.[56,57] Besides quantitative readings which reveal cardiac symptoms, markers of heart diseases can also be visualized. Atherosclerotic plagues can be easily detected via CT imaging as they contain highly attenuating calcium deposits.[58] Furthermore the calcification levels of these plaques can be quantified via thresholding.[58–60] CT imaging is also used in the follow up of corrective procedures such as the implantation of grafts and stents.[58]

Cerebro–vasculature disorders are associated with high morbidity and mortality but these outcomes can be avoided with early detection via neuro CT imaging. Cranial aneurgsms and vascular calcifications are readily observed on CT scans thus prompting early medical therapies.[61] Thrombrolysis is a stroke treatment and its effectiveness is dependent on the temporal development of the ischemic penumbra.[62] Wintermark *et al.* advocated the use of CT data which informs clinicians of the locations of the occlusion sites and ischemia coverage so that they can optimize thromobrolysis.[62] Quantitative cerebro–vasculature measurements are also accessible as blood volume and flow rates can be studied from the time serial scans, thus shedding light on neuro-physiology. An alternative neuro-imaging method is MRI, but being time consuming and costly, it is a less appealing technique.[62]

5.3. *Clinical imaging: respiratory system*

The tissue — air interface of the respiratory tract provides good contrast in CT screening.[63] From inhalation and exhalation scans, lung volumes are deduced and the results can be confirmed by plethysmographic measurements.[64] Respiratory bronchiolitis, pneumonia,[65] silicosis[66] and tracheobronchomalacia[67] can be diagnosed from the CT data. Through thresholding measurements, ventilation inhomogeneity due to bronchiolar obstruction[68] is observed. This non-invasive radiographic method is also used in the study of asthma. It was observed that the mean lung density increases with the narrowing of airways during an asthmatic reaction[69] and prolong thickening of the airway wall was noted by Niimi *et al.*[70] which is indicative of airway remodeling. Besides understanding the pathological developments in asthma, CT imaging can also be used to quantify the effects of asthmatic treatments.

5.4. *Clinical imaging: gastroinstinal tract*

In the past, endoscopy is the preferred technique for diagnosing abdominal problems as non-invasive means are lacking. A mere 5% sensitivity is noted for ultrasound scan, while plain film radiography has inadequate resolution.[39] Clinical CT imaging is not hampered by these weaknesses and it has a diagnostic sensitivity of 92% with ability to conduct full body imaging at single breath hold. Upon its introduction, CT imaging is commonly used in the detection of small intestinal aliments[71] such as polyp-like lesions, abscesses and ischemia.[39] In fact, CT imaging of the gastrointestinal tract has become so much of a mainstream approach that CT colonography is fast displacing endoscopy as the initial screening of colon malignancies.[72] CT colonography does away with sedatives and its impeccable safety record appeals to both frail and reluctant patients. Pickhardt's CT colonography clinical trials were shown to be highly effective and the method can be upgraded with advanced 3D polyp detection.[73]

Immediate medical attention is warranted for sudden abdominal pains and a speedy but accurate diagnosis is pertinent. CT screening excels in this aspect by providing near instantaneous results thereby triaging patients into the appropriate therapies.[74] This is shown in the case of appendicitis. Despite being a common and trivial aliment, diagnosis for appendicitis proves to be difficult and erroneous judgment would either lead to unnecessary operations[75] or a delay in surgical interventions.[76] These ambiguities are cleared up by checking for an inflamed appendix, perforation and abscesses through CT imaging.[76] If an operation is required, a safe access route which avoids the vital organs can be decided with the scans. Besides appendicitis, other acute abdominal aliments such as diverticulitis and bowel obstruction can be diagnosed with CT scans.[74]

5.5. *Clinical imaging: tumor detection*

Cancers are prevalent in the modern society and public cancer screening is promoted to address this health issue. The rationale behind such a move would be to improve the patient's outcome by detecting and treating tumors while they are still small and potentially curable.[16] However, a highly sensitive diagnosis is needed as initial lesions are small and sometimes undetectable. CT imaging is a competent technique for this application. Furthermore, short imaging time[77] and accessible facilities[27] make CT screening a feasible option in cancer detection programs.[78]

Lung cancer is a leading cause of death in the America and it can be attributed to cigarette smoking.[19,79] To counter this public health problem, early lung cancer detection via CT imaging is encouraged. The key strength of this method is the ability to identify and quantify potentially cancerous nodules. A malignancy estimation is derived from this procedure[80] while follow up scans monitor the aliment.[81] Discretion is needed when vetting through the scan data as the method susceptible to false positives. Minute nodules which go undetected in chest radiography are highlighted while non-cancerous infections are wrongly diagnosed as observed by Kazerooni, thus other confirmation methods such as sputum tests are required.[19]

Pancreatic and hepatic carcinomas are screened using similar methods. With the appropriate use of contrast agents, McNulty and co-workers have shown that CT analysis is an excellent technique in diagnosing such tumors.[82] This is reinforced by the fact that a diagnostic accuracy of 88–97% is noted for tumors bigger than 9 mm.[36,83] Being a quantitative method, cystic and solid lesions are differentiated[55] while the involvement of vasculature in carcinogenesis is detected. CT evaluation assisted Freeny *et al.* in the classification of tumors which is necessary for the selection of therapies.[84]

5.6. *Clinical imaging: urography*

Radiopaque contrast agents are used to assist in the CT screening of the urinary system. Potential urinary abnormalities such as infections, urinary tract calculi and urothelial lesions can be detected and treated promptly.[85,86] Clinical CT imaging is favored as an urography technique because it is sensitive[87] and non-invasive. It is widely used in the screening of kidney stones[85] and its advantage stems from the fact that these accumulations of calcium and phosphate show up easily on the CT scans.

5.7. *Clinical imaging: emergency and trauma*

Accidents and emergencies demand immediate medical response and hospitals devote resources to cater for such sudden needs. Life threatening situations necessitates prompt and accurate diagnosis which in turn determines the treatment. CT imaging is frequently adopted as the first stage of screening[88] as it provides a though and quick body scan which allows clinicians to ascertain the full extent of injuries.[89] This approach is helpful in the evaluation of blunt traumas resulting from traffic accidents where multiple organ injury is a possibility. Fatal wounds such as splenic rupture,[90] renal[91] and intracanial[62] haemorrhages may be difficult to diagnose with conventional means but are easily deduced from the CT scans. Moreover, contrast enhanced imaging reveals gastrointestinal and vasculature complications. By facilitating precise and speedy diagnosis, the CT imager is an indispensable tool to emergency personnel.

5.8. *Surgical planning*

Very often, surgeons are expected to be familiar with complex anatomies so that an effective surgical method can be chosen. In the past, they are assisted by plain film radiography but complicated 3D anatomical structures are poorly represented on the 2D medium. CT imaging replaces such traditional methods as 3D visualizations and surgical simulations are available.[92] One of such an example would be the removal of liver tumors. Leeuwen *et al.* advocated pre procedural imaging so that the extent of tumor growth and the proximity of hepatic vasculature can be gauged.[93] The practicality of the resection can be judged from the remaining liver volume as observed in simulations. In the case of craniofacial and maxillofacial reconstructions, surgeons are even furbished with physical models fabricated out using CT data so that they would be well acquainted with the anatomical complexities.[94,95]

The next phase in the development of surgery is real time guided operations. Gronomeyer *et al.* suggested the coupling of CT scanning in minimal invasive operations[54] such as biopsy collection. Tumor samples meant for chemotherapeutic tests can be extracted with live CT monitoring. CT-guided interventions would also enable precise drug deliveries to cancerous sites which minimize the undesirable effects on the surrounding tissue. Besides CT imaging, endoscopy, MRI and ultrasound are capable of such real time data acquisition, but there are limitations. Only proximal visualization at the surgical site is obtained via endoscopy, while imaging noise is predominant in ultrasound.[96] Furthermore, only compatible surgical instruments are allowed in MRI as it uses a strong magnetic field.[97,98] CT imaging is not constrained by these factors thus it is an attractive option in image-guided surgeries.

Operations in the central nervous systems are risky especially so when surgeons have to perform complex neuro-navigation in order to access specific sites. Zernov and Horsley *et al.* have proposed the use of external markers[99] and Cartesian maps[100] to assist surgeons in this challenging task, but the accuracy of these methods is compromised by brain shifts arising from cerebrospinal fluid leakage.[101] CT neuro-mapping deals with this complication with a live imaging procedure and a computerized navigation system. In this technique, the physical positioning of the instrument tip is referenced back on the updated CT images thus guiding surgeons to the appropriate site. Moreover surgeons are better able to differentiate cancerous growth from normal tissues on the scans[101] and Grunert *et al.* has observed that with this approach, residual lesions which are often overlooked can be excised.[101] CT-guided neurosurgery is a significant medical development as it reduces the reliance on the surgeon's experience while improving the patient's chances of recovery.[102]

5.9. *Prosthetic and implant design*

In the use of implants and prostheses, customized engineering is preferred because every patient is unique. Custom designed orthopedic implants have superior geometrical compatibility which optimizes the bone interface contact and this improves host integration.[94] To cater for such outcomes, plain film radiographs and cadavers are studied. But these methods are unsatisfactory because plain film data is two dimensional while a large number of cadaveric samples is needed to address population variation. CT-guided design does not have these restrictions and Robertson *et al.* have harnessed it in the design of total hip implants which precisely fit and fill the femoral canal of specific patients.[103] Moreover a proposed hip implant which suits *in vivo* demands can be engineered with biomechanical considerations.[104,105]

Fixation methods benefit from CT imaging. For example, in dental surgeries, CT imaging would highlight the dense bone regions which are required as secure anchoring sites for dental implants. Furthermore drilling templates can be fabricated using the scan data so that screws can be guided precisely into the desired locations. This technique can also be adopted for spinal fixation procedures.[94] Surgical procedures are streamlined with improved fixation techniques.

In the transition from biomedical research to clinical bedside applications, CT imaging can be exploited for its ability to provide precise anatomical information for the custom design of biological constructs. This is demonstrated in Hutmacher *et al.*'s attempt to create a human ear implant.[106] The anatomical details of the external ear were captured by CT imaging to create a virtual 3D model.

This digital representation is subsequently decomposed into 2D slices which were used as material deposition paths for rapid prototyping.[107] The resultant porous scaffold resembled the natural ear and it provided a substrate for later cell seeding procedures.

6. Micro CT

Research and industrial players express interest in CT analysis for non-clinical applications. The micro CT is one particular invention which caught their attention because it is capable of high resolution imaging. This innovation came about in the early 1980s when Feldkamp was trying to study engine ceramics at high resolutions.[108] His bench top scanner comprised of a microfocus X-ray source and a fluorescent screen coupled to a video camera. After diverging out from the microfocus spot, the cone beam casts a magnified X-ray shadow which amplifies the specimen details (Fig. 5). This data would be captured and processed by a specialized reconstruction algorithm. Feldkamp collaborated with the Henry Ford hospital in the landmark study of trabeculae bone and he managed to obtain images at a spatial resolution of $70 \, \mu$m.[109] Subsequently, engineers sought various ways to improve the rudimentary design. Kalender *et al.* discovered that the imaging time can be shortened by translating and rotating the specimen simultaneously during the scan.[110,111] To increase the resolution, X-ray sources with higher heat tolerances and smaller focal spots are chosen. Moreover, X-ray emission of narrow energy bandwidth is preferred.[14] Sensitive detector arrays consisting of smaller elements[6] and smarter reconstruction algorithms[14] are introduced. Alternative beam magnification set ups such as optical lens and diffraction systems are also available.[108]

Micro CT is a popular technique in biomedical sciences because it is more versatile than traditional methods which include histology, Scanning Electron Microscopy (SEM) and confocal laser microscopy. Histology is a destructive time consuming process which requires samples to be sectioned and stained.[112] The alignment of the resultant 2D sections is problematic and complete data acquisition

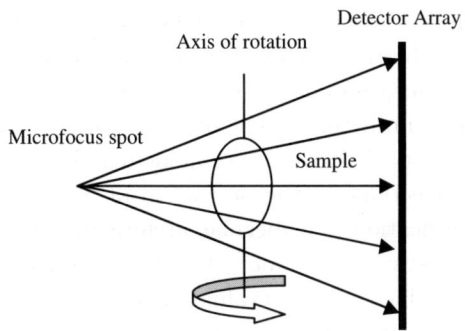

Fig. 5.   Cone beam geometry in a micro CT setup.

is impossible due to the missing parts of the sectioned sample.[113] SEM and confocal laser microscopy are also found lacking as they are only capable of superficial assessments. Micro CT is not hampered by such hassles.[6,7,48] From the digital representation of the sample, selected features can be extracted and studied while the intact specimen can be reserved for later assays.[1] Biomedical researchers have used micro CT in the investigation of trabeculae architectures, vascular networks and tissue engineered constructs.

6.1. *The differences between micro CT and clinical CT*

The micro CT and clinical CT operate on the same general principle but they differ from each other technically. Micro CT is meant for research purposes while the clinical CT caters to the patient's needs and safety. To achieve optimal resolution, high radiation exposures can be selected especially so for the imaging of inanimate objects. The micro CT achieves this with the microfocus spot and long exposure times. This is not feasible in clinical imaging as excessive radiation is detrimental to the patient. Patients are imaged using short exposures of low intensity X-rays and the signal decline is compensated by large detector arrays.[1] A resolution of $100-10,000\,\mu$m is sufficient for clinical scans while higher resolution of $0.15-100\,\mu$m is of interest in research.[1] Table 1 elaborates on the technical differences between the micro CT and the clinical CT.

6.2. *Micro CT imaging: bone research*

When the first micro CT imager was built, it was meant primarily for bone research. Even till now, imaging applications are still dominated by bone studies and researchers have harnessed this non-destructive approach to further the understanding of bone physiology. One of the first few research groups which pioneered the micro CT study of bone is Muller and Ruegsegger. They characterized trabeculae architecture through 3D modeling and parameters such as trabeculae thickness and separation were measured.[29,112,114] Histomorphometry is a conventional approach in trabeculae studies which requires specimen sectioning.[115] In this technique, the trabeculae architecture is modeled as a simplified network of rods and plates. This inaccurate model is widely accepted[116,117] and incorporated into micro CT modeling until the advent of precise digital methods which model the actual trabeculae struts.[118] With better modeling algorithms, Hildebrand *et al.* initiated a series of corrections to the derivation of morphological parameters so that an accurate quantification of trabeculae architecture was possible.[119]

Bone research mostly center on skeletal disorders. Osteoporosis is a prevalent bone disease which can be evaluated by Bone Mineral Density (BMD) measurements. However, investigators such as Keaveny *et al.* have noted a discrepancy between BMD and bone strength.[120,121] This arises because trabeculae architecture plays a significant role and parameters such as anisotropy affect bone

Table 1.   Differences between micro CT and clinical CT.

	Clinical CT	Micro CT
1. Dimensions of X-ray source	0.5 to 2 mm	< 100 μm
2. X-ray emission	Pulsed	Continuous
3. X-ray dosage	No restrictions for inanimate samples. Optimization required for *in vivo* scans.	0.05 Sv per year for an individual
4. Scanning time	In seconds	Minutes to an hour
5. Resolution	100–10,000 μm	0.15–100 μm
6. Size of setup	A room is required for installation	Most setups are bench top units
7. Other differences	The X-ray source–detector pair rotates around the patient.	The specimen rotates while the X-ray source–detector pair remains stationary. However the *in vivo* imager rotates the source–detector pair.
	The position of the patient between the source and detector is fixed.	The position of the specimen between the source and detector can be altered so as to adjust the imaging resolution.

strength.[122,123] This hypothesis is supported by Chappard *et al.*'s observation that a change in architectural parameters precedes BMD reduction in osteoporosis.[124] Besides quantifying pathological conditions, micro CT evaluation is also an effective gauge for the efficacies of bone therapies.[125]

A plethora of possibilities awaits bone researchers who use micro CT imaging. Wong *et al.* observed the hydroxyapatite concentration profile of the rat femur on micro CT scans.[126] On the other hand, Bagi *et al.* derived the moment of inertia to predict the ultimate bending strength of bone.[127] The progression of osteolysis can also be monitored by using this radiographic method.[128] Amidst the myriad of applications, a few seem promising. One of them involves correlating the clinical data of patients with micro CT analysis when bone biopsies are unavailable. This is demonstrated by Guggenbuhl *et al.* when he matched micro CT bone architectural data to plain X-ray images. His aim was to quantify bone architecture from ordinary X-ray images.[124] Showalter *et al.* and Teo *et al.* have shown similar results by using low resolution clinical CT scans. Without resorting to high resolution imaging, they approximated the trabeculae parameters which tally well with micro CT results.[115,129] These applications can be anticipated in the future clinical diagnosis of bone disorders.

6.3. *Micro CT imaging: vasculature studies*

Molecular transport is an integral part of biological systems as it ensures gaseous exchange, waste removal and a constant supply of nutrients. Vasculature networks aid molecular transport and very often vasculature developments accompany tissue growth and healing.[43] Therefore, vasculature studies are commonly employed in the investigation of tumor growth and tissue regeneration. Histology, laser doppler perfusion and Positron Emission Tomography (PET) can be used to probe vascular networks, but they are found to be lacking in one way or another.[43] 3D quantitative analysis is not achievable in histology, while laser doppler perfusion provides superficial information which is not representative of the entire sample. Moreover, PET is incapable of high resolution scans. Micro CT imaging is not plagued by these problems but it has shortcomings. Guldberg and co-workers discovered that their results were constrained by the imaging resolution[43] as fine arterioles were omitted at a resolution of 36 urn. This problem was only alleviated at a resolution of 8–16 μm.

Vasculature studies of the liver,[130] lung[131] and heart[132,133] are frequently reported in current literature. Some of these articles report on vascular abnormalities as a result of infirmities. One example would be Simopoulos *et al.*'s work on diabetes.[134] Through quantitative micro CT analysis, a significant drop in corporeal vascular volume and luminal area were observed with on set of diabetes. Ritman and co-workers have centered their work on renal vasculature and its response to kidney failure.[46] They estimated the vascular volume with respect to the tissue volume from the scan data. At high resolution imaging, morphological details such as vessel length, connectivity and the branching angles were investigated.[135] With micro CT imaging, vascular pathology and physiology can be studied.

6.4. *Micro CT imaging: scaffold characterization*

Scaffolds are often employed in tissue engineering applications because they serve as cellular adhesion stratums and mechanical supports systems. The eventual success of biological constructs depends on the mechanical and biological properties of the scaffold and these are intertwined with the scaffold architecture. Scaffold architecture is defined by parameters such as porosity, surface area to volume ratio, strut thickness, anisotropy and pore interconnectivity.[136] Porosity and pore interconnectivity affect molecular transport, which in turn influences cellular survival and proliferation.[137] The mechanical strength of the scaffold is dependent on anisotropy and strut thickness while surface area to volume ratio determines cellular adhesion. To achieve viable tissue engineered constructs, architecture evaluations are required for scaffold optimizations.[138,139]

Architectural parameters can be derived via various techniques which include micro CT imaging, gas pycnometry, mercury intrusion porosimetry, Archimedes and liquid displacement techniques.[136] Micro CT imaging is preferred[140] because it achieves 3D visualization and precise quantification non-destructively.[139] Closed pores which are entrapped within the scaffold go undetected with conventional means.[136] But with micro CT scans, these elusive pores can be clearly visualized and measured. Being semiquantitative or inaccurate, traditional scaffold assessment techniques are incapable of a comprehensive architectural evaluation,[136] thus they are less appealing when compared to micro CT analysis.

Research groups specializing in scaffold applications have incorporated micro CT evaluations in their scaffold optimizations. Using micro CT scans, Guldberg *et al.* derived parameters such as porosity, strut dimensions and anisotropy. These measurements were used to correlate the porogen composition to the physical features of a porous poly (L-lactide-co-DL-lactide) scaffold.[118] Fragile hydrogel matrices can also be examined using this technique.[141] With digital manipulation, regions of interest within complex architectures can be extracted out for close ups. This advantage is demonstrated in Hollister *et al.*'s evaluation of a biphasic scaffold which comprises of a top poly-L-lactic acid sponge and a bottom hydroapatite matrix. The internal structures of the two phases and the interface region were visualized using micro CT imaging.[142] From these investigations, the micro CT technique is shown to be a versatile scaffold characterization method.

6.5. *Micro CT imaging: tissue engineering*

The efficacy in tissue regeneration determines the performance of tissue engineered constructs. Therefore, tissue engineers seek to isolate and ascertain the viability of the new tissues. In view of this, the author's group implemented a novel approach of using micro CT imaging in the *in vivo* study of osteochondral implants.[143,144] These implants are grafted into the critical size defects of the medial condyle in the rabbit model. Animal samples from various time points were imaged and subsequently the implants were isolated out via digital means.[145] Specific thresholds were later applied to visualize and quantify the regenerated bone.[144] Following that, the bone volume fraction of the regenerated bone was derived and compared to that of the native site, thereby providing a quantitative indicator of recovery. Host bone integration and growth patterns were examined using 3D visualization, and the results were in excellent agreement with histological findings. Therefore, micro CT imaging is demonstrated to be a reliable approach in tissue restoration studies.

The functionality of the regenerated tissue is determined by its quantity and quality. For example, functional bone constructs are not just assessed by bone volume but also bone mineralization. This is because the mechanical strength of the new tissue is dependent on mineralization. Schantz *et al.* encountered this when he noted a wide variance in the thresholds of the regenerated calverial bone.[146] This could be attributed to the different mineralization levels. In a similar experiment, Verna *et al.* was able to formulate a mineralization profile based on the different thresholds.[145] This phenomenon was also observed by Jones *et al.* when the micro structure of the regenerated bone was examined at a resolution of $2\,\mu m$.[147] Besides *in vivo* studies, mineralization in cultured constructs can also be analyzed via micro CT imaging. In a dynamic culturing experiment, Meinel *et al.* quantified the size and distribution of mineralized nodules located within scaffolds.[148] Micro CT analysis assists bone researchers and with time, other biomedical researchers will harness this technique to evaluate various regenerated tissues.

6.6. *Micro CT imaging: soft tissue analysis*

There are emerging applications in micro CT imaging which go beyond just bone research. One of which is soft tissue analysis. The imaging of soft tissue proves to be problematic due to the lack of contrast, but this outlook is set to change with contrast enhancement agents and high resolution imaging. Watz *et al.* took on the challenging task of imaging alveolar architectures which collapse easily after tissue extraction.[47] The poor X-ray attenuation of the lung tissue added further complication. To overcome such difficulties, Watz *et al.* devised a method of preparing the lung samples before micro CT scanning. To preserve the delicate alveolar structures, the soft tissue was inflated and fixed with formalin vapor, while a silver nitrate stain was applied to improve the contrast. With this unique technique, virtual endoscopic imaging of the airspaces was obtained.

A wealth of information can be derived from the micro CT studies of soft tissue. Easterly *et al.* employed it as a phenotypic evaluation of the fat and muscle in mice screening.[149] Ritman *et al.* used the scan data to study the spiral arrangement of the myocardium fibers and attempted to correlate this unique muscle fiber distribution to stress transmission.[132] Besides physiological interpretations, quantitative analysis can also be carried out in the imaging of soft tissues. Wehmeyer *et al.* recognized the affinity between gadolinium and proteoglycan and went on to improve the imaging contrast of cartilage by treating the samples with the heavy metal.[49] Moreover the intensity measurements were correlated to the proteoglycan content. Thus the proteoglycan concentration could be measured while visualizing the cartilage morphology.

6.7. *Micro CT imaging: In vivo imaging*

Longitudinal studies involve the following up of the responses to drugs, therapies and treatments. As the progression of the condition in the individual animals is of utmost importance, animal survival must be ensured throughout the experiment. Being a non-invasive approach, micro CT *in vivo* imaging can be used for these time serial studies. But there are concerns regarding X-ray exposure. Excessive radiation is lethal moreover physiology alterations at non lethal levels might introduce experimental errors. Hence low dosage scans are encouraged but that would comprise the imaging resolution. One must be mindful that high resolution *in vivo* imaging is necessary for the optimal observation in small animals. To resolve this constraint, signal loss at low dosage scanning is compensated by the use of sensitive detector arrays[29] and improved algorithms.[108] A real time reconstruction program was even devised by Brasse *et al.* for this purpose.[150] To prevent unnecessary exposure, Van der Sloten resorted to lead shielding for the animal.[30,151] Physiological motion is also a concern for *in vivo* scanning because that leads to blur images. These movements are attributed to normal cardiac pulsation and respiration. To reduce image blurring, synchronized data acquisition is carried out with gating techniques. However these measures are not effective with regards to non cyclic events such as the accumulation and flow of contrast agents.[14]

In vivo micro CT imaging allows follow up animal studies. Waarsing *et al.* exploited this advantage in the assessment of bone remodeling.[29] Trabeculae scans at different time points were mathematically matched using 3D registration programs so that bone resorption and formation at the level of single trabeculae could be visualized. Moreover the *in vivo* scan data became an input for computer simulation and the results were verified by follow up scans. This computational technique evaluates the factors involved in bone remodeling. Besides bone research, soft tissue investigations can be done with micro CT imaging. Su *et al.* studied the role of Matrix Metalloproteinase (MMP) in myocardial remodeling with a MMP targeted intravenous radiotracer.[152] Anatomical data from micro CT imaging was matched with that from micro Single Photon Emission Computed Tomography (SPECT) which detected the presence of the tracer. Therefore the spatial and temporal changes in MMP activity due cardiac infarction could be measured from the *in vivo* micro CT/SPECT scan.

6.8. *Micro CT imaging: finite element modeling (FEM)*

In finite element modeling (FEM), the physical interactions within a region of interest are simulated mathematically. Parameters which describe the external conditions and inherent properties are applied onto virtual models which represent the interacting bodies. Micro CT scanning provides detailed digital representations of the specimens which can be loaded onto the FEM platform. FEM models which resemble the actual samples can also be created via algorithms but they are unreliable as they are only approximations. The feasibility of a micro CT–FEM analysis was demonstrated by Muller *et al.* in the biomechanical evaluation of trabeculae samples which examined the effects of age and disease on bone strength.[153]

Since the reliability of FEM hinges on the accuracy of the models, caution should be exercised when using micro CT data. In the study of trabeculae architecture, Pistoia *et al.* noted a decline in simulation accuracy at low imaging resolutions.[154] Moreover imaging noise and contrast were concerns. FEM studies base on 2D micro CT images are found to be inadequate as the 3D aspect of the specimen is poorly represented. Hence the usage of 3D micro CT models is encouraged.[113]

Biomechanical interactions can studied in live animal models with *in vivo* micro CT–FEM analysis. The scanning process captures the differences between the individual animals which influence the mechanical interactions. Such a scenario was noted in Van der Sloten *et al.*'s work on the peri-implant bone adaptation in guinea pigs.[30] In his project, bone geometry, implant position and bone density differed from animal to animal even though the same implantation site was used. These factors affected the stress and strain distributions in the host bone, thus *in vivo* micro CT imaging was carried out with a FEM assessment for each animal. As temporal progression was critical to the experiment, histology was deemed to be an unsuitable follow up method since it necessitated animal sacrifice at each time point.

Micro CT–FEM analysis offers flexibility in biomechanical studies as the strengths of non-destructive imaging is combined with virtual modeling, thus numerous avenues of applications can be explored. One of these avenues would be the functional evaluation of regenerated tissues as demonstrated by Jones *et al.* when he predicted the Young's modulus of bone in growth located within implants.[155] Moreover, with micro CT–FEM, implant design can be optimized by matching the mechanical properties of the construct with that of the native tissue.[30] Fracture and flow dynamics studies are also exciting possibilities. Takada *et al.* examined the effects of the third molar on the mandibular fracture angle.[156] The stress concentration and transmission measurements corresponded well with clinical findings. Cioffi and co-workers employed a novel approach in the dynamic culturing of tissue engineered cartilage constructs.[157] Computational fluid dynamic modeling was carried out with 3D models of porous polyurethane scaffolds which were derived via micro CT imaging. Flow fields and excessive internal shear stresses with respect to the input flow parameters were quantified via FEM, thus optimal flow conditions could be selected for the actual culturing experiment. These are just examples in the wide range of biomedical applications in micro CT–FEM.

7. Future Development in Clinical and Micro CT

The performance of CT is dictated by two factors, and they are the hardware and software components of the system. Advancements in these two areas would lead to better scanners. Cost reduction is brought about by streamlining the hardware aspect, thus enhancing the commercial availability of clinical and micro CT setups. Currently, clinical CT facilities are only accessible in affluent countries. Hence health care in developing nations would definitely benefit from the introduction of cheaper clinical CT facilities. Being a computation method, digital bottlenecks and data storage limitations are commonplace. Therefore improved data management is needed and scientists envision the day when the common desktop is capable of complex CT data processing.

There are two emerging trends in the development of CT systems. First, multimodality matching which combines CT with other imaging methods is anticipated.[152,158] These imaging techniques would include MRI and PET. Second, there is a move from mere visualization to detailed quantifications which allows a more in depth evaluation.[159] These trends are noted in clinical and research applications.

A next phase of development in clinical CT would not just witness better imaging resolutions but also smart imaging techniques. Multimodal imaging can be achieved by using dual PET/CT scanners which detect the biochemical events with positron emitting radiotracers.[158] These tracers target tumors, specific cellular receptors and activities within the patient's body. The acquisition of PET image is followed by CT scanning and subsequently the two data sets are merged. CT complements PET with anatomical data, while the PET highlights the subtle abnormalities which go undetected in CT.[160] Co-registration of PET and CT images from separate scanners is another possibility if the dual scanner is not available. Medical practitioners foresee much promise of this new technique in cancer diagnosis.[158] Besides multimodal imaging, another exciting area is the development of CT diagnostic programs. In the screening of heart aliments, Gaspar *et al.* demonstrated the feasibility of the automated detection of carotid plaques and stenosis in patients who have undergone a heart CT scan.[58] Soon similar diagnostic software coupled to CT imaging would be tested in the screening of various disorders.

Imaging resolution continues to be a top priority in research because of the need for more accurate data acquisitions. Hence advancements in micro CT technology would continue to be dominated by developments in this feature. Set ups equipped with high heat tolerance X-ray sources and sensitive detector arrays are capable of high resolution imaging.[14] To achieve submicrometer resolution, zone plates and diffraction optics which magnify the X-ray projection are recommended.[108] Non-attenuating imaging approaches based on the fundamental principles of K-edge subtraction, X-ray phase delay and X-ray scatter are options which lead to improved image sensitivity and contrast.[14] Besides improving the data acquisition process, there is also a demand for upgraded data processing methods. Precise digital analysis can be facilitated by efficient algorithms which speed up computations while reducing imaging noise and artifacts.[14] Moreover, user friendliness and the range of quantitative assessments are also areas of considerations in software design. With these developments, one would envision the micro CT imager being an integral part of future biomedical laboratories.

8. Conclusion

Biomedical science has witness quantum leaps in the last few decades with successes in the human genome project, animal cloning and stem cell research. CT technology is also part of this scientific advancement and despite being a relatively new technique, it already has a wide range of clinical and research applications. Clinical CT is appealing because it is a non-invasive method which can be supplemented with 3D quantitative analysis. The main limitation of clinical CT is the use of ionizing X-rays, and caution is warranted in administering the radiation dosage. A majority of micro CT applications centre on bone research as it was primarily developed for this purpose. But there are increasing reports of its use in tissue engineering, soft tissue and vasculature imaging. This indicates the potential of the technique in novel areas of research. With the current interest in non–invasive and non–destructive evaluation approaches, CT technology is set to become increasingly popular and dominant in biomedical sciences.

References

1. R. A. Ketcham and W. D. Carlson, Acquisition, optimization and interpretation of X-ray computed tomographic imagery: Applications to the geosciences, *Computers and Geosci.* **27** (2001) 381–400.
2. V. K. Gerhard and D. Stefan, Computed tomography in various fields outside medicine, *Eur. Radiol.* **15**(Supplement 4) (2005) D74–D81.
3. F. McLaughlin, J. Mackintosh, B. P. Hayes, A. McLaren, I. J. Uings, P. Salmon, J. Humphreys, E. Meldrum and S. N. Farrow, Glucocorticoid-induced osteopenia in the mouse as assessed by histomorphometry, microcomputed tomography, and biochemical markers, *Bone* **30**(6) (2002) 924–930.
4. R. Müller, H. Van Campenhout, B. Van Damme, G. Van der Perre, J. Dequeker, T. Hildebrand and P. Rüegsegger, Morphometric analysis of human bone biopsies: A quantitative structural comparison of histological sections and micro-computed tomography, *Bone* **23**(1) (1998) 59–66.

5. G. N. Hounsfield, Computed transverse axial scanning (tomography): Part 1, Description of system, *British J. Radiol.* **46** (1973) 1016–1022.
6. D. W. Holdsworth and M. M. Thornton, Micro-CT in small animal and specimen imaging, *Trends Biotechnol.* **20**(8) Supplement (2002) S34–S39.
7. U. Bonse and F. Busch, X-ray computed microtomography (μCT) using synchrotron radiation (SR), *Prog. Biophys. Molecul. Biol.* **65**(1/2) (1996) 133–169.
8. G. Wang and M. W. Vannier, Computerized tomography. *Encyclopedia Electric. Electro. Eng.* (1998) 1–22.
9. F. Spoor, N. Jeffery and F. Zonneveld, Imaging skeletal growth and evolution, *Development, Growth and Evolution.* Chapter 6, (2000) 124–161.
10. W. C. Hayes, L. M. Keer, G. Herrmann and L. F. Mockros, A mathematical analysis for indentation tests of articular cartilage, *J. Biomech.* **5** (1972) 541–551.
11. W. Andrew, X-ray imaging and computed tomography, *Introduction to Biomedical Imaging.* Chapter 1 (2003) 1–56.
12. D. J. Dowseth, P. A. Kenny and R. E. Johnston, *The Physics of Diagnostic Imaging* (Chapman and Hall Medical, London, 1998).
13. C. B. Stewart, Quality control, *Computed Tomography.* Chapter 10, (2000) 141–142.
14. E. L. Ritman, Molecular imaging ion small animals–roles for micro-CT, *J. Cellul. Biochem. Suppl.* **39** (2002) 116–124.
15. D. A. Chesler, S. J. Riederer and N. J. Pelc, Noise due to photon counting statistics in computed X-ray tomography, *J. Comput. Assisted Tomograp.* **1** (1977) 64–77.
16. P. Mathias, Cancer screening with CT: Dose controversy, *Eur. Radiol.* **15** (Supplement 4) (2005) D55–D61.
17. National research council, Committee on the biological effects of ionizing radiations, *Health Effects of Exposure to Low Levels of Ionizing Radiation: BEIR VII* (National Academy Press, Washington, DC, 2005).
18. D. J. Brenner and M. A. Georgsson, Mass screening with CT colonography: Should the radiation exposure be of concern? *Gastroenterology* **129** (2005) 328–337.
19. A. K. Ella, Lung cancer screening, *Eur. Radiol.* **15**(Supplement 4) (2005) D48–D51.
20. National research council, Committee on the biological effects of ionizing radiations, *Health Effects of Exposure to Low Levels of Ionizing Radiation: BEIR V* (National Academy Press, Washington, DC, 1990).
21. B. L. Cohen, Cancer risk from low-level radiation, *Am. J. Roentgenol.* **179** (2002) 1137–1143.
22. J. S. Marilyn, Pediatric CT angiography, *Eur. Radiol.* **15**(Supplement 4) (2005) D32–D36.
23. M. Kachelriess, O. Watzke and W. A. Kalender, Generalized multi-dimensional adaptive filtering for conventional and spiral single-slice, multi-slice, and cone-beam CT. *Med. Phys.* **28** (2001) 475–490.
24. T. H. Mulkens, P. Bellinck, M. Baeyaert, D. Ghysen, X. Van Dijck, E. Mussen, C. Venstermans and J. L. Termote, Use of an automatic exposure control mechanism for dose optimization in multi-detector row CT examinations: Clinical evaluation, *Radiology* **237** (2005) 213–223.
25. W. A. Kalender, H. Wolf, C. Suess, M. Gies, H. Greess and W. A. Bautz, Dose reduction in CT by on-line tube current control: Principles and validation on phantoms and cadavers, *Eur. Radiol.* **9** (1999) 323–328.
26. M. K. Kalra, S. Rizzo, M. M. Maher, E. F. Halpern, T. L. Toth, J. A. Shepard and S. L. Aquino, Chest CT performed with z-axis modulation: Scanning protocol and radiation dose, *Radiology* **237** (2005) 303–308.

27. W. K. Jurgen and W. Simon, Multidetector–row CT angiography of upper and lower extremity peripheral arteries, *Eur. Radiol.* **15**(Supplement 4) (2005) D3–D9.
28. I. Zein, D. W. Hutmacher, K. C. Tan, S. H. Teoh, Fused deposition modeling of novel scaffold architectures for tissue engineering applications, *Biomaterials* **23** (2002) 1169–1185.
29. J. H. Waarsing, J. S. Day and H. Weinans, Longitudinal micro-CT scans to evaluate bone architecture. *J. Musculoskeletal Neuronal Interact*, **5**(4) (2005) 310–312.
30. S. V. N. Jaecques, H. Van Oosterwyck, L. Muraru, T. Van Cleynenbreugel, E. De Smet, M. Wevers, I. Naert and J. V. Sloten, Individualised, micro CT-based finite element modeling as a tool for biomechanical analysis related to tissue engineering of bone, *Biomaterials* **25** (2004) 1683–1696.
31. J. H. Kinney, N. E. Lane and D. L. Haupt, *In vivo*, three-dimensional microscopy of trabeculae bone, *J. Bone Mineral Res.* **10** (1995) 264–270.
32. A. A. Johnsson, T. Sawaii, M. Jacobsson, G. Granstrom, C. B. Johansson, K. G. Strid and I. Turesson, A microradiographic investigation of cancellous bone healing after irradiation and hyperbaric oxygenation: A rabbit study, *Int J. Radiation Oncol. Biol. Phys.* **48** (2000) 555–563.
33. J. D. Bisgard and J. B. Hunt, Influence of roentgen rays and radium on epiphyseal growth of long bones, *Radiology* **26** (1936) 56–68.
34. A. B. Michael, Contrast media: Safety, viscosity and volume, *Eur. Radiol.* **15** (Supplement 4) (2005) D62–D64.
35. C. B. Stewart, Radiation safety, *Computed Tomography*. Chapter 9 (2000), pp. 133–136.
36. V. Valerie, Tumour detection in the liver: Role of multidetector–row CT, *Eur. Radiol.* **15**(Supplement 4) (2005) D85–D88.
37. S. P. Cornelia and P. Mathias, MDCT for the diagnosis of acute pulmonary embolism, *Eur. Radiol.* **15**(Supplement 4) (2005) D37–D41.
38. Z. Paroz, R. Moncada and Sovak M, *Contrast Media: Biological Effects and Clinical Applications*, Vols 1–3. (CRC Press, Boca Raton, Florida, 1987).
39. R. Patrik. CT of the small intestine, *Eur. Radiol.* **15**(Supplement 4) (2005) D142–D148.
40. E. L. Ritman, Myocardial capillary permeability to iohexol: evaluation with fast X-ray computed tomography, *Investigative Radiol.* **29** (1994) 612–617.
41. L. O. Lerman, M. Rodriguez-Porcel and J. C. Romero, The development of X-ray imaging to study renal function, *Kidney Int.* **55** (1999) 400–416.
42. J. A. Webb, F. Stacul, H. Thomsen and S. K. Morcos, Late adverse reactions to intravascular iodinated contrast media, *Eur. Radiol.* **13** (2003) 181–184.
43. C. L. Duvall, W. R. Taylor, D. Weiss and R. E. Guldberg, Quantitative micro-computed tomography analysis of collateral vessel development after ischemic injury, *Am. J. Physiol. Heart Circulatory Physiol.* **287** (2004) H302–H310.
44. N. Maehara, Experimental microcomputed tomography study of the 3D micro-angioarchitecture of tumors, *Eur. Radiol.* **13** (2003) 1559–1565.
45. D. C. Moore, C. W. Leblanc, R. Muller, J. J. Crisco III and M. G. Ehrlich, Physiologic weightbearing increases new vessel formation during distraction osteogenesis: a microtomographic imaging study, *J. Orthoped. Res.* **21** (2003) 489–496.
46. M. D. Bentley, M. C. Ortiz, E. L. Ritman and J. C. Romero, The use of microcomputed tomography to study microvasculature in small rodents, *Am J. Physiol. Regulatory, Integrative and Comparative Physiology* **202** (2002) R1267–R1279.

47. W. Henrik, A. Breithecker, W. S. Rau and A. Kriete, Micro-CT of the human lung: Imaging of alveoli and virtual endoscopy of an alveolar duct in a normal lung and in a lung with centrilobular emphysema–initial observations, *Radiol.* **236** (2005) 1053–1058.

48. H. D. Litzlbauer, C. Neuhaeuser, A. Moell, S. Greschus, A. Breithecker, F. E. Franke, W. Kummer and W. S. Rau, Three–dimensional imaging and morphometic analysis of alveolar tissue from microfocal X-ray computed tomography, *Am. J. Physiol. Lung Cellular and Molecul. Physiol.* **291**(3) (2006) L535–L545.

49. M. D. Cockman, C. A. Blanton, P. A. Chmielewski, L. Dong, T. E. Dufresne, E. B. Hookfin, M. J. Karb, S. Liu and K. R. Wehmeyer, Quantitative imaging of proteoglycan in cartilage using a gadolinium probe and micro CT, *Osteoarthritis Cartilage* **14** (2006) 210–214.

50. N. Godfrey. Hounsfield, Computed Medical Imaging, Nobel Lecture, 8th of Decemeber 1979. http://nobelprize.org/medicine/laureates.

51. C. B. Stewart, Historical perspective, *Computed Tomography*, Essentials of Medical Imaging Series, Chapter 1 (McGraw-Hill, 2000), pp. 1–3.

52. C. B. Stewart, Operational modes, *Computed Tomography*, Essentials of Medical Imaging Series, Chapter 2 (McGraw-Hill, 2000), pp. 9–13.

53. G. Wang, *Computed Tomography Principles* http://dolphin.radiology.uiowa.edu/ge/teaching.html.

54. D. Gronemeyer, A. Gevargez, R. Seibel and A. Melzer, Tomographic microtherapy, *Comput. Aided Surg.* **3** (1998) 188–193.

55. C. B. Stewart, Special imaging techniques, *Computed Tomography.* Chapter 6, (2000), pp. 99–103.

56. F. K. Andreas, H. Martin, R. Anja, K. Axel, B. Thorsten, O. Martin, B. Christoph, B. Harald, D. C. Claus and S. Stephen, Evaluation of cardiac function and myocardial viability with 16 and 64 slice multidetector computed tomography, *Eur. Radiol.* **15**(Supplement 4) (2005) D15–D20.

57. Y. Masuda, T. Uda and K. Yoshida, Diagnosis of myocardial infarction by CT: The study of an initial filling defect and late enhancement of the infarcted myocardium after injection of contrast material, *J. Cardiograp.* **13** (1983) 809–819.

58. G. Tamar, H. David, R. Ronen and P. Nathan, Clinical applications and future trends in cardiac CTA, *Eur. Radiol.* **15**(Supplement 4) (2005) D10–D14.

59. S. Achenbach, D. Ropers, U. Hoffmann, B. MacNeill, U. Baum and K. Pohle, Assessment of coronary remodeling in stenotic and nonstenotic coronary atherosclerotic lesions by multidetector spiral computed tomography, *J. Am. College Cardiol.* **43** (2004) 842–847.

60. Y. Koyama, H. Matsuoka and H. Higashino, Myocardial perfusion defect in acute myocardial infarction on enhanced helical CT after successful reperfusion therapy: A prognostic value, *Radiology* **221** (2001) 195.

61. J. K. Willmann, D. Mayer, M. Banyai, L. M. Desbiolles, F. R. Verdun, M. Seifert, B. Marincek and D. Weishaupt, Evaluation of peripheral arterial bypass grafts with multi-detector row CT angiography: Comparison with duplex US and digital subtraction angiography, *Radiology* **229** (2003) 465–474.

62. W. Max, Brain perfusion-CT in acute stroke patients, *Eur. Radiol.* **15**(Supplement 4) (2005) D28–D31.

63. A. G. Philippe, Detection of altered lung physiology, *Eur. Radiol.* **15**(Supplement 4) (2005) D42–D47.

64. H. U. Kauczor, *Functional Imaging of the Chest* (Springer, Berlin, Heidelberg, New York, 2004).

65. L. E. Heyneman, S. Ward, D. A. Lynch, M. Remy-Jardin, T. Johkoh and N. L. Muller, Respiratory bronchiolitis, respiratory bronchiolitis-associated interstitial lung disease, and desquamative interstitial pneumonia: Different entities or part of the spectrum of the same disease process? *Am. J. Roentgenol.* **173** (1994) 1617–1622.

66. H. Arakawa, P. A. Gevenois, Y. Saito, H. Shida, V. D. Maertelaer, H. Moikubo and M. Fujioka, Silicosis: Expiratory thin–section CT assessment of airway obstruction, *Radiology* **236** (2005) 1059–1066.

67. R. H. Baroni, D. Feller-Kopman, M. Nishino, H. Hatabu, S. H. Loring, A. Ernst and P. M. Boiselle, Tracheobronchomalacia: Comparison between end-expiratory and dynamic expiratory CT for evaluation of central airway collapse, *Radiology* **233** (2005) 635–641.

68. P. A. Grenier, C. Beigelman-Aubry, C. Fetita, F. Preteux, M. W. Brauner and S. Lenoir, New frontiers in CT imaging of airway disease, *Eur. Radiol.* **12** (2002) 1022–1044.

69. J. G. Goldin, M. F. McNitt-Gray and S. M. Sorensen, Airway hyperreactivity: Assessment with helical thin-section CT, *Radiology* **208** (1998) 321–329.

70. A. Niimi, H. Matsumoto, R. Amitani, Y. Nakano, M. Mishima and M. Minakuchi, Airway wall thickness in asthma assessed by computed tomography. Relation to clinical indices, *Am. J. Respir. Crit. Care Med.* **162** (2000) 1518–1523.

71. S. James, D. M. Balfe, J. K. Lee and D. Picus, Small-bowel disease: Categorization by CT examination, *Am. J. Roentgenol.* **148** (1987) 863–868.

72. D. J. Vining, D. W. Gelfand and R. E. Bechtold, Technical feasibility of colon imaging with helical CT and virtual reality, *Am. J. Roentgenol.* **62**(Supplement) (1994) 104.

73. J. P. Perry, Virtual colonoscopy: Issues related to primary screening, *Eur. Radiol.* **15**(Supplement 4) (2005) D133–D137.

74. P. F. Michael, CT of the acute (emergency) abdomen, *Eur. Radiol.* **15**(Supplement 4) (2005) D100–D104.

75. S. S. Raman, D. S. K. Lu, B. M. Kadell, D. J. Vodopich, J. Sayro and H. Cryer, Accuracy of nonfocused helical CT for the diagnosis of acute appendicitis: A 5–year review, *Am. J. Roentgenol.* **178** (2002) 1319–1325.

76. J. B. C. M. Puylaert, Imaging and intervention in patients with acute right lower quadrant disease, *Bailliere's Clin. Gastroenterol.* **9**(1) (1995) 37–51.

77. Radiological society of North America, Whole-body MR screening found feasible, *Radiolog. Soc. North Am. News* **14**(2) (2004) 10–11.

78. N. B. Z. Michael, The role of computed tomography in screening for cancer, *Eur. Radiol.* **15**(Supplement 4) (2005) D52–D54.

79. Centers for disease control, Cigarette smoking among adults-United States 2003, Morbidity, Mortality Weekly Report **54** (2005) 509–513.

80. C. I. Henschke, D. F. Yankelevitz, D. P. Naidich, D. I. McCauley, F. McGuinness, D. M. Libby, J. P. Smith, M. W. Pasmantier and O. S. Miettinen, CT screening for lung cancer: Suspiciousness of nodules according to size on baseline scans, *Radiology* **231** (2004) 164–168.

81. D. F. Yankelevitz, A. P. Reeves, W. J. Kostis, B. Zhao and C. I. Henschke, Small pulmonary nodules: Volumetrically determined growth rates based on CT evaluation, *Radiology* **217** (2000) 251–256.

82. N. McNulty, I. Francis, J. Platt, R. Cohan, M. Korobkin and A. Gebremariam, Multidetector row helical CT of the pancreas: Effects of contrast-enhanced multiphasic 41 imaging on enhancement of the pancreas, peripancreatic vasculature, and pancreatic adenocarcinoma, *Radiology* **220** (2001) 97–102.

83. P. Freeny, L. Traverso and J. Ryan, Diagnosis and staging of pancreatic adenocarcinoma with dynamic computed tomography, *Am. J. Surg.* **165** (1993) 600–606.

84. C. F. Patrick, CT diagnosis and staging of pancreatic carcinoma, *Eur. Radiol.* **15**(Supplement 4) (2005) D96–D99.

85. K. Melvyn, CT urography, *Eur. Radiol.* **15**(Supplement 4) (2005) D82–D84.

86. E. M. Caoili, R. H. Cohan, M. Korobkin, J. F. Platt, I. R. Francis, G. J. Faerber, J. E. Montie and J. H. Ellis, Urinary tract abnormalities: Initial experience with multi-detector row CT urography, *Radiology* **222** (2002) 353–360.

87. N. C. Dalrymple, M. Verga and K. R. Anderson, The value of unenhanced helical computerized tomography in the management of acute flank pain, *J. Urol.* **159** (1998) 735–740.

88. D. B. Christoph and A. P. Pierre, The trauma concept: The role of MDCT in the diagnosis and management of visceral injuries, *Eur. Radiol.* **15**(Supplement 4) (2005) D105–D109.

89. U. Linsenmaier, M. Krotz and H. Hauser, Whole-body computed tomography in polytrauma: Techniques and management, *Eur. Radiol.* **12** (2002) 1728–1740.

90. C. D. Becker, P. Spring, A. Glattli and W. Schweizer, Blunt splenic trauma in adults: Can CT findings be used to determine the need for surgery, *Am. J. Roentgenol.* **162** (1994) 343–347.

91. K. S. Miller and J. W. McAninch, Radiographic assessment of renal trauma: Our 15–year experience, *J. Urol.* **154** (1995) 352–355.

92. G. Schlondorff, Computer-assisted surgery: Historical remarks, *Comput. Aided Surg.* **3** (1998) 150–152.

93. M. Van Leeuwen, H. Obertop, A. H. Hennipman and M. A. Fernandez, 3-D reconstruction of hepatic neoplasms: A preoperative planning procedure, *Bailliere's Clin. Gastroenterol.* **9**(1) (1995) 121–133.

94. M. Michiel, A system for intra-operative manufacturing of stems of total hip replacements, in *Computer Technology in Biomaterials Science and Engineering.* Jos Vander Sloten, ed., Chapter 7a, (2000), pp. 262–300.

95. J. J. Beaman, Solid Freeform Fabrication: A new direction in manufacturing, J. J. Beamann, J. W. Barlow, D. L. Bourell, R. H. Crawford, H. L. Marcus and K. P. McAlea (Eds). (Kluwer Boston, MA, 1997), p. 1.

96. J. S. Lewin, J. L. Duerk, V. R. Jain, C. A. Petersilge, C. P. Chao and J. R. Haaga, Needle localization in MR-guided biopsy and aspiration: Effects of field strength, sequence 42 design, and magnetic field orientation, *Am. J. Roentgenol.* **166** (1996) 1337–1345.

97. E. Alexander III, T. M. Moriarty, R. Kikinis, P. Black and F. M. Jolesz, The present and future role of intraoperative MRI in neurosurgical procedures, *Stereotactic Func. Neurosurg.* **68** (1997) 10–17.

98. T. M. Moriarty, R. Kikinis, F. A. Jolesz, P. M. Black and E. Alexander III, Magnetic resonance imaging therapy: Intraoperative MR imaging, *Neurosurg. Clin. North Am.* **7** (1996) 323–331.

99. G. H. Barnett and D. W. Miller, Brain biopsy and related procedures, *Image-Guided Neurosurgery*, eds. G. H. Barnett, D. W. Roberts and R. J. Maciunas (QMP Inc, St Louis, MO, 1998), pp. 181–191.

100. V. Horsley and R. H. Clarke, The structure and functions of the cerebellum examined by a new method, *Brain* **31** (1908) 45–124.

101. P. Grunert, W. Muller-Forell, K. Darabi, R. Reisch, C. Busert, N. Hopf and A. Perneczky, Basic principles and clinical applications of neuronavigation and intraoperative computed tomography, *Comput. Aided Surg.* **3** (1998) 166–173.

102. C. Matula, K. Rossler, M. Reddy, E. Schindler and W. T. Koos, Intraoperative computed tomography guided neuronavigation: Concepts, efficiency and work flow, *Comput. Aided Surg.* **3** (1998) 174–183.

103. D. D. Roberson, P. S. Walker, J. W. Granholm, P. C. Nelson, P. J. Weiss, E. K. Fishman and D. Magid, Design of custom hip stem prostheses using three-dimensional CT modeling, *J. Comput. Assisted Tomograp.* **11**(5) (1987) 804–809.

104. N. N. Arturo, Numerical simulation of load-bearing dental implants, in *Computer Technology in Biomaterials Science and Engineering*, ed. Jos Vander Sloten, 1st edn., Chapter 3b (2000) 132–148.

105. A. P. Josep, Towards an integrated lifetime prediction software for biomaterials systems, in *Computer Technology in Biomaterials Science and Engineering*, ed. Jos Vander Sloten, 1st edn., Chapter 3c (2000) 149–177.

106. D. W. Hutmacher, K. W. Ng, C. Kaps, M. Sittinger and S. Klaring, Elastic cartilage engineering using novel scaffold architectures in combination with a biomimetic cell carrier, *Biomaterials* **24** (2003) 4445–4458.

107. D. W. Hutmacher, Scaffolds in tissue engineering bone and cartilage, *Biomaterials* **21** (2000) 2529–2543.

108. E. L. Ritman, Micro-computed tomography-current status and developments, *Ann. Rev. Biomed. Eng.* **6** (2004) 185–208.

109. L. A. Feldkamp, S. A. Goldstein, A. M. Parfitt, G. Jesion and M. Kleerekoper, The direct examination of three-dimensional bone architecture in vitro by computed tomography, *J. Bone Mineral Res.* **4** (1989) 3–11.

110. W. Kalendar, W. Klotz and E. Vock, Spiral volumetric CT with single-breathhold technique, continuous transport and continuous scanner rotation, *Radiology* **176** (1990) 181–183.

111. G. Wang, T. H. Lin, P. C. Cheng, D. M. Shinozaki and H. G. Kim, Scanning cone-beam reconstruction algorithms for X-ray microtomography, *Proc. Int. Soc. Optical Eng.* **1556** (1991) 99–112.

112. R. Muller, T. Hildebrand and P. Ruegsegger, Non-invasive bone biopsy: A new method to analyse and display the three-dimensional structure of trabecular bone, *Phys. Med. Biol.* **39** (1994) 145–164.

113. H. Van Oosterwyck, J. Duyck, J. Vander Sloten, G. Van der Perre, J. Jansen, M. Wever and I. Naert, The use of microfocus computerized tomography as a new technique for characterizing bone tissue around oral implants, *J. Oral Implantol.* **26**(1) (2000) 5–12.

114. R. Muller, M. Hahn, M. Vogel, G. Delling and P. Ruegsegge, Morphometric analysis of non-invasively assessed bone biopsies: Comparison of high-resolution computed tomography and histologic sections, *Bone* **18** (1996) 215–220.

115. C. Showalter, B. D. Clymer, B. Richmond and K. Powell, Three-dimensional texture analysis of cancellous bone cores evaluated at clinical CT resolutions, *Osteoporosis Int.* **17** (2006) 259–266.

116. J. S. Day, M. Ding, A. Odgaard, D. R. Sumner, I. Hvid and H. Weinans, Parallel plate model for trabecular bone exhibits volume fraction-dependent bias, *Bone* **27**(5) (2000) 715–720.

117. W. J. Whitehouse, The quantitative morphology of anisotropic trabecular bone, *J. Microsc.* **101** (1974) 153–168.

118. T. Hildebrand, A. Liab, R. Muller, J. Dequeker and P. Ruegsegger, Direct threedimensional morphometric analysis of human cancellous bone: Microstructural data from spine, iliac crest, and calcaneus, *J. Bone Min. Res.* **14**(7) (1999) 1167–1174.

119. T. Hildebrand and P. Ruegsegger, A new method for the model-independent assessment of thickness in three-dimensional images, *J. Microsc.* **185**(1) (1997) 67–75.
120. T. M. Keaveny and O. C. Yeh, Architecture and trabecular bone–towards an improved understanding of the biomechanical effects of age, sex and osteoporosis, *J. Musculoskeletal Neuronal Interact.* **2** (2002) 205–208.
121. E. Legrand, D. Chappard, C. Pascaretti, M. Duquenne, C. Rondeau, Y. simon, V. Rohmer, M. F. Basle and M. Audran, Bone mineral density and vertebral fractures in men, *Osteoporosis Int.* **10** (1999) 265–270.
122. S. A. Goldstein, R. Goulet and D. McCubbrey, Measurement and significance of threedimensional architecture to the mechanical integrity of trabecular bone, *Calcified Tissue Int.* **53** (1993) S127–S133.
123. R. W. Goulet, S. A. Goldstein and M. J. Ciarelli, The relationship between structural and orthogonal compressive properties of trabecular bone, *J. Biomech.* **27** (1994) 375–389.
124. P. Guggenbuhl, F. Bodic, L. Hamel, M. F. Basle and D. Chappard, Texture analysis of X-ray radiographs of iliac bone is correlated with bone micro-CT, *Osteoporosis Int.* **17** (2006) 447–454.
125. J. H. Hu, M. Ding, K. Søballe, J. E. Bechtold, C. C. Danielsen, J. S. Day and I. Hvid, Effects of short-term alendronate treatment on the three-dimensional microstructural, physical, and mechanical properties of dog trabecular bone, *Bone* **31**(5) (2002) 591–597.
126. F. S. L. Wong, J. C. Elliott, P. Anderson and G. R. Davis, Mineral concentration gradients in rat femoral diaphyses measured by X-ray microtomography, *Calcified Tissue Int.* **56** (1995) 62–70.
127. C. M. Bagi, N. Hanson, C. Andresen, R. Pero, R. Lariviere, C. H. Turner and A. Laib, The use of micro-CT to evaluate cortical bone geometry and strength in nude rats: Correlation with mechanical testing, pQCT and DXA, *Bone* **38** (2006) 136–144.
128. S. A. Arrington, J. E. Schoonmaker, T. A. Damron, K. A. Mann and M. J. Allen, Temporal changes in bone mass and mechanical properties in a murine model of tumor osteolysis, *Bone* **38** (2006) 359–367.
129. J. C. M. Teo, K. M. Si-Hoe, J. E. L. Keh and S. H. Teoh, Relationship between CT intensity, micro-architecture and mechanical properties of porcine vertebral cancellous bone, *Clin. Biomech.* **21** (2006) 235–244.
130. S. Y. Wan, A. P. Kiraly, E. L. Ritman and W. E. Higgins, Extraction of the hepatic vasculature in rats using 3D micro-CT images, *IEEE Trans. Med. Imaging* **19** (2000) 964–971.
131. R. H. Johnson, H. Hu, S. T. Haworth, P. S. Cho, C. A. Dawson and J. H. Linehan, Feldkamp and circle-and-line cone-beam reconstruction for 3D micro-CT of vascular networks, *Phys. Med. Biol.* **43** (1998) 929–940.
132. S. M. Jorgensen, O. Demirkaya and E. L. Ritman, Three-dimensional imaging of vasculature and parenchyma in intact rodent organs with X-ray micro-CT, *Am. J. Physiol. Heart Circulat. Physiol.* **44** (1998) H1103–H1114.
133. B. Kantor, E. L. Ritman, D. R. Holmes and R. S. Schwartz, Imaging angiogenesis with three-dimensional microscopic computed tomography, *Current Interven. Cardiol. Report* **2** (2000) 204–212.
134. D. N. Simopoulos, S. J. Gibbons, J. Malysz, J. H. Szurszewski, G. Farrugia, E. L. Ritman, R. B. Moreland and A. Nehra, Corporeal structural and vascular micro architecture with X-ray micro computerized tomography in normal and diabetic rabbits: Histopathological correlation, *J. Urol.* **165** (2000) 1776–1782.

135. D. A. Nordsletten, S. Blackett, M. D. Bentley, E. L. Ritman and N. P. Smith, Structural morphoplogy of renal vasculature, *Am. J. Physiol. Heart Circulat. Physiol.* **291**(1) (2006) H296–309.
136. S. T. Ho and D.W. Hutmacher, A comparison of micro CT with other techniques used in the characterization of scaffolds, *Biomaterials* **27** (2006) 1362–1376.
137. V. Karageorgiou and K. Kaplan, Porosity of 3D biomaterial scaffolds and osteogenesis, *Biomaterials* **26** (2005) 5474–5491.
138. A. S. P. Lin, T. H. Barrows, S. H. Cartmell and R. E. Guldberg, Microarchitecture and mechanical characterization of oriented porous polymer scaffolds, *Biomaterials* **24** (2003) 481–489.
139. F. Wang, L. Shor, A. Darling, S. Khalil, W. Sun, S. Guceri and A. Lau, Precision extruding deposition and characterization of cellular poly-E-caprolactone tissue scaffolds, *Rapid Prototyp. J.* **10**(1) (2004) 42–49.
140. T. S. Karande, J. L. Ong and C. M. Agrawal, Diffusion in musculoskeletal tissue engineering scaffolds: Design issues related to porosity, permeability, architecture, and nutrient mixing, *Ann. Biomed. Eng.* **32**(12) (2004) 1728–1743.
141. R. Landers, U. Hubner, R. Schmelzeisen and R. Mulhaupt, Rapid prototyping of scaffolds derived from thermoreversible hydrogels and tailored for applications in tissue engineering, *Biomaterials* **23** (2002) 4437–4447.
142. R. M. Schek, J. M. Taboas, S. J. Segvich, S. J. Hollister and P. H. Krebsbach, Engineered osteochondral grafts using biphasic composite solid free-form fabricated scaffolds, *Tissue Eng.* **10**(9/10) (2004) 1376–1385.
143. S. T. Ho and D. W. Hutmacher, Application of micro CT and computational modeling in tissue engineering applications, *Computer-Aided Design* **37**(11) (2005) 1151–1161.
144. X. X. Shao, D. W. Hutmacher, S. T. Ho, J. C. H. Goh and E. H. Lee, Evaluation of a hybrid scaffold/cell construct in repair of high loading-bearing osteochondral defects in rabbits, *Biomaterials* **27**(7) (2006) 1071–1080.
145. C. Verna, C. Bosch, M. Dalstra, U. M. E. Wikesjo and L. Trombelli, Healing patterns in calvarial bone defects following guided bone regeneration in rats, *J. Clin. Periodontol.* **29** (2002) 865–870.
146. J. T. Schantz, W. H. Dietmar, C. X. F. Lam, M. Brinkman, K. M. Wong, T. C. Lim, N. Chou, R. E. Guldberg and S. H. Teoh, Repair of calvarial defects with customized tissueengineered bone grafts II. Evaluation of cellular efficiency and efficacy *in vivo*, *Tissue Eng.* **9** (S1) (2003) S127-S139.
147. A. C. Jones, B. Milthorpe, H. Averdunk, A. Limaye, T. J. Senden, A. Sakellariou, A. P. Sheppard, R. M. Sok, M. A. Knackstedt, A. Brandwood, D. Rohner and D. W. Hutmacher, Analysis of 3D bone ingrowth into polymer scaffolds via micro-computed tomography imaging, *Biomaterials* **25** (2004) 4947–4954.
148. L. Meinel, V. Karageorgiou, R. Fajardo, B. Snyder, V. Shinde-Patil, L. Zichner, D. Kaplan, R. Langer and G. Vunjak-Novakovic, Bone tissue engineering using human mesenchymal stem cells: Effects of scaffold material and medium flow, *Ann. Biomed. Eng.* **32**(1) (2004) 112–122.
149. M. E. Easterly, Body condition scoring: Comparing newly trained scorers and microcomputed tomography imaging, *Lab Animals* **30** (2001) 46–49.
150. D. Brasse, B. Humbert, C. Mathelin, M. C. Rio and J. L. Guyonnet, Towards an inline reconstruction architecture for micro-CT systems, *Phys. Med. Biol.* **50** (2005) 5799–5811.
151. S. V. N. Jaecques, E. De Smet, M. Wevers, J. Van der Sloten, G. Van der Perre and I. Naert, Feasibility of monitoring bone remodeling around loaded percutaneous tibial implants in guinea pigs by *in vivo* microfocus computed tomography, *Int. Cong. Ser.* **1230** (2001) 422–428.

152. H. L. Su, F. G. Spinale, L. W. Dobrucki, J. Song, J. Hua, S. Sweterlitsch, Dione D. P, P. Cavaliere, C. Chow, B. N. Bourke, X. Y. Hu, M. Azure, P. Yalamanchili, R. Liu, E. H. Cheesman, S. Robinson, S. Edwards and J. Sinusas, Noninvasive targeted imaging of matrix metalloproteinase activation in a murine model of postinfarction remodeling, *Circulation* **112** (2005) 3157–3167.

153. M. Ralph, High resolution QCT-based models of bone architecture, in *Computer Technology in Biomaterials Science and Engineering*. Jos Vander Sloten, eds. Chapter 2a (2000), pp. 20–44.

154. W. Pistoia, B. Van Rietbergen, A. Laib and P. Ruegsegger, High-resolution threedimensional-pQCT images can be an adequate basis for *in-vivo* μFE analysis of bone, *J. Biomech. Eng.* **123** (2001) 176–183.

155. A. C. Jones, A. Sakellariou, A. Limaye, C. H. Arns, T. J. Senden, T. Sawkins and M. A. Knackstedt, Investigation of microstructural features in regenerating bone using micro computed tomography, *J. Mater. Sci.: Mater. Med.* **15** (2004) 529–532.

156. H. Takada, S. Abe, Y. Tamatsu, S. Mitarashi, H. Saka and Y. Ide, Threedimensional bone microstructures of the mandibular angle using micro-CT and finite element analysis: Relationship between partially impacted mandibular third molars and angle fractures, *Dental Traumatol.* **22** (2006) 18–24.

157. M. Cioffi, F. Boschetti, M. T. Raimondi and G. Dubini, Modeling evaluation of the fluid–dynamic microenvironment in tissue–engineered constructs: A micro–CT based model, *Biotechnol. Bioeng.* **93**(3) (2006) 500–510.

158. A. S. Barry and D. Farrokh, Oncologic PET/CT: Current status and controversies, *Eur. Radiol.* **15**(Supplement 4) (2005) D127–D132.

159. R. E. Guldberg, A. S. P. Lin, R. Coleman, G. Robertson and C. Duvall, Micro-computed tomography imaging of skeletal development and growth, *Birth Defects Res. (Part C)* **72** (2004) 250–259.

160. R. H. John, Interventional CT: 30 years' experience, *Eur. Radiol.* **15**(Supplement 4) (2005) D116–D120.

CHAPTER 7

METHODS IN COMBINED COMPRESSION AND ELONGATION OF LIVER TISSUE AND THEIR APPLICATION IN SURGICAL SIMULATION

ICHIRO SAKUMA

Department of Precision Engineering
School of Engineering, The University of Tokyo
7-3-1 Hongo Bunkyo-ku, Tokyo 113-8656, Japan
sakuma@miki.pe.u-tokyo.ac.jp

CHEEKONG CHUI

Institute of Environmental Studies
Graduate School of Frontier Sciences, University of Tokyo
7-3-1 Hongo Bunkyo-ku, Tokyo 113-8656, Japan
and
Department of Mechanical Engineering
National University of Singapore, E3-05-23 Engineering Drive 3
Singapore 119260, Singapore
mpecck@nus.edu.sg

A fundamental problem in computer aided surgical simulation is soft tissue modeling. It is difficult to represent the complex biomechanical properties and yet computational efficient for fast simulation. This paper reviews the methodologies for determination of the elastic properties of porcine liver tissues. The combined compression and elongation test is used as a unified framework to study the liver biomechanics for computer aided surgical simulation. At a length scale of approximately $10\,\text{mm}$, liver tissue is incompressible, anisotropic and nonlinear viscoelastic. It is stiffer during compression. The tissue sample will buckle under a mean stress of $2.313 \times 10^5\,\text{Pa}$ under compression. The Poisson's ratio was 0.466 ± 0.147 during compression and 0.431 ± 0.155 during elongation. Constitutive laws including strain energy based combined energy equation and equivalent stress and stain based multi-linear model were used in modeling the nonlinear stress-strain behavior of liver tissues under compression and elongation. Application of the experimental data and theoretical models is demonstrated via finite element simulation of liver organ deformation.

1. Introduction

Computer aided surgery (or computer integrated and robot assisted surgery) is performed to satisfy unmet complex needs in surgeries such as image guided surgeries. Image guided surgeries or minimally invasive surgeries are becoming increasingly popular. In an image guided surgery, the surgical procedure is facilitated by a real time correlation of the operative field to a monitor, which shows the precise location of a selected surgical instrument to the surrounding structures. This is different from the conventional open surgery in which the surgeons can see the tissue being operated on directly. The image guided surgery is both beneficial to patients and cost-effective, and is fast becoming the standard of care for various surgeries.[1]

A computer aided surgery process is complex. In a typical process shown in Fig. 1, its components include preoperative imaging, modeling and segmentation, simulation, then registering sources of data and applying these to the intervention on the patient. The interventions are monitored, corrected, or extended, according to the results of intraoperative imaging. Virtual reality-based simulation of image guided surgery has been reported by various investigators. Virtual reality techniques[2] and the emergence of automatic surgical tools and robots[3] have been driving an exciting area of research–computer simulation of surgical procedures or computer aided surgical simulation.

Virtual reality and simulator-based technology systems have significant practical value in training and in evaluating user responses in situation-specific problem solving for both the military and industrial sectors.[4,5] It is only natural that this technology be utilized for medical applications. For example, the various surgical simulation systems for interventional radiology, cardiology and neuro-radiology reported in Anderson *et al.*[6] and references cited therein focus on training of user skills, improving hand-eye coordination, training of specific patient management decision-making skills, training of very specific specialized skills, and evaluating treatment approaches for patient specific pretreatment planning. There are on-going research efforts to develop patient specific catheterization devices using simulation-based design technology.[7,8] Another application of computer programs enabling accurate modeling of soft tissue deformation is in surgical robot control systems for neurosurgery[9] as well as treatment of liver cancers.[10] Nevertheless, clinical applications of this surgical simulation technology are currently limited.

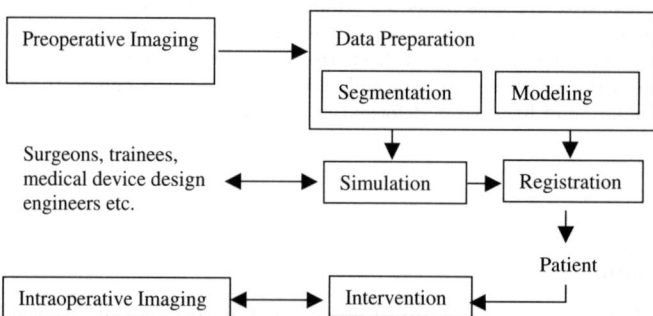

Fig. 1.   Typical computer aided surgery process: The focus of this study is on surgical simulation, in particular the biomechanical modeling of liver tissue. Outcome of simulation may be used for training as well as medical device design and evaluation.

As of today, virtual reality is not likely to be found in the operating room.[11] The underlying computer-based anatomical models are not quite realistic enough. There should be a faithful representation of geometry, boundary and loading conditions as well as mechanical properties of the organ. The fundamental problem in anatomical modeling is the lack of "physics" in particular soft tissue modeling of liver, kidney and brain. It is desirable to have the behavior of the object depend on the constitutive properties of the object being simulated. The mechanical properties of liver, kidney and brain tissues are also different. Brain tissue is apparently softer and is more viscous compared to that of liver tissue. Several studies have underlined the importance of duly considering elastic tissue deformation.[12]

Precise information about the elastic properties and corresponding constitutive laws of biological soft tissues determines the performance of surgical simulators. These tissues are highly nonlinear and complex. Quantitative data about the biomechanical properties of soft tissues are few. It is a challenge to derive a representative constitutive law that is clinically relevant as well as computationally efficient for computer aided surgical systems. Basic research and measurement experiments are required to understand and model the biomechanics of soft tissue. The field of biomechanics which is defined as the research and analysis of the mechanics of living organisms places great emphasis on the physiological correctness of the mathematical model. On the other hand, computational efficiency is essential for practical clinical application. The approach employed here involves refining the conventional approaches based on continuum mechanics to measure and model the biomechanics of liver tissue for computer aided surgical simulation.

This paper is organized as follows. In Sec. 2, we discuss the various methods in measuring the mechanical properties of liver tissues with particular focus on the combined compression and elongation test. The combined compression and elongation test enabled zero stress state of the tissue sample to be precisely determined for the tensile test. In Sec. 3, we characterize the mechanical properties of liver tissue. When deformed, kidney and brain will behave differently from liver. It is necessary to have an in-depth investigation on the biomechanical properties of liver on its own. In Sec. 4, the strength and elastic modulus of liver tissues are investigated. Mathematical modeling of liver tissue mechanics is discussed in Sec. 5. It is more beneficial to model the stress–strain behavior from combined compression and elongation test than that of simply compression or simply elongation. Organ deformation involves both compressible and tensile displacement. Depending on the specific applications, the constitutive model used is a trade off between computational accuracy and interactivity. Section 6 describes biomechanical modeling of liver organ and surgical simulation of organ deformation. In surgical simulation, the biomechanical model has to be computationally efficient so that the computer simulation could provide a timely solution. Concludes Sec. 7 with a brief discussion on the future work.

2. Measurement of Liver Tissue Elasticity

The developments in computer aided surgery where precise information about the elastic properties of living tissues are desired fuels the recent interest and progress in measuring the mechanical properties of biological tissues. The emphasis of these measurement methods is on low speed loading condition.

Surgical instruments had been equipped with force-sensing capabilities allowing elasticity measurement during surgeries.[13,14] Pathak et al.[15] applied indentation methods for *in vivo* experiments on the skin. However, these techniques lacked well-defined boundary conditions during experiment and often failed to address the complex material properties of tissue with nonlinear constitutive equations. MR elastography[16] was a possible method for non-invasive imaging of elastic properties in non-homogeneous organs. This method spatially maps and quantifies small displacements caused by propagating harmonic mechanical waves. Nevertheless, the resulting very small displacements and frequency range could not predict the tissue behavior in the range of strains and strain rates observed during surgical interventions. Kauer et al.[17] presented a tissue aspiration method for *in vivo* determination of the material parameters of biological soft tissue. An explicit axisymmetric finite element simulation of the aspiration experiment is used together with a Levenberge-Marquardt algorithm to estimate the material model parameters in an inverse parameter determination process. This tissue aspiration method with inverse finite element characterization has well defined mechanical boundary conditions and could induce relatively large tissue deformation. However, the condition of axisymmetry assumed in this method could not be met in the measurement experiments since soft tissues are in general anisotropic. Generally, it will be too expensive even if it is possible to generate enough data using *in vivo* measurement experiments to obtain adequate statistical interpretation of the mechanical properties of soft tissue. This is primarily due to the extreme technical and ethical demands on such experiments, and vast diversity in mechanical properties of biological tissues.

Indentation tests were used in Davies et al.[18] to determine the mechanical properties of spleen tissue. Tie and Desai[19] reported their indentation experiments to characterize the biomechanical properties of porcine liver tissue. Indentation experiment on whole liver organ with inverse finite element parameters estimation was reported in Onodera et al.[20] Inverse finite element parameters estimation has increasingly been used in measurement experiments[21] to help determine the mechanical properties of biological tissues. The tissue indentation equipment is generally customary designed and developed by the investigators. In Onodera et al.[20] an exponential strain energy function from Fung[22] was implemented into MARC 7 (MSC Software Corporation, USA), a commercially available finite element package popular for nonlinear analysis to perform inverse finite element parameters estimation. However, tissue indentation could be a complex mathematical problem involving both compressive and tensile properties of tissue. If at all possible, it is difficult to separate the compressive and tensile properties of the tissue samples.

Uniaxial load testing has long been used to measure the mechanical properties of both soft and hard tissues.[23] Miller and Chinzei[24] described a uniaxial compression test to measure the mechanical properties of brain tissue. Uniaxial compression and elongation experiments with porcine liver were reported in Chui *et al.*[25] and Sakuma *et al.*[26] Uniaxial load testing is simple but, nevertheless, provides us with basic and useful information on the mechanical properties of liver tissue. There are extensive reports on uniaxial testing with arterial elasticity, e.g. see Ref. 27 and references cited therein. Extensive uniaxial testing with liver tissue is relatively few. The zero stress state of the tissue sample must be identified for testing. However, this identification may not be easy since the neighborhood of the zero stress state of a soft tissue is soft and difficult to handle. The combined compression and elongation test[25,26] enabled the zero stress state to be precisely determined for the tensile test after the compression cycle. The combined compression and elongation cycle was clearly a simpler method compared to other more elaborated approaches for example the use of laser for initial state estimation.[9,24]

2.1. *Preparation of tissue sample*

Careful tissue sample preparation is necessary because cutting the samples possibly affects the results obtained. For example, particular attention should be paid to the orientation of tissue samples because biological tissues are mostly anisotropic, and their mechanical properties depend on direction. In order to determine a mechanical property as close as possible to that of *in vivo*, it is important to test the tissue fresh and maintain its freshness during experiments.

Fresh porcine livers were purchased from a local slaughterhouse for our measurement experiments. Rat liver organs were used in experiments in the "Virtual Rat" project.[28] However, it is generally believed that the mechanical properties of pig liver are close to those of human liver. The weight of a whole porcine liver was 1.5 ± 0.2 kg. The liver was approximately 210 mm by 330 mm with a thickness of 35 mm. Test samples were cylindrical in shape with a fixed diameter of 7 mm and height ranging from 4.5 mm to 11 mm. Figure 2 illustrates the preparation of cylindrical test sample. To establish maximum bonding between the tissue and the attachment unit, we tested the adhesion between liver tissue and various surfaces including wood, steel, cloth and rubber. Adhesion to the rubber plate was maintained with the highest tension used in our experiments. This was twice that obtained using wood, which had the lowest value. At a temperature of $20 \pm 3°C$, the surgical bond was able to sustain a stress of up to $380 \, \text{kg/cm}^2$.

Before testing, liver tissue samples were visually inspected for visible vessels and large porous. Samples with vessel or obvious porous were discarded. Since the samples were rather small at 7 mm diameter and generally less than 10 mm in height, and the fact that they were extracted near the liver surface, we were quite certain that the presence of vessel in sample was not significant.

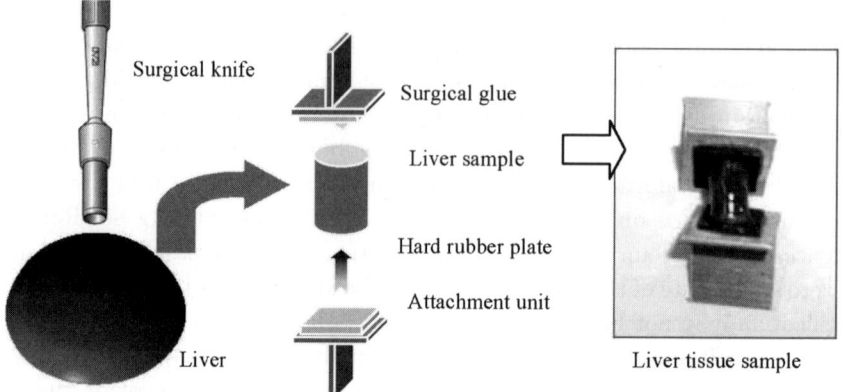

Fig. 2. Overview of cylindrical liver tissue sample preparation:[25] a circular surgical knife is used to extract the tissue sample, and then cut to the desired length using normal surgical knife. Surgical bond (Adhesive A, Sankyo Co. Ltd., Tokyo, Japan) was used to glue the sample to the attachments.

2.2. *Experimental setup*

The test unit was made and placed under a testing machine for experiments. Force and displacement were measured during the loading test by the precision instrument, Eztest, from Shimadzu Co Ltd. of Japan. This instrument had a resolution of $\pm 1\%$, and could support loading rates ranged from 0.5 to 1000 mm/min. A load cell that was capable of measuring a force up to 20 N was used. A video camera was placed in front of the test sample to record the deformation. The environmental temperature was maintained at about 22°C. Humidity was kept between 60% and 70% to prevent drying of the test pieces.

2.3. *Uniaxial loading tests*

The tests could be classified into following categories: elongation/compression tests, creep tests and relaxation tests. In uniaxial tests, an increasing force is steadily applied to a tissue sample in one direction, and the resulting sample deformation is measured, which gives relations between stress and strain (or stretch ratio). For theoretical treatment, stress and strain in the Lagrangian sense was reference. The tensile or compressive stress T is the load F divided by the cross sectional area A of the sample at zero stress state. The "stretch ratio" or "compression ratio" λ is the ratio of the length or height L of the sample stretched or compressed under the load divided by the initial length L_0 at the zero stress state. Strain ε is the ratio of the displacement $(L - L_0)$ divided by L_0, or $\varepsilon = \lambda + 1$.

Creep and relaxation tests are used for the evaluation of the viscoelasticity or inelastic properties of materials. In the creep tests, tissue sample elongation or compression is measured while a constant static or cyclic force is applied to the sample. In the relaxation test, stress reduction is observed while a tissue sample is elongated or compressed to a constant length and maintained at that length. Uniaxial tensile or compression testing is the most fundamental method for the determination of the elastic properties of materials, which are evaluated primarily on the basis of stress–strain relations.

In addition to performing the conventional uniaxial elongation and compression tests on liver tissue, force–displacement could be measured during a cycle of compression and elongation. In the combined compression and elongation test, the tissue sample is first compressed and then elongated at the same rate to its stress free position and beyond as illustrated in Fig. 3.

Based on the experimental results, by compressing a cylindrical liver sample of diameter 7 mm by a force of less than 1 N, the tensile test could be started at the zero stress and strain state. Figure 4 compares the measured force–strain data from the elongation only experiments and that of the elongation in the combined

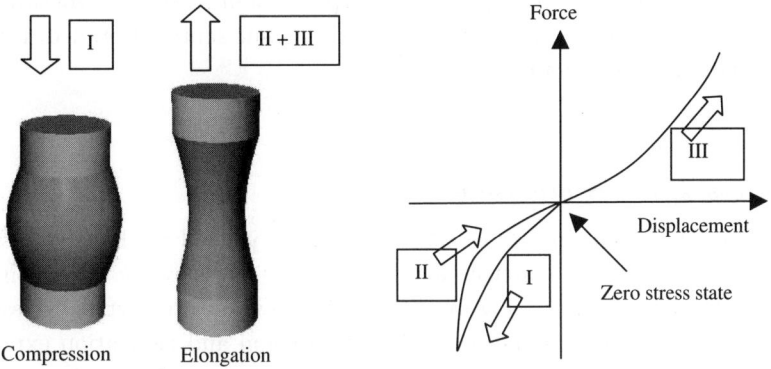

Fig. 3.   Illustration of combined compression and elongation test: I — compression phrase; II — return to stress free state; III — elongation phrase.

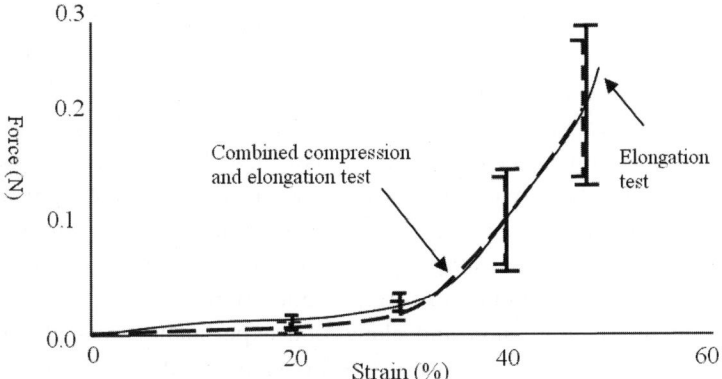

Fig. 4.   Comparison of experimental force–strain data from elongation only test and combined compression and elongation test: number of samples = 8, diameter = 7 mm; loading rate = 10 mm/min. Error bar indicates the standard deviation from the average experimental data.

compression and elongation test. The liver tissue samples were compressed up to
0.4 N in the combined compression and elongation test. The measured data between
the two experiments are compatible.

3. Characteristics of Liver Tissue

Liver is the second largest organ of the body after the skin. The surface of the liver
is covered by a membrane called the visceral peritoneum, also commonly referred
to as liver capsule. The liver capsule extends into the substance of liver as highly
branched septae. The human liver is comprised of 4 lobes, with the largest two, the
right and left lobe, separated by the falciform ligament. The liver lobes are made up
of many functional units called lobules. Each hepatic lobule, which is about 1–2 mm
in diameter, is a roughly hexagonal arrangement of plates of hepatocytes radiating
outward from a central vein in the center. Hepatic lobules are the structural unit of
the liver. They are delineated by the connective tissue septae. Detailed description
of liver anatomy can be found in Tortora.[29]

3.1. Stress–strain relationship

All the liver specimens in our *in vitro* experiment yielded nonlinear stress–strain
behavior, having higher distensibility in the low stress range and losing it at
progressively higher stresses. Figures 5(a) and 5(b) illustrated typical stress–strain
curves of a porcine liver tissue tested in compression and elongation experiments
respectively. Each curve could be divided into three parts. In the first part, from
O to A (toe region), the load increases exponentially with increasing compression.
This is the physiological range in which the tissue normally functions. In the second
part, from A to B (linear region), the stress–strain relationship is fairly linear. In the
third part, from B to C, the relationship is nonlinear and ends with rupture. B is the
yield point. At point C the maximum load is reached, corresponding to the ultimate
stress and strain. D is the break point. The slope defined by points A and B is the
elastic stiffness from which Young's modulus of liver tissue during compression and
elongation are derived respectively if linear elastic model is assumed in computation.
Young's modulus or elastic modulus is a measure of the stiffness of a given material.
Figure 5(c) shows the average stress–strain curve from combined compression and
elongation test of liver tissue samples. The average stress–strain curve is typically
used for biomechanical modeling in surgical simulation.

The combined compression and elongation experiments were also performed
on kidney and brain tissues. The stress–strain behaviors of liver, kidney and brain
tissues are different. Figure 6 compares the average stress–strain data. The brain
tissue is significantly softer compared to liver and kidney tissues. Kidney tissue is
stiffer than liver tissue.

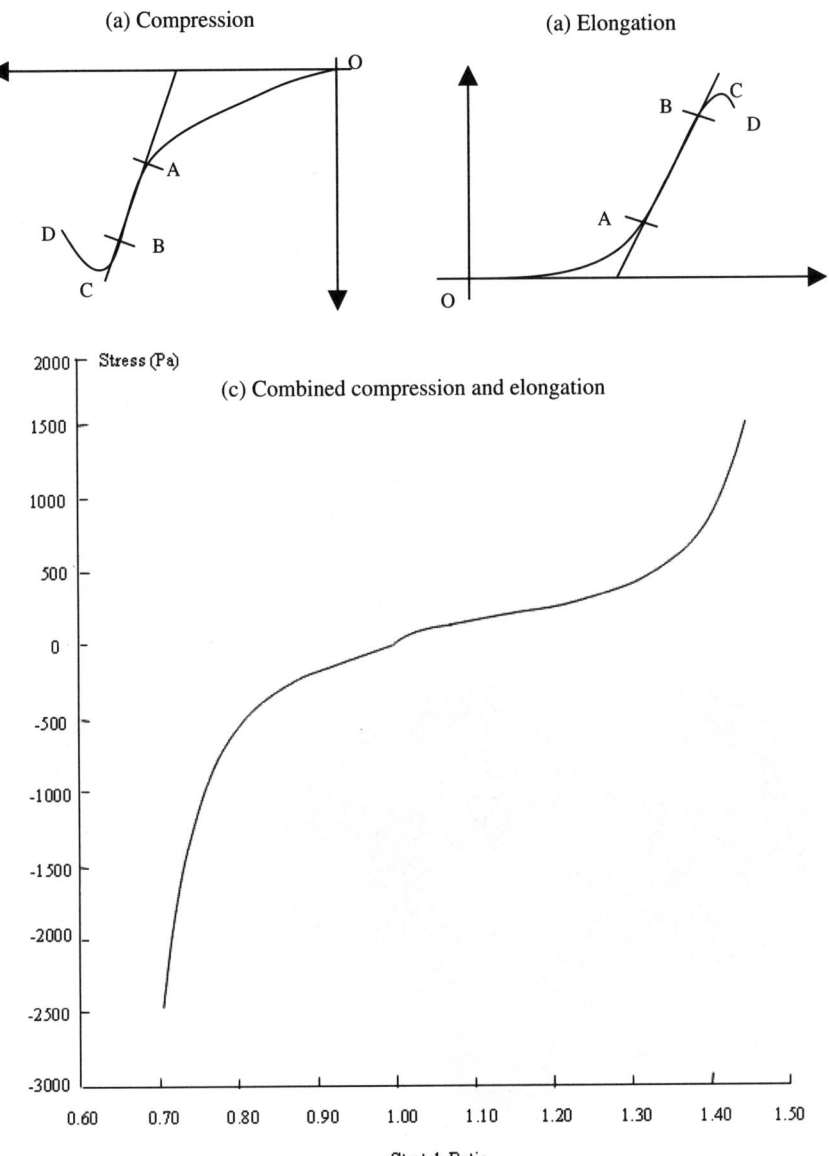

Fig. 5. Typical load–displacement curves of porcine liver tissue until fail during (a) compression and (b) elongation respectively. (c) Average stress–strain curve of combined compression and elongation experiment. Number of samples: 65 from 18 livers. Note that constant loading rate at 10 mm/min is used in all experiments.

3.2. *Nonhomogeneity*

Figure 7 compares the mass density of tissue samples extracted from various parts of a liver organ. Eight groups of samples were extracted from the surface at different locations (A1, A2, B1, B2, C1, C2, D1, D2) in the liver. Mass density is determined

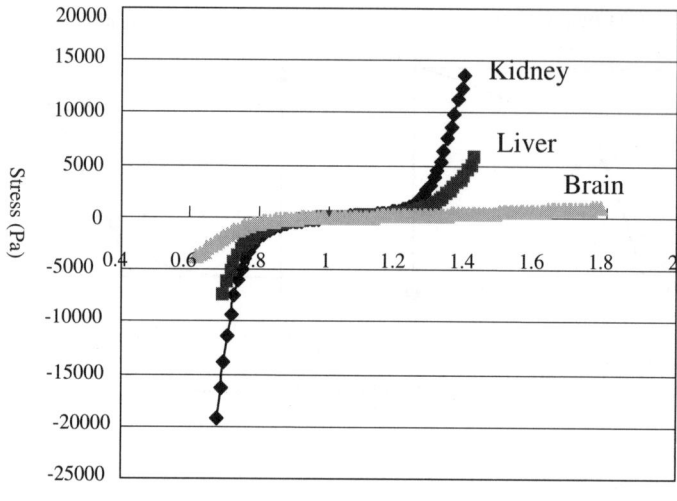

Fig. 6.   Comparison of experimental stress–strain data from combined compression and elongation tests of liver, kidney and brain tissues: number of samples = 5 for each tissue type; diameter: 7 mm; loading rate: 10 mm/min.

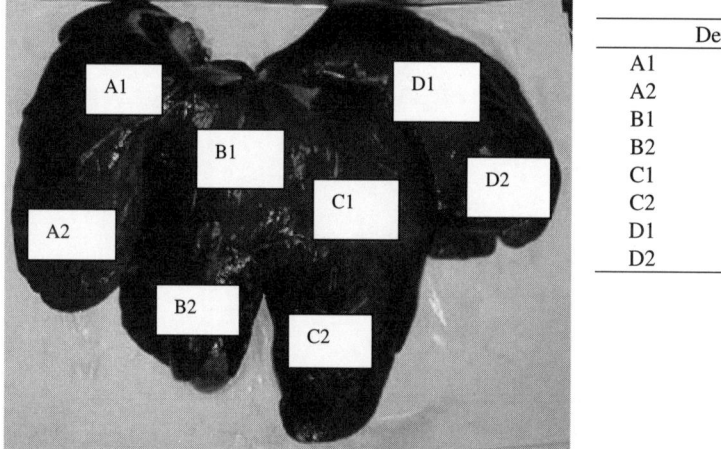

	Density (g/cm^3)
A1	1.070
A2	1.078
B1	1.030
B2	1.074
C1	1.058
C2	1.074
D1	1.074
D2	1.057

Fig. 7.   Mass densities of tissue samples extracted from different parts of the liver.

by dividing the measured weight by the volume of the tissue sample. There is no apparent different in the stress–strain relationship of these tissue samples in uniaxial loading tests.

From the comparison of the stress–strain curves from visceral side, diaphragmatic side and edge of the liver organs, it was observed that samples extracted from the upper surface (diaphragmatic side) of liver were noticeably harder than those from other parts of the liver. In the experiment,[25] a total of 21 samples were extracted from two porcine livers. Height of the cylindrical samples was about 5 mm. The loading rate was 10 mm/min. The presence of a thin capsular layer on the liver surface may help contribute to the stiffness. Since we were mainly interested in computer aided surgical simulation, with surgical devices such as needles approaching liver from the top, samples extracted from the diaphragmatic side of liver were used in our bio-mechanical analyses of liver properties.

3.3. *Effects of temperature*

The effect of temperature on the mechanical properties of liver is clinically important. Diseased liver organ is heated in RF ablation procedure, and cooled in cryosurgery for cancer cell destruction. Figure 8 compares the stress–strain behavior of liver tissue at different temperature (22°C, 37°C, 60°C and 80°C). The material behavior of liver tissue was essentially the same at 22°C and 37°C. At 60°C, the nonlinear shape of stress–strain curve remains although the tissue is softer. At 80°C, the liver tissue was heat-denatured. This agrees with the observation from Haemunerich et al.[30] that water loss from the samples was significant at temperature above 70°C. Haemunerich et al. reported an *in vitro* heating of liver samples using two electrodes. In our cooling experiments, we found that freezing has significant effects on the mechanical properties of porcine liver tissue. Chua et al.[31] reported an analytical study on the thermal effects of cryosurgery.

The temperature of tissue samples could be maintained with Ringer solution circulated at a constant rate during experiments. Ringer solution is a solution that is isotonic with blood. One liter of ringer solution contains 130 mEq of sodium ion, 109 mEq of choride ion, 28 mEq of lactate, 4 mEq of potassium ion and 3 mEq of calcium ion.

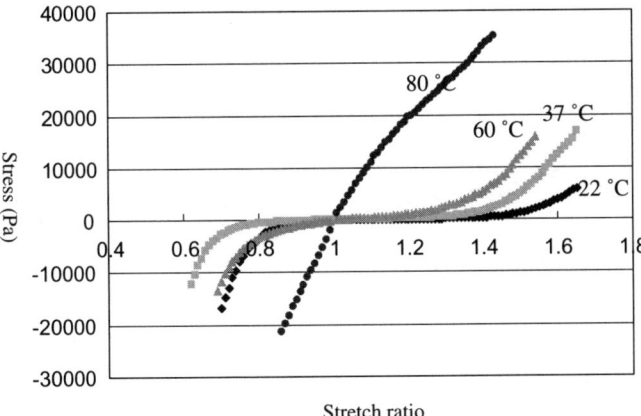

Fig. 8.   Comparison of experimental stress–strain data from combined compression and elongation tests of liver tissues at different temperature: number of samples: 12 (3 at each temperature); diameter: 7 mm; loading rate: 10 mm/min.

3.4. *Strain rate dependency*

The effect of strain rate on porcine liver tissue was shown to be relatively insignificant from various experiments (e.g. Refs. 19 and 25). Constant speed of elongation/compression of 1, 2, 5, 10, 20, 50, 100 and 200 mm/min are corresponded to strain rates of 0.003, 0.006 0.030, 0.061, 0.151, 0.303 and 0.606 per second respectively. Varying strain rate has little effect on hysteresis from the stress–strain curves obtained from compression and then elongation testing. Hysteresis is the energy dissipation between the loading and unloading of the tissue during mechanical tests. Figure 9 shows the hysteresis measured during the cycle of compression and elongation to zero stress state in combined compression and elongation experiments with varying loading rates. There is little change in hysteresis when the loading rates range between 5 and 50 mm/min.

As was also reported for other animal tissues,[22] porcine liver exhibited tissue relaxation. During the relaxation experiments, the liver tissue sample was compressed, and then the compression was maintained, the amount of force measured gradually decreased.[26] At low loading rates (1–2 mm/min), some tissue relaxation was observed, while very fast rates (50–200 mm/min) resulted in large increments between data points. Liver tissue is not linear viscoelastic when the loading rates are between 5 and 50 mm/min. The loading rate of 10 mm/min was found to be the most suitable for extensive measurement experiments. This corresponded to a strain rate of between 0.041 per second and 0.015 per second since our samples ranged in height from 4 to 11 mm. This was consistent with values required for our targeted application, that is, computer aided surgical simulation for

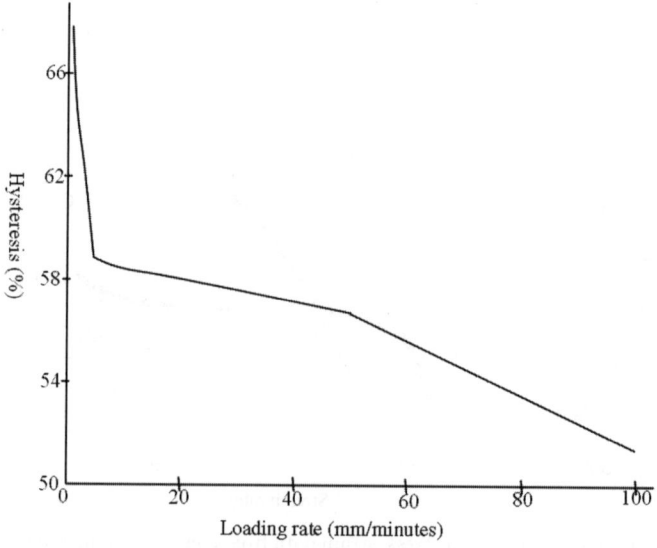

Fig. 9.   Strain rate dependency of liver tissue sample: number of samples = 54 from 9 porcine livers; diameter and height of the samples were 7 mm and 5.5–10 mm respectively.

abdominal surgery. Slightly higher strain rates were included in our study because we needed to predict the initial response of liver to a surgical probe. By testing all samples at the same rate, confounding effects of tissue viscoelasticity could be minimized.

3.5. *Incompressibility and Poisson's ratio*

When a solid is subjected to load, it deforms and changes its shape and volume. The volume of an incompressible material remains constant when deform. Biological soft tissues including liver have often been assumed to be incompressible. Liver tissue incompressibility can be studied via measurement of Poisson's ratio. The values of Poisson's ratio for most engineering materials are constant and range between 0.25 and 0.35.

With reference to a cylindrical sample of height H and diameter D under a load τ, elastic elongation or compression in the direction of the applied load (known as axial strain ε_a) is accompanied by contraction or expansion in the perpendicular direction (known as transverse strain ε_t). Poisson's ratio is defined as the negative ratio of transverse strain to axial strain ($\varepsilon_t/\varepsilon_a$). Poisson's ratio is a material property that has received relatively less attention. This parameter is difficult to measure experimentally particularly for biological soft tissue which is generally heterogeneous and anisotropic, in addition to its softness which makes handling difficult.

To determine Poisson's ratio, a digital video camera was used to record the compression and elongation process with force at each instant measured and noted. The video was then processed, and broken into individual frames. Each frame was processed to determine the mean diameter of the tissue samples D, and this value was compared with the previous frame to determine ΔD. The Poisson's ratios during compression and elongation were readily determined since the axial displacement ΔH is known. Figure 10(a) illustrates the experimental setup used to determine the Poisson's ratio of liver tissue, and a typical frame captured using the digital camera was shown in Fig. 10(b).

In theory, Poisson's ratio for a biological material can vary from less than zero to over one half. This is in contrast to the 0–0.5 range for isotropic continua. Consistent with the theory, we have determined that the Poisson's ratio for compression and elongation were 0.466 ± 0.147 and 0.431 ± 0.155 respectively. The values were measured from a size of 15 tissue samples for compression and 24 tissue samples for elongation. Figure 11 compares the Poisson's ratio for compression and elongation.

3.6. *Anisotropy*

Markers on the test sample were prepared and deformation of the sample during experiment was recorded via a digital video camera described above. Figure 12 was snap shots in the middle and end of the tension experiment. We observed that

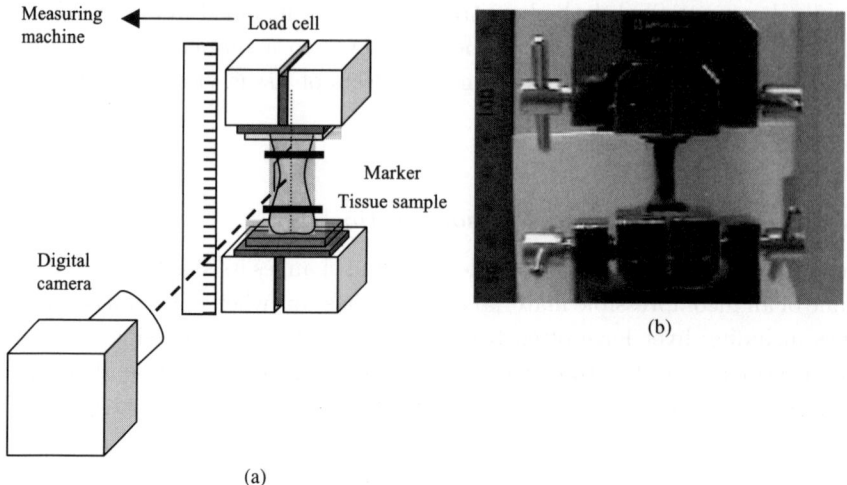

(a)

(b)

Fig. 10. Overview of experiments to determine Poisson's ratio of porcine liver tissues: (a) experimental setup for Poisson's ratio measurement; (b) snap shot of tissue sample during experiment.

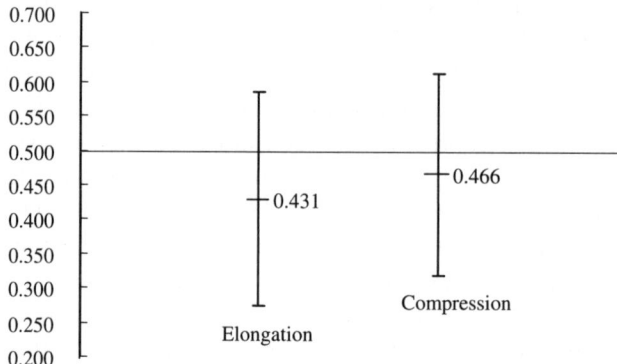

Fig. 11. Comparison of Poisson's ratio during elongation and compression experiments of liver tissue samples. Number of samples: 15 for compression; 24 for elongation.

there was a tendency for liver to displace in the direction of the force, which was acting perpendicular to the cross sectional x–y or horizontal plane. The originally horizontal marker placed on the specimen remained roughly horizontal at the middle and end of elongation. If there is no plane of symmetry or transverse, the marker will fail to remain horizontal. The horizontal displacement from necking differs from the vertical displacement. We did not observe any change in the shape of the cross sectional plane of the sample. The porcine liver tissue sample is likely to be a transversely isotropic material with the principal axis along the z direction or vertical plane. Investigation on the anisotropy properties of porcine liver tissue has been reported in Ref. 74.

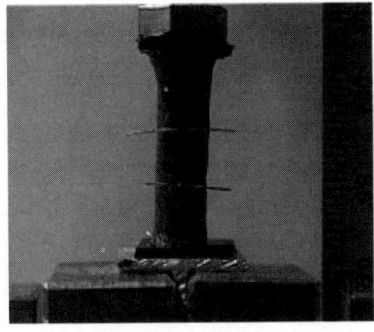 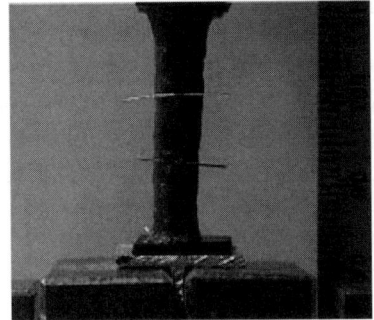

(a) During elongation test　　　　　　　　(b) End of elongation test

Fig. 12. Snap shots of deformation of liver tissue sample during experiment.

In summary, liver tissue is incompressible and is not isotropic at the length scale of approximately 10 mm. The liver tissue also possesses a nonlinear stress–strain behavior. It is not quite strain rate dependent. Linear viscoelasticity is not significant at moderate strain rate experienced during surgery. The liver tissue samples can be considered as a homogeneous material if they are extracted from the surface of the liver organ. They are noticeably harder than brain tissue and softer than kidney tissue.

4. Strength and Elastic Modulus of Liver Tissues

From investigation on the strength of liver tissue, the yield stress and strain were approximately 2.5×10^5 Pa and 69.5% for compression. With this yield stress, the compressive stress achieved by 1 N was one order of magnitude less than the yield stress. The resultant force–displacement relationship before and after preconditioning was found to have not change with 1 N of preconditioning load. Precondition may not be necessary since surgeon interacts with non preconditioned tissues and/or organ.

Assuming a linear elastic model, we determined that the mean modulus was 1355 kPa with a standard deviation of 0.7811×10^5 Pa. The mean yield stress was $-2.478 \pm 0.7811 \times 10^5$ Pa. The ultimate stress lies in the range of -1364×10^5 to -4.054×10^5 Pa. The maximum compression at rupture was between 61% and 79%. The measured parameters of the 13 *in vitro* destructive compression tests are listed in Table 1.

Determining Young's modulus of the liver tissue during elongation proved to be harder than compared with that of compression. This was due to our experimental method using surgical bond in attaching the specimen to the measuring instrument. As described in Sakuma *et al.*[26] this method had an advantage in stress concentration and possessed no slipping as in conventional uniaxial tests using clamps. However, the bond adhesiveness was weaker compared

Table 1. Material parameters measured from compression of liver specimens. The diameter and height of each specimen was 7 mm and 5 mm respectively. Stress is in terms of 1×10^5 N/m^2 and Young's modulus is in terms of 1×10^6 N/m.^{2}

Specimen	Yield		Maximum		Break		Young's modulus
	Stress	Strain (%)	Stress	Strain (%)	Stress	Strain (%)	
1	−3.118	−71	−3.352	−74	−3.066	−76	1.299
2	−3.637	−71	−3.767	−73	−3.611	−75	2.055
3	−3.118	−73	−3.507	−75	−3.170	−76	1.359
4	−2.910	−69	−3.144	−72	−2.858	−74	1.336
5	−1.948	−72	−2.104	−74	−1.974	−75	1.006
6	−2.468	−75	−2.754	−77	−2.442	−79	1.862
7	−1.922	−72	−2.130	−74	−1.689	−75	1.380
8	−2.546	−75	−2.754	−77	−2.598	−78	1.110
9	−2.468	−75	−2.754	−77	−2.442	−79	1.862
10	−3.637	−71	−4.053	−74	—	—	1.707
11	−1.546	−59	−1.689	−61	—	—	0.707
12	−1.533	−58	−1.611	−60.5	−1.585	−61	0.890
13	−1.351	−63	−1.364	−64	−1.039	−70	1.039
Mean	−2.478	−69.54	−2.691	−71.82	−2.313	−74.36	1.355
Standard deviation	0.781	5.825	0.862	5.988	0.805	5.104	0.413
Range	(−1.351, −3.638)	(58, 75)	(−1.364, −4.054)	(60.5, 77.4)	(−1.039, −3.612)	(61, 79)	(0.707, 2.055)

to the liver tissue. The attachment gave way prior to the break point of the liver tissue during elongation. In order to overcome this problem, separate tests using clamps were conducted to measure the ultimate stress and strain. The measured material parameters of all the seven tests are listed in Table 2. We determined that the mean value of ultimate stress and ultimate strain were 6.9×10^4 Pa and 79% respectively. Young's modulus was 227 kPa. This is significantly smaller than that determined during compression.

For comparison, liver tissue was stiffer than the muscular tissue and somewhat close to artery tissue. The artery tissue can withstand a larger strain compared to that of liver tissue. It was reported in the literature that Young's modulus, maximum stress and strain of artery were 200 kPa, 2×10^6 N/m^2 and 100% respectively during elongation. For muscular tissue, the corresponding values were 30 kPa, 2×10^5 N/m^2 and 60%.

Note that engineering stress and strain were referenced in the above discussions. For comparison, Young's modulus was measured from true stress and true strain during elongation experiments. The Young's modulus ranged from 500 to 750 kPa. This was consistent with the value of 650 kPa from experiments by Toyota Co, Japan reported in Chui et al.[31] It was typical for Young's modulus calculated from

Table 2. Material parameters measured from elongation of liver specimens. Height is between 7 and 9.5 mm, stress is in 1×10^4 N/m,^{2} and Young's modulus is in 1×10^5 N/m.^{2} All specimens have the same initial cross sectional area with diameter $= 0.007$ m.

Specimen	Yield		Maximum		Young's modulus
	Stress	Strain (%)	Stress	Strain (%)	
1	4.9	68.89	6.756	86.67	2.046
2	4.9	68.75	5.847	86.25	2.161
3	2.9	71.76	3.378	77.06	1.822
4	5.8	59.50	7.2	68.0	2.620
5	8.4	70.00	10.0	82.0	2.695
6	8.0	60.00	8.6	65.0	2.857
7	5.8	82.00	6.7	88.0	1.727
Mean	5.826	68.7	6.926	79.0	2.276
Standard deviation	1.89	7.61	2.088	9.32	0.448
Range	(2.91, 8.4)	(59.5, 82)	(3.378, 10.0)	(65.0, 88.0)	(1.727, 2.857)

true stress to be higher than that calculated using engineering stress. Nevertheless, the different was significant.

5. Mathematical Description of Liver Tissue Elasticity

A constitutive equation describes a physical property of a material. Its derivation should begin with empirical measurements. There are two alternatives for constitutive modeling: the continuum approach and the microstructure approach. With the first approach, the material is assumed to be a continuum. The relevant variables are identified, and these are related in a framework that ensures invariance under a change of frames. This was our approach in this paper.

One of the earliest reported mathematical/experimental treatments of biologic materials in the context of large deformation and modern continuum mechanics was that of Ticker and Sacks, 1964 and 1967, according to Vossoughi.[33] Since then, a number of constitutive models have appeared that described the passive material properties of both hard and soft tissues. However, few deal with abdominal tissues such as the liver. If the material is linear and the deformation is limited and infinitesimal, then a simple linear relationship derived according to Hooke's law might be sufficient to uniquely describe the stress–strain relationship. The formulation is not unique for a nonlinear material capable of undergoing large deformations. One constitutive model may well represent one type of soft tissue but not the others, or a model may well approximate a portion of the stress–strain curve, but not the entire space. The numerical complexity of these nonlinear functions is also an issue for interactive computing using currently available computer hardware and software.

In Carter *et al.*[13] and Davies *et al.*[18,34] the authors described biomechanical modeling with experimental indentations of animal abdominal organs, including liver. Their study assumed that the tissues were isotropic, homogeneous and incompressible. A nonlinear constitutive model based on a strain energy polynomial function was used in Miller[35] to model liver and kidney, using experimental results from *in vivo* experiments on Rhesus monkeys by Melvin *et al.*[36] The experiments approximated uniaxial compression under high strain rates typical for car crashes. These nonlinear models were numerically complex, and not suitable for fast medical simulation.

A well-known approach for studying nonlinear constitutive relations of bodies capable of finite deformation is to postulate that elasticity has the form of an elastic potential, or strain energy function, W. A number of constitutive models based on strain energy have already been proposed to describe the passive material properties of soft tissues. For solid biomechanics, most of the work has concentrated on blood vessels and myocardium. There are fewer reports of work on lung, skin, ligament, tendon, cartilage and bone tissue. Chui *et al.*[25] reports strain energy based constitutive relation that is derived from extensive measurements on liver tissue samples. There are also some recent reports on empirical expressions for fitting uniaxial tensile stress–strain relationship of soft tissue. These expressions are generally computational efficient and do not reduce to the form of strain energy. We tried to determine a constitutive equation that could fit the experimental data. The theoretical curve should follow the shape of the average curve with small standard error. Standard error is defined as root means square errors (RMSE), and is calculated from the difference between the theoretical estimate and the experimental measurement. To estimate the coefficients for the nonlinear functions, software for nonlinear least-square data fitting using the Gauss–Newton method could be used. Generally, models with few material parameters are preferred for the purpose of computational efficiency. Numerical stability of the parameters is desired for finite element computation. Depending on the specific applications, the constitutive model used is a trade off between computational accuracy and interactivity. Stress–strain graphs of compression, elongation and combined compression and elongation experiments can be found in Chui *et al.*[25]

5.1. *Empirical expressions*

The most popular expression that is not reduced to the form of strain energy is the exponential function by Tanaka and Fung.[37,38] Tanaka and Fung proposed a constitutive relation for soft tissue for simple uniaxial state of stress–strain as:

$$\sigma = (\sigma^* + \beta)e^{C_1(\lambda - \lambda^*)} - C_2$$

where σ and λ are the stress and stretch ratio, $\sigma*$ and $\lambda*$ corresponds to a point on the stress–strain curve, C_1 and C_2 are the material constants. A variant from

Fung[22] with an additional material constant is,

$$T = C_1 e^{C_2 \lambda} - C_3$$

where T is the engineering stress, C_1, C_2 and C_3 are the material constants. The other empirical formulae proposed to fit experimental stress–strain data include Kenedi *et al.*[39] and Ridge and Wright.[40] The former with two material constants is,

$$T = C_1 \lambda^{C_2 - 1} - \frac{1}{\lambda}.$$

The empirical formulae are simple. However, they are limited to a uniaxial state of stress–strain. These equations could model the stress–strain curve of elongation reasonably well. Generally, they do not fit the experimental data on compression of liver tissues well. All of these equations could not model the stress–strain curve from combined compression and elongation experiments. A more general multi-axial based formulation is preferred for medical simulation.

5.2. *Strain energy functions*

The strain energy for an elastic body is a function of the state of deformation. Let $\mathbf{X}$ denotes a point in the reference configuration. The current position of the point is denoted by $\mathbf{x}$, where $\mathbf{x}$ is a function of time. The gradient of $\mathbf{x}$ with respect to $\mathbf{X}$ is called the deformation gradient,

$$\mathbf{F} = \left(\frac{\partial \mathbf{x}}{\partial \mathbf{X}} \right)^T.$$

The right Cauchy–Green tensor, $\mathbf{C}$ is a measure of the strain the body experiences and is given by

$$\mathbf{C} = \mathbf{F}^T \mathbf{F}.$$

The constitutive assumption of nonlinear elasticity is that the stress tensor at point $\mathbf{x}$ depends only on the material and the deformation gradient at $\mathbf{x}$. If the mechanical properties do not depend explicitly on the particular point $\mathbf{x}$, the material is said to be homogeneous. The liver tissue is assumed to be homogeneous and incompressible in this investigation.

When a quantity is unchanged with a frame rotation, it is said to be invariant. From $\mathbf{C}$, which is a second order tensor, three scalar invariants can be formed by taking the trace of $\mathbf{C}$, $\mathbf{C}^2$ and $\mathbf{C}^3$. They are

$$I = \text{trace}(\mathbf{C}) = C_{ii}, \quad II = \text{trace}(\mathbf{C}^2) = C_{ij}C_{ji} \text{ and } III = \text{trace}(\mathbf{C}^3) = C_{ij}C_{jk}C_{ki}.$$

However, it is customary to use strain invariants

$$I_1 = I, \quad I_2 = \frac{1}{2}(I^2 - II) \quad \text{and} \quad I_3 = \frac{1}{6}(I^3 - 3I \cdot II + 2III) = \det(\mathbf{C}).$$

Assuming that liver tissue is isotropic, the strain energy function can be expressed as a function of the above strain invariants, $W(I_1, I_2, I_3)$. We denote λ_i as the principal values of $\mathbf{F}$ and I_i is a function of λ_i.

$$\mathbf{F} = \begin{pmatrix} \lambda_1 & & \\ & \lambda_2 & \\ & & \lambda_3 \end{pmatrix}$$

Since liver is known to comprise highly incompressible material, $\det \mathbf{F} = \lambda_1 \lambda_2 \lambda_3 = 1$. Under uniaxial deformation, the cross-sectional area of the cylindrical sample reduces by $1/\lambda$ when the height of the sample is increased by a factor of λ. By setting $\lambda = \lambda_3$, we have $\lambda_1 = \lambda_2 = \frac{1}{\sqrt{\lambda_3}}$. Invariants I_1, I_2 and I_3 under uniaxial deformation can be evaluated as $I_1 = \lambda^2 + 2/\lambda$, $I_2 = 2\lambda + 1/\lambda^2$ and $I_3 = 1$, respectively.

For an elastic material, the second Piola-Kirchhoff stress tensor $\mathbf{S}$ can be expressed in terms of strain energy W and Green–Lagrange strain tensor $\mathbf{E}$ as

$$\mathbf{S} = \frac{\partial W}{\partial \mathbf{E}} = 2\frac{\partial W}{\partial \mathbf{C}}.$$

The Cauchy stress $\boldsymbol{\sigma}$ is related to $\mathbf{S}$ by

$$\boldsymbol{\sigma} = \frac{1}{J}\mathbf{F} \cdot \mathbf{S} \cdot \mathbf{F}^T$$

where $J = \det \mathbf{F}$. Component of $\boldsymbol{\sigma}$ in the tensile or compressive direction could now be expressed as partial derivative of W by the invariants.

$$\sigma = 2\frac{\partial W}{\partial I_1}\left(\lambda^2 - \frac{1}{\lambda}\right) + 2\frac{\partial W}{\partial I_2}\left(\lambda - \frac{1}{\lambda^2}\right). \tag{1}$$

Cauchy stress $\boldsymbol{\sigma}$ is related to the first Piola-Kirchhoff stress tensor $\mathbf{T}$ by

$$\boldsymbol{\sigma} = \frac{1}{J}\mathbf{F} \cdot \mathbf{T}.$$

Since $\sigma = \lambda T$, we can deduce from Eq. (1) that

$$T = \frac{2}{\lambda}\frac{\partial W}{\partial I_1}\left(\lambda^2 - \frac{1}{\lambda}\right) + \frac{2}{\lambda}\frac{\partial W}{\partial I_2}\left(\lambda - \frac{1}{\lambda^2}\right). \tag{2}$$

Suppose that the original cross sectional area of the cylindrical sample used in our experiment is A_0 and the tensile or compressive load is F,

$$T = \frac{F}{A_0}.$$

Suppose that the original length of the cylindrical sample is L_0, the displacement is $\Delta L = L_0(\lambda - 1)$.

T and ΔL are concurrently measured in the experiments. By comparing the experimental curve obtained by plotting T against λ with the theoretical curve from Eq. (2) obtained using various strain energy functions, the strain energy function that can best represent the material behavior of porcine liver tissue could be determined. For example, with the following Mooney–Rivlin energy function with nine material constants (known as the 9-constant theory),[43]

$$W = C_1(I_1 - 3) + C_2(I_2 - 3) + C_3(I_3 - 3)^2 + C_4(I_1 - 3)(I_2 - 3)$$
$$+ C_5(I_2 - 3)^2 + C_6(I_1 - 3)^3 + C_7(I_1 - 3)^2(I_2 - 3)$$
$$+ C_8(I_1 - 3)(I_2 - 3)^2 + C_9(I_2 - 3)^3$$

where C_1, C_2, C_3, C_4, C_5, C_6, C_7, C_8 and C_9 are material constants. The stress–strain relationship could be derived by substituting W into Eq. (2). The resulting equation was highly complex, with the highest order term having a power of 6 and the lowest order term having a power of -5.

Equation (3) is the 2-constant version of the energy function for the Mooney–Rivlin material.

$$W = \frac{C_1}{2}(I_1 - 3) + \frac{C_2}{2}(I_2 - 3) \tag{3}$$

where C_1 and C_2 are material constants and C_1, $C_2 > 0$. Similarly, partial differentiation of W, with I_1 and I_2 obtained from Eq. (2) yielded the following stress–strain relation.

$$T = C_1\lambda + C_2 - \frac{C_1}{\lambda^2} - \frac{C_2}{\lambda^3}$$

where λ is equal to strain plus one. For ease of discussion, we simply refer to $T = f(\lambda)$ as stress–strain relation. How well this stress–strain relation represented the experimental data could be evaluated using this stress–strain relation. Our assumption on isotropic, homogeneous and incompressible liver model is consistent with recent literature[13,18,35,41,42] on modeling of abdominal organs for surgical simulation.

There are several types of strain energy functions: polynomial, exponential, logarithmic and power. The Mooney–Rivlin material is an example of a strain energy function with polynomial form. The simplest polynomial-based energy function is the neo-Hookean model, which was originally applied to incompressible nonlinear elastic engineering materials. The neo-Hookean model is a subset of the Mooney–Rivlin model with $C_2 = 0$. There is only one material constant C_1 in this equation shown below:

$$W = C_1(I_1 - 3).$$

An exponential form of strain energy due to Fung[38] and Demiray[54] is shown as follows,

$$W = \frac{C_1}{2C_2}(e^{C_2(I_1-3)} - 1)$$

where C_1 and C_2 are material constants, and $C_1, C_2 > 0$.

Other exponential strain energy function includes Veronda and Westmann[44] shown as follows,

$$W = C_1(e^{C_3(I_1-3)} - 1) + C_2(I_2 - 3) + g(I_3).$$

If liver tissue is assumed as incompressible, $g(I_3) = 0$.

A related class of exponential equations with logarithmic form was proposed by Hayashi and Takamizawa.[45,46] The equation was intended for transversely anisotropic material:

$$W = -C_1\ln\left(1 - \frac{1}{2}C_2(I_1 - 3)^2 + \frac{1}{2}C_3(I_4 - 1)^2 + C_4(I_1 - 3)(I_4 - 1)\right).$$

The corresponding logarithmic equation for isotropic material is as follows,

$$W = -C_1\ln(1 - C_2(I_1 - 3)).$$

The main difference between isotropic version and the original Hayashi equation is the absent of invariant I_4 in the former. This invariant was not applicable with an isotropic material.

The fourth type of commonly used constitutive relation is the power law of the form $T = KS^n$ where T is the Lagrangian stress tensor, S is the strain or strain rate tensor, and K and n are the material constants. The advantage of power law stress–strain function is its simplicity. The following equation originally proposed by Tanaka and Fung[37] was used to model the zero-stress state of blood vessel walls in Xie et al.[47]

$$T = C_1(\lambda - 1)^{C_2}.$$

Other applications of the power law energy function include the formulation of extrafibrillar matrix of tendor material as a hyperelastic material using Odgen form of strain energy function[49] expressed by,

$$W = \sum_{n=1}^{3} \frac{C_n}{\alpha_n}(\lambda_1^{0.5\alpha_n} + \lambda_2^{0.5\alpha_n} + \lambda_3^{0.5\alpha_n}),$$

$$T = \sum_{n-1}^{3} \frac{C_n}{2}(\lambda^{\alpha_n} - \lambda^{0.5\alpha_n-1}).$$

A variant of Odgen model was proposed in Bogen et al.[50] to describe passive myocardial behavior, where C_1 and C_2 are material constants. The equations were as follows,

$$W = \frac{C_1}{C_2}(\lambda_1^{C_2} + \lambda_2^{C_2} + \lambda_3^{C_2} - 1),$$

$$\sigma = C_1(\lambda^{C_2} + \lambda^{-2C_2}).$$

The corresponding first Piola-Kirchhoff form of Bogen equation is

$$T = C_1(\lambda^{C_2-1} + \lambda^{-2C_2-1}).$$

The combined logarithmic and polynomial model[25] can be derived in the same spirit as the derivation of combined exponential and polynomial model in Fung *et al.*[51] At low strain, the logarithmic component in the combined model was small, and the polynomial component was the dominant one. Their roles were reversed at high strain. The combined logarithmic and polynomial model is therefore advantageous in describing the entire stress–strain curve. Note that the Veronda and Westmann model also has both exponential and polynomial terms. The Veronda and Westmann model was a sum of an exponential function and a polynomial originally for constitutive modeling of the skin. The combined logarithmic and polynomial equation for isotropic materials is as follows,

$$W = \frac{-C_1}{2}\ln(1 - C_2(I_1 - 3)) + C_3(I_1 - 3).$$

To simplify the discussion, we referred to this equation as the combined logarithmic and polynomial model or combined energy model.

Almost all the constitutive models provided good fits for the experimental data over the elongation region. The fits for the neo-Hookean and the Mooney–Rivlin (2-constants) were not acceptable for the purpose of fitting the entire curves. Not all equations provided good fits for the experimental compression data. The Tanaka model could not match the compression stress–strain curve since a power equation could not represent compression since the theoretical stress computed using this equation was always positive for all positive stretch ratios. Failure of these equations to match the experimental data of combined compression and elongation test was partly due the difficulties in representing both negative and positive domains numerically. A RMSE of greater than 120 Pa is considered a bad fit. The combined energy model and Mooney–Rivlin (9-constant) model were the only models that could adequately represent these data.

The best constitutive model appeared to be the combined logarithmic and polynomial equation.[25] The combined energy equation provided a good fit for the stress–strain relationships in the tests involving compression followed by elongation, as well as consistently matching the independent compression and elongation data. Although the combined model has larger RMSE than that of Mooney–Rivlin (9-constant, the former has smaller number of material constants and the parameters are numerically more stable. With Mooney–Rivlin (9-constant) model, the material parameters varied widely — a parameter could be positive in one

Table 3. Material parameters of combined energy model in representing elongation, compression and combined compression and then elongation experimental data.

$$W = \frac{C_1}{2} \ln(1 - C_2(I_1 - 3)) + C_3(I_1 - 3)$$

	Elongation	Compression	Combined Compression and Elongation
C_1	−337.7	−7881.1	−342.4
C_2	2.2	1.6	1.9
C_3	−287.7	−3941.4	−136.0

representation and negative in another. This pitfall was typical with polynomial-based constitutive equation. It could cause very different mechanical behavior in 3D cases and pose serious accuracy issues during numerical analysis such as finite element method.[48] Table 3 lists the material constants used in the combined energy model to fit the average stress–strain curve respectively from elongation, compression and combined compression and elongation experiments. More details on the curve fitting results can be found in Chui *et al.*[25]

We repeated the analyses for liver tissue with porcine kidney and brain tissues. The experimental conditions and procedures were the same for all three types of soft tissues. A close fit was possible with the combined logarithmic and polynomial model. The combined logarithmic and polynomial model could model these tissues with similar errors, and small deviations in material parameters. The polarity of the parameters did not change in the combined model. This demonstrates the suitability of our combined logarithmic and polynomial energy function as the model of choice for soft tissues in general and liver tissue in particular. The experiments with porcine kidney and brain tissues were conducted preliminary with five test samples each.

5.3. *Image based inverse finite element parameter estimation*

Although the strain energy based constitutive equations are generally valid for three-dimensional stress state, the material parameters determined in this section are limited by the uniaxial loading experiments. Typical multi-axial experiments involve frozen tissue. This will inevitably alter the biomechanics of underlying tissue. Image based inverse finite element parameter estimation could be used in conjunction with uniaxial combined compression and elongation experiments to determine the material parameters of liver tissue in three-dimensional stress state.

Figure 13(a) is a flow chart that illustrates the process. Input to the method was video images of the deformation. The video was processed and separated into individual frames of deformation with known force and time. A displacement driven axisymmetric finite element model of the tissue sample was developed to determine mechanical properties of liver tissue (Figure 13(b)). This generic model was adjusted to represent liver tissue sample height measured during experiments. The diameter of the sample was set at 7 mm. The planar surface was assumed to be flat and bonded to the hard rubber plates. Due to asymmetry, only 1/8 of the tissue sample is required to be modelled. The model comprises of eight nodes brick elements. MARC 7 a commercially available finite element solver is used in conjunction with Patran 2001 (MSC Software Corporation, USA), a pre- and post processor for CAE simulation, in the solution process as well as material properties assignment. From the list of instantaneous parameters, a set of parameters is selected based on its ability to model the stress–strain curve.

Recall that Piola-Kirchhoff stress can be expressed in terms of energy W and Green–Lagrange strain E_{ij} as follows:

$$S_{ij} = \frac{\partial(W)}{\partial E_{ij}}.$$

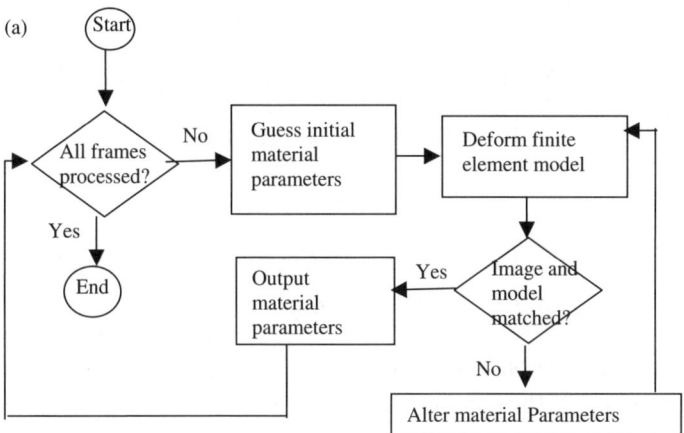

Fig. 13(a). Overview of image based inverse finite element parameters estimation: flow chart for estimation of material parameters for instantaneous deformation.

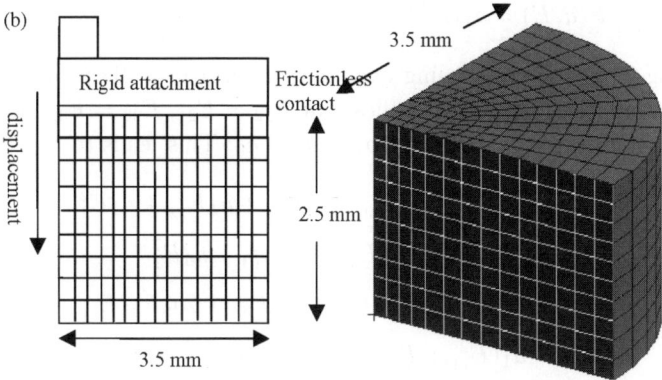

Fig. 13(b). Overview of image based inverse finite element parameters estimation: finite element modeling.

For modeling of biological soft tissue, a popular constitutive equation was the pseudo-strain-energy function proposed by Fung.[52] Following is the original generalized exponential equation where α_{ijk}, β_0, β_{mnpq}, γ_{ij} and κ_{ijkl} are constants to be determined empirically,

$$W = \frac{1}{2}\alpha_{ijk}E_{ij}E_{kl} + (\beta_0 + \beta_{mnpq}E_{mn}E_{pq})\exp(\nu_{ij}E_{ij} + \kappa_{ijk}E_{ij}E_{kl} + \cdots).$$

The derivation could be illustrated by first considering a two dimension problem space. Following equation is the simplified 2D version that is valid for the physiological range. Note that E_{12} is the shear.

$$W = \frac{1}{2}(\alpha_1 E_{11}^2 + \alpha_2 E_{22}^2 + \alpha_3 E_{12}^2 + \alpha_3 E_{21}^2 + 2\alpha_4 E_{11}E_{22})$$
$$+ \frac{1}{2}C\exp(a_1 E_{11}^2 + a_2 E_{22}^2 + a_3 E_{12}^2 + a_3 E_{21}^2 + 2a_4 E_{11}E_{22}$$
$$+ \nu_1 E_{11}^3 + \nu_2 E_{22}^3 + \nu_4 E_{11}^2 E_{22} + \nu_5 E_{11}E_{11}^2).$$

By having ν's terms equal to 0, the equation can be simplified further to

$$W = f(\alpha, E) + C\exp(F(a, E)),$$

where

$$f(\alpha, E) = \alpha_1 E_{11}^2 + \alpha_2 E_{22}^2 + \alpha_3 E_{12}^2 + \alpha_3 E_{21}^2 + 2\alpha_4 E_{11}E_{22},$$
$$F(a, E) = a_1 E_{11}^2 + a_2 E_{22}^2 + a_3 E_{12}^2 + a_3 E_{21}^2 + 2a_4 E_{11}E_{22}.$$

If we are considering physiological range only and have no concern on very small strain, we can simplify the exponential energy function further to

$$W = C\exp(F(a, E)).$$

Assuming that liver tissue is isotropic ($E_{12} = E_{21}$),

$$F(a, E) = a_1(E_{11}^2 + E_{22}^2) + 2a_3 E_{12}^2 + 2a_4 E_{11}E_{22}.$$

Following is the corresponding exponential term in a 3D problem space. The assumption on material isotropy implies that $E_{12} = E_{21}$, $E_{23} = E_{32}$ and $E_{13} = E_{31}$. Also $a_1 = a_2 = a_3$, $a_4 = a_5 = a_6$ and $a_7 = a_8 = a_9$. This leads to

$$F(a, E) = a_1 E_{11}^2 + a_2 E_{22}^2 + a_3 E_{33}^2 + a_4 E_{12}^2 + a_4 E_{21}^2$$
$$+ a_5 E_{23}^2 + a_5 E_{32}^2 + a_6 E_{13}^2 + a_6 E_{31}^2$$
$$+ 2a_7 E_{11}E_{22} + 2a_8 E_{22}E_{33} + 2a_9 E_{33}E_{11}$$
$$= a_1(E_{11}^2 + E_{22}^2 + E_{33}^2) + 2a_4(E_{12}^2 + E_{23}^2 + E_{31}^2)$$
$$+ 2a_7(E_{11}E_{12} + E_{22}E_{23} + E_{33}E_{31}).$$

Hence,

$$W = C \exp(F(a, E)),$$

where

$$F(a, E) = a_1(E_{11}^2 + E_{22}^2 + E_{33}^2) + 2a_4(E_{12}^2 + E_{23}^2 + E_{31}^2)$$
$$+ 2a_7(E_{11}E_{12} + E_{22}E_{23} + E_{33}E_{31})$$

Note that if effect from shear is not considered then $a_4 = a_5 = a_6 = 0$. If the effect similar to Poisson's ratio is negligible, $a_7 = a_8 = a_9 = 0$.

Equivalent logarithmic energy function is given as follows:

$$W = -C \ln(F(a, E)),$$

where

$$F(a, E) = \frac{a_1}{2}(E_{11}^2 + E_{22}^2 + E_{33}^2) + a_4(E_{12}^2 + E_{23}^2 + E_{31}^2)$$
$$+ a_7(E_{11}E_{12} + E_{22}E_{23} + E_{33}E_{31}).$$

The corresponding combined logarithmic and polynomial energy function is as follows:

$$W = -\frac{C}{2}\ln(1 - F(a, E)) - \frac{C}{2}F(a, E) + \frac{F_1(a, E)}{2},$$

where

$$F(a, E) = \frac{a_1}{2}(E_{11}^2 + E_{22}^2 + E_{33}^2) + a_4(E_{12}^2 + E_{23}^2 + E_{31}^2)$$
$$+ a_7(E_{11}E_{12} + E_{22}E_{23} + E_{33}E_{31})$$
$$F_1(a, E) = \frac{a_{10}}{2}(E_{11}^2 + E_{22}^2 + E_{33}^2) + a_{11}(E_{12}^2 + E_{23}^2 + E_{31}^2)$$
$$+ a_{12}(E_{11}E_{12} + E_{22}E_{23} + E_{33}E_{31}).$$

In modeling the uniaxial tension/compression tests that we performed, the shear terms are ignored. The exponential strain energy functions in 2D problem spaces become

$$W = C \exp(F(a, E)),$$

where

$$F(a, E) = a_1(E_{11}^2 + E_{22}^2) + 2a_4 E_{11} E_{22}.$$

The corresponding equation in 3D is

$$W = C \exp(F(a, E)),$$

where

$$F(a, E) = a_1(E_{11}^2 + E_{22}^2 + E_{33}^2) + 2a_7(E_{11}E_{12} + E_{22}E_{23} + E_{33}E_{31}).$$

The equivalent logarithmic energy functions in 2D and 3D problem spaces are respectively,

$$W = -C\ln(F(a, E)),$$

where

$$F(a, E) = \frac{a_1}{2}(E_{11}^2 + E_{22}^2) + a_4 E_{11} E_{22}$$

and

$$W = -C\ln(F(a, E)),$$

where

$$F(a, E) = \frac{a_1}{2}(E_{11}^2 + E_{22}^2 + E_{33}^2) + a_7(E_{11}E_{12} + E_{22}E_{23} + E_{33}E_{31}).$$

The combined logarithmic and polynomial energy function for non isotropic material in 3D space is

$$W = -\frac{C}{2}\ln(1 - F(a, E)) - \frac{C}{2}F(a, E) + \frac{F_1(a, E)}{2},$$

where

$$F(a, E) = \frac{a_1}{2}(E_{11}^2 + E_{22}^2 + E_{33}^2) + a_7(E_{11}E_{12} + E_{22}E_{23} + E_{33}E_{31}),$$

$$F_1(a, E) = \frac{a_{10}}{2}(E_{11}^2 + E_{22}^2 + E_{33}^2) + a_{12}(E_{11}E_{12} + E_{22}E_{23} + E_{33}E_{31}).$$

The inverse approach to determine liver material properties involve comparing the experimental data with theoretical stress and strain calculated using finite element method. The liver material properties are expressed in terms of material constants in various energy functions.

Figure 14(a) illustrates the comparison of images of experiments and finite element deformation of the liver tissue sample at six regular intervals. It is possible to obtain a good fit with the stress–strain curve from elongation test using appropriate material parameters as shown in Fig. 14(b).

(a)

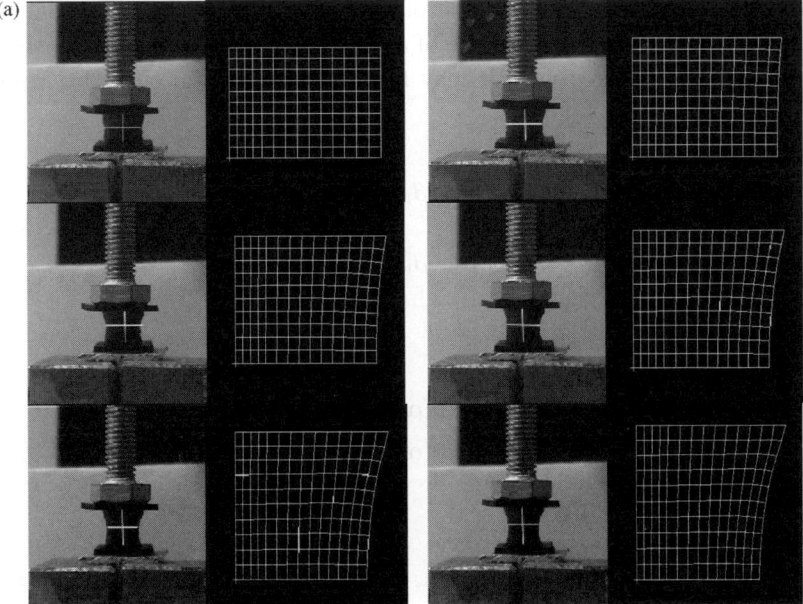

Fig. 14(a). Results from inverse finite element parameters estimation: matching of deformed model and images of experiment.

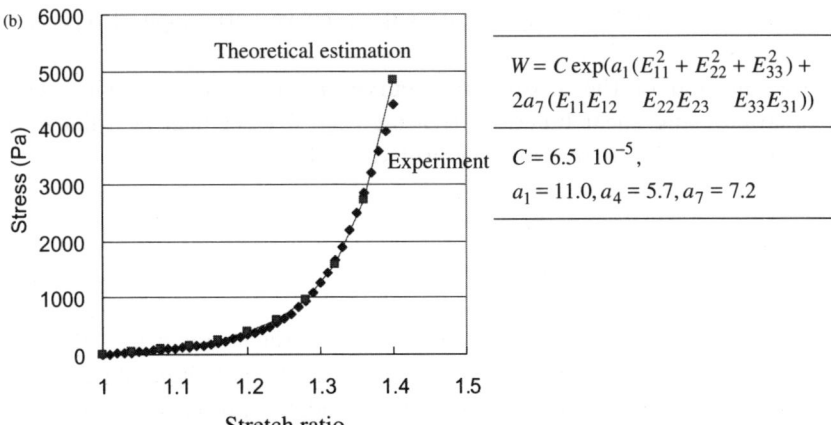

Fig. 14(b). Results from inverse finite element parameters estimation: curve fitting of experimental stress–strain curve.

5.4. *Multi-linear constitutive equation*

Fast computation with reasonable accuracy is desired in computer aided surgical simulation. A multi-linear constitutive equation defined on the concept of equivalent stress may be appropriate for such applications. The constitutive model assumes that the mechanical properties of liver tissue are isotropic and could be defined using instantiated elastic modulus and Poisson's ratio from stress–strain curve.

We refer to a cylindrical sample of liver tissue undergoing uniaxial tension and/or compression test. If the slope of σ versus ε is plotted against σ, the result was a roughly straight curve. We may fit this experimental curve by a series of straight lines, i.e.

$$\frac{d\sigma}{d\varepsilon} = \alpha_1(\sigma + \beta_1), \quad 0 \leq \sigma \leq \sigma_1$$

$$\frac{d\sigma}{d\varepsilon} = \alpha_2(\sigma + \beta_1), \quad \sigma_1 \leq \sigma \leq \sigma_2$$

An integration gives

$$\sigma + \beta_1 = c_1 \exp(\alpha_1 \varepsilon), \quad 0 \leq \sigma \leq \sigma_1$$
$$\sigma + \beta_2 = c_2 \exp(\alpha_2 \varepsilon), \quad \sigma_1 \leq \sigma \leq \sigma_2$$

and

$$\begin{aligned}\sigma &= c_1 \exp(\alpha_1 \varepsilon) - \beta_1, \quad 0 \leq \sigma \leq \sigma_1 \\ \sigma &= c_2 \exp(\alpha_2 \varepsilon) - \beta_2, \quad \sigma_1 \leq \sigma \leq \sigma_2 \end{aligned} \qquad (4)$$

The integration constants can be determined by curve fitting this equation with the original experimental stress–strain curve. Stress is used to define the intervals. Strain can also be used by simply start with a curve with slope of σ versus ε is plotted against ε.

Representation of the stress–strain curve can also be done via piece-wise approximation using linear functions treating each line segment as a linear elastic material. Following is the bilinear constitutive model:

$$\begin{aligned}\sigma &= E_0\varepsilon_0, \quad \varepsilon \leq \varepsilon^* \\ \sigma &= E(\varepsilon - \varepsilon^*) + E_0\varepsilon^*, \quad \varepsilon > \varepsilon^*,\end{aligned}$$

where E_0 is Young's modulus at the toe region, ε^* is the strain at toe-linear region. An issue with this model is that it is very sensitive to the definition of the maximum stress. The following multi-linear constitutive model is proposed to represent the nonlinear material model.

$$\sigma = E_0\varepsilon_0, \quad \varepsilon \leq \varepsilon^*$$

$$\sigma = E_i \left(\varepsilon_i - \sum_{j=0}^{i-1} \varepsilon_j \right) + \sum_{j=0}^{i-1} E_j\varepsilon_j, \quad \varepsilon > \varepsilon_i^*,$$

To define the intervals ε_i, curve fitting was applied on the $d\varepsilon - \sigma$ curve with Eq. (4). A region/interval was established when the residual error from the fitting was greater than a tolerance. In this study, a very small tolerance of 0.00001 was used.

$$\sigma = C_1(\varepsilon + C_2) = C_1\varepsilon + C_3$$

where C_1, C_2 and $C_3 = C_1C_2$ are constants, and $d\varepsilon$ is the Young's modulus. Hence, the relation at each interval is expressed in terms of straight lines. The parameter C_1 represents the rate of increase of the elastic modulus with respect to increasing tension or compression corresponding to the slope of the curve. The parameter C_3 is the intercept of the straight-line segment extended to zero stress.

Note that unloading at the same strain rate results in similar straight lines with different slopes. In view of the significant difference during loading and unloading of liver tissue, loading and unloading should be in fact considered as two different materials. Only loading curve is considered. The multi-linear constitutive model is a more direct approach compared to the exponential based method and is the focus of this section. Multi-linear constitutive model is also applicable to Poisson's ratio. However, the Poisson's ratio of liver tissue was found to vary around 0.5, and considering the infusion of blood in patient's liver organ, we assume that liver tissue is incompressible.

5.4.1. *Equivalent stress and strain for multi-axial state*

The constitutive equations described above are often good practical choices for fast surgical simulation with less emphasis on accuracy. They do not reduce to the form of strain energy and generally are not valid for three dimensional stress states. To relate the uniaxial stress–strain relationship represented by these constitutive equations with the general multi-axial stress–strain relationship, equivalent stress and strain is proposed as the "bridge" for this correlation.

The engineering stress T is the load F divided by the cross-sectional area of the specimen at zero stress state, A_0. The engineering strain e is defined as the ratio between displacement $(L_f - L_0)$ and the original length of the specimen L_0. T and e were measured in our experiments. As was described earlier, liver tissue being a nonlinear material, true or nature stress σ and strain ε should be used since we seek to model large strain deformation. The following definitions for true stress and strain are used.

$$\varepsilon = \int_0^\varepsilon dE = \int_{L_0}^{L_f} \frac{dL}{L} = \ln\frac{L_d}{L_0} \tag{5}$$

where dL is the incremental change and L is the length at beginning of increment.

$$\sigma = \frac{F}{A}$$

where A is the instantaneous cross sectional area of the deformed specimen. From Eq. (5) and definition of engineering strain, we arrived at the following relationship between engineering and true strain,

$$\varepsilon = \ln(1 + e). \tag{6}$$

Similarly, the following relationship between engineering and true stress can be established,

$$\sigma = T(1 + e).$$

After determining the true stress and stress from uniaxial experiment, it is necessary to relate this uniaxial observation to stress and strain in the general state. For this purpose, we assume that for any given stress state, there exists an equivalent uniaxial stress state generally associated with plastic deformation.[51] For realistic simulation of 3D deformation, it is suffice to define six stress components $(\sigma_x, \sigma_y, \sigma_z, \tau_{zy}, \tau_{yz}, \tau_{zx})$ and six strain components $(\varepsilon_x, \varepsilon_y, \varepsilon_z, \nu_{zy}, \nu_{yz}, \nu_{zx})$ under multi-axial stress–strain state. The equivalent stress σ_e, also known as von Mises stress and equivalent strain ε_e are defined as follows

$$\sigma_e = \frac{1}{\sqrt{2}}((\sigma_x - \sigma_y)^2 + (\sigma_y - \sigma_z)^2 + (\sigma_z - \sigma_x)^2 + 6(\tau_{xy}^2 + \tau_{yz}^2 + \tau_{zx}^2)).$$

$$\varepsilon = \int d\varepsilon_e,$$

where $d\varepsilon_e$ is the strain increment defined as follows

$$d\varepsilon_e = \frac{\sqrt{2}}{3}((d\varepsilon_x - d\varepsilon_y)^2 + (d\varepsilon_y - d\varepsilon_z)^2 + (d\varepsilon_z - d\varepsilon_x)^2 + 6(d\nu_{xy}^2 + d\nu_{yz}^2 + d\nu_{zx}^2)).$$

During finite element simulation with multi-axial state of stress, the computed stress of the finite element will be first converted to the equivalent stress. This is to select the appropriate region in the multi-linear constitutive model for representation of the material properties of the soft tissue at the finite element. Under uniaxial state of stress,

$$\sigma_z = \sigma$$

$$\sigma_x = \sigma_y = \tau_{xy} = \tau_{yz} = \tau_{zx} = 0.$$

We assume that liver is isotropic and incompressible. Hence,

$$\varepsilon_z = \varepsilon$$

$$\varepsilon_x = \varepsilon_y = -\frac{\varepsilon}{2}$$

$$\nu_{xy} = \nu_{yz} = \nu_{zx} = 0.$$

Since $\sigma_e = \sigma_z = \sigma$ and similarly for strain, followed by integration by parts,

$$\varepsilon_e = \int d\varepsilon = \varepsilon.$$

Hence, it is suffice for us to assume that the equivalent stress is the true stress and equivalent strain is the true strain under uniaxial state of stress and strain.

Figure 15 illustrated the variation of elastic modulus calculated from average true stress and strain curves with true stress during compression and elongation test. The variation in elongation was relatively smaller and could be represented using several straight lines. Nevertheless, in the case of compression, we observed much disparity in the fitting the experiment data with straight lines. More straight lines were required to fit this experimental data. The variations defined the intervals where elastic modulus is desired.

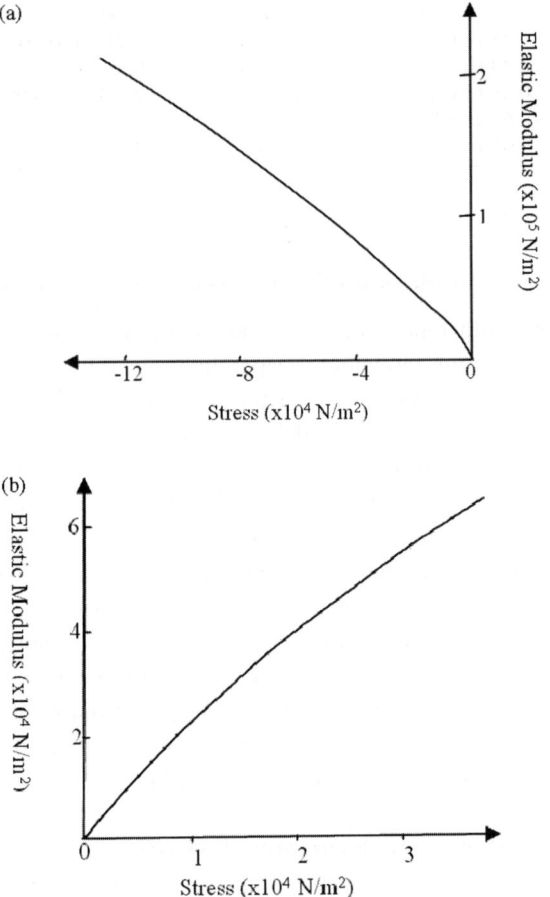

Fig. 15. Variation of elastic modulus with stress for (a) elongation and (b) compression. The stress for elongation and compression was an average of the data listed in Table 1 and Table 2 respectively.

Table 4. Material parameters of equivalent stress and strain based multi-linear constitutive model.

$$\sigma = E_0\varepsilon_0, \quad \varepsilon \le \varepsilon_0$$

$$\sigma = E_i\left(\varepsilon_i - \sum_{j=0}^{i-1}\varepsilon_j\right) + \sum_{j=0}^{i-1}E_j\varepsilon_j, \quad \varepsilon > \varepsilon_i$$

Strain Intervals, ε_i	Elastic Modulus, $E_i(\times 10^4\,\mathrm{N/m^2})$	Stress Intervals $(\times 10^4\,\mathrm{N/m^2})$
−0.57 to −0.60	−424.133	−11.067 to −12.724
−0.55 to −0.57	−553.350	−9.180 to −11.067
−0.52 to −0.55	−305.999	−6.348 to −9.180
−0.48 to −0.52	−158.699	−4.887 to −6.348
−0.46 to −0.48	−244.380	−3.404 to −4.887
−0.42 to −0.46	−85.112	−2.101 to −3.404
−0.36 to −0.42	−35.018	−0.887 to −2.101
0.00 to −0.36	−2.465	0.00 to −0.887
0.00 to 0.38	1.176	0.00 to 0.447
0.38 to 0.43	17.600	0.447 to 0.880
0.43 to 0.48	34.740	0.880 to 1.737
0.48 to 0.52	63.699	1.737 to 2.548
0.52 to 0.54	148.154	2.548 to 2.963
0.54 to 0.58	95.502	2.963 to 3.820

6. Finite Element Simulation of Soft Tissue Deformation

Accuracy and computational time are two main constraints in the practical application of soft tissue modeling. Depending on the applications, there are different requirements in these two criteria. Typically, simulation for surgical planning may have from 30 s to 1 h to deliver a clinically relevant result for outcome prediction. A surgical procedure training system will have computational time in the order of 0.1 s to achieve smooth user interaction whereas accuracy of deformation is not necessary of primary important. There were interactive computer simulations based on techniques in biomechanical engineering and computer graphics, e.g.[55]

An approach in simulation of soft tissue deformation is via finite element method. Finite element based simulation of soft tissue deformation have been applied both in surgical simulators[6,56,57] as well as elastic image registration.[58,59] The multi-linear constitutive equation is an appropriate material model for surgical training application that demands fast computation with reasonable accuracy. The strain energy based constitutive equations should be used when higher accuracy is desired.

The main motivation of employing von Mises stress in multi-linear constitutive model is its ability to predict nonlinear stress–strain relationship at and after yield point. In order to validate the hypothesis of our scheme in relating the multi-axial stress and strain with that measured during uniaxial experiments, independent experiments were conducted, and the recorded experimental deformation were

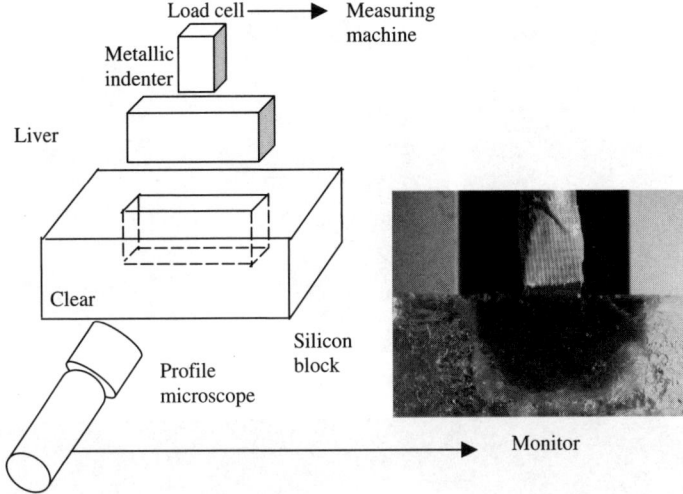

Fig. 16. *In vitro* experiment with multi-axial deformation. Tissue of rectangular shape was extracted from porcine liver organ and placed inside a hole of the same size in a silicon block. The deformation of the liver tissue was recorded using a profile microscope. Insert is snap shot of experimental tissue sample at zero stress state.

compared with that of the corresponding finite element simulation using the multi-linear constitutive equation described above. The experimental setup (Fig. 16) was similar to that of our uniaxial experiment described earlier. A rectangular block of porcine liver tissue sample with dimension 30 mm × 10 mm × 10 mm was used in an indentation test. The test resembles the multi-axial structure problem involving local load on half space. A uniform load from an indenter with a square base (10 mm × 10mm) was applied on the top surface of the sample. The sample was placed in a transparent silicon block with dimension 30 mm × 10 mm × 10 mm. Recording of the deformation was done using a profile microscope. The loading rate and other conditions were the same as that of the compression and elongation tests at 10 mm/min.

Figure 17 shows finite element simulation of the rectangular block sample, and corresponding deformation on the X–Y plane recorded at various time steps. In this simulation, we use MARC 7 for finite element analysis and Patran 2001 as pre- and post processor. There were a total of 657 TETRA4 elements and 208 nodes in the model. The material was represented using the multi-linear constitutive model. Boundary conditions are imposed at the bottom and the four sides. Since the deformation is relatively large at 1 mm, 2 mm and 3 mm, geometrical nonlinear condition was imposed and hence, a nonlinear solver was used in the solution process. The simulated deformations were compared with the recorded images during the experiment. It was observed that the deformation from finite element simulation consistently smaller than that of the recorded images by an almost

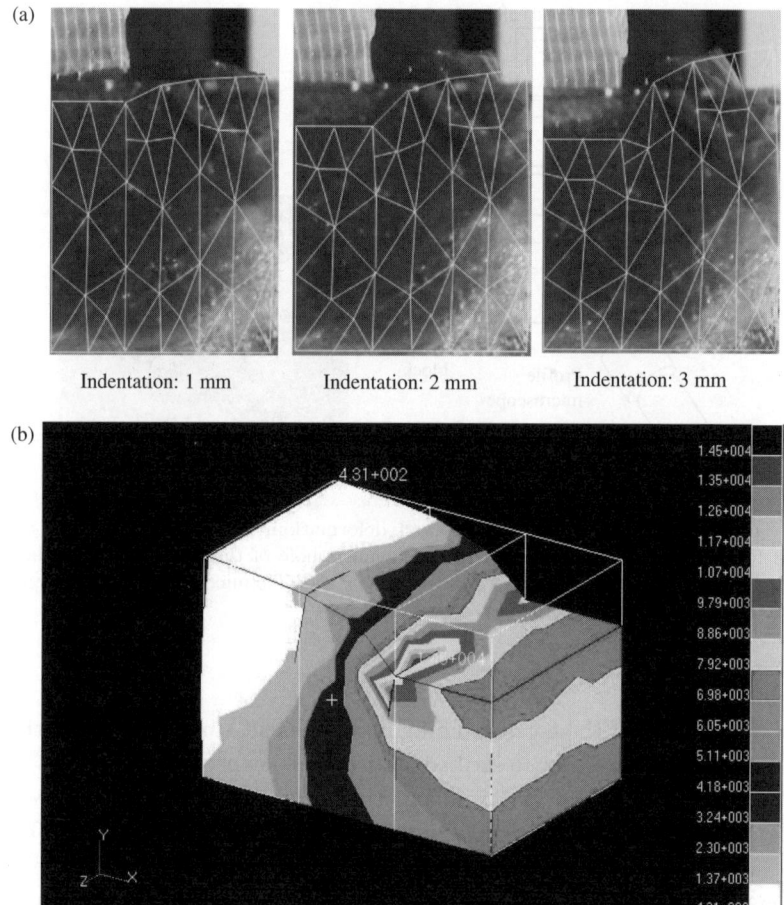

Fig. 17. Finite element simulation of multi-axial deformation experiment. (a) The simulated deformation (drawn with mesh lines) is compared with the recorded deformation at various instants. (b) Equivalent stress distribution at 3 mm indentation.

constant area. This inconsistency was possibly due to the imperfect condition of the experiments. For example, friction was not considered in the computational study. Although precaution have been taken to avoid the liver tissue becoming dry, friction was inevitable. Nevertheless, this shortfall is rather consistent. The simulation is reasonably accurate if this offset is considered.

To quantitatively evaluate the "match" between the computational and experimental deformation, we use the root-mean-square value of the residual as the quantitative standard error indicator for the match. Residual can be defined as the difference between the observed and predicted data. Suppose that A is the residual of deformed contors predicted by the computational method and experimental method. The root-mean-square value is equal to $\mathrm{norm}(A)/\sqrt{n}$ where n is the number of elements in A, and $\text{norm}(A) = \sqrt{\sum A^2}$. The standard error for the deformation at deformation 1 mm, 2 mm and 3 mm are: in x direction — 0.48 mm, 1.15 mm and 2.02 mm; in y direction — 0.63 mm, 1.11 mm and 0.22 mm. The average percentage of error is 8% and 4 % respectively. The relatively small error prompted us to believe that the computational deformation will match the corresponding experimental deformation if the rather consistent shortfall described in previous paragraph has been taken care off. Hence, the validity of using equivalent stress and strain as the "bridge" to transform the uniaxial experiment and constitutive model to the general multi-axial state was demonstrated.

The strain is generally greater than 10% during surgical simulation. This is large deformation by definition. Numerically, static finite element method, also known as small strain theory, does not apply here. In this case, finite element method based on finite deformation should be used. In the previous paragraph, the nonlinear solver takes an average CPU time of 0.1 s for a 17 steps deformation analysis on an Intel Pentium III 1.2 GHz notebook computer. This is equivalent to about 10 frames per second. Figure 18(a) is a high resolution finite element model of human liver organ. Figure 18(b) shows the corresponding low resolution finite element model deformed under force applied from the front with a large probe. The deformation is near real time with approximately 12 frames per second using a customized nonlinear finite element code. It might be possible to achieve real time interaction for the high resolution model if deformation can be considered local and small strain theory is applicable.

The requirement of fast computation prompted many investigators to exploit the possible use of small strain theory in medical simulation. For application of small strain theory, we can divide the large deformation into a number of much smaller displacement steps. For each small displacement step, the strain components are computed using Cauchy's infinitesimal strain tensor formula. Note that in this case, the incremental errors introduced by small strain formulation were assumed to be

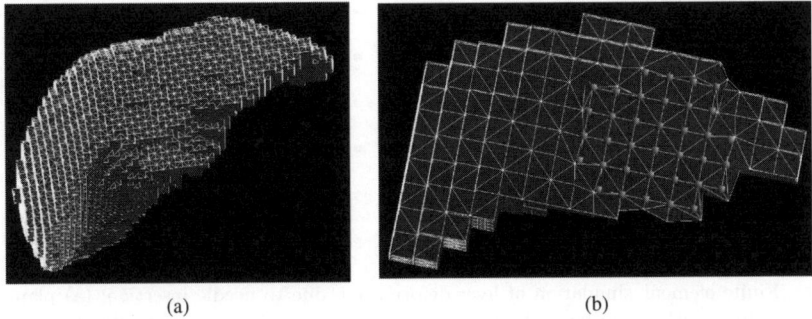

(a)　　　　　　　　　　　　　　(b)

Fig. 18.　Finite element modeling and simulation of human liver organ. (a) High resolution finite element model; (b) deformation of low resolution finite element model of liver with 3470 linear tetrahedral elements and 1079 nodes.

small and can be neglected

$$\varepsilon_x = \frac{\partial u}{\partial x}, \quad \varepsilon_y = \frac{\partial v}{\partial y}, \quad \varepsilon_z = \frac{\partial w}{\partial z}$$

$$\nu_{xy} = \frac{1}{2}\left(\frac{\partial u}{\partial y} + \frac{\partial v}{\partial x}\right), \quad \nu_{yz} = \frac{1}{2}\left(\frac{\partial v}{\partial z} + \frac{\partial w}{\partial y}\right), \quad \nu_{zx} = \frac{1}{2}\left(\frac{\partial u}{\partial z} + \frac{\partial w}{\partial x}\right),$$

where $u = u(x,y,z)$, $v = v(x,y,z)$ and $w = w(x,y,z)$ are the displacement fields in the x, y and z directions respectively, from one small displacement iteration to another. Nodal stress in the finite element is then computed using conventional linear finite element method.

Figure 19 illustrates a 2D deformation of the liver due to needle insertion using the small strain theory and the multi-linear constitute model. A frictionless contact was assumed. We also assume that a node fails when the stress at the node is greater

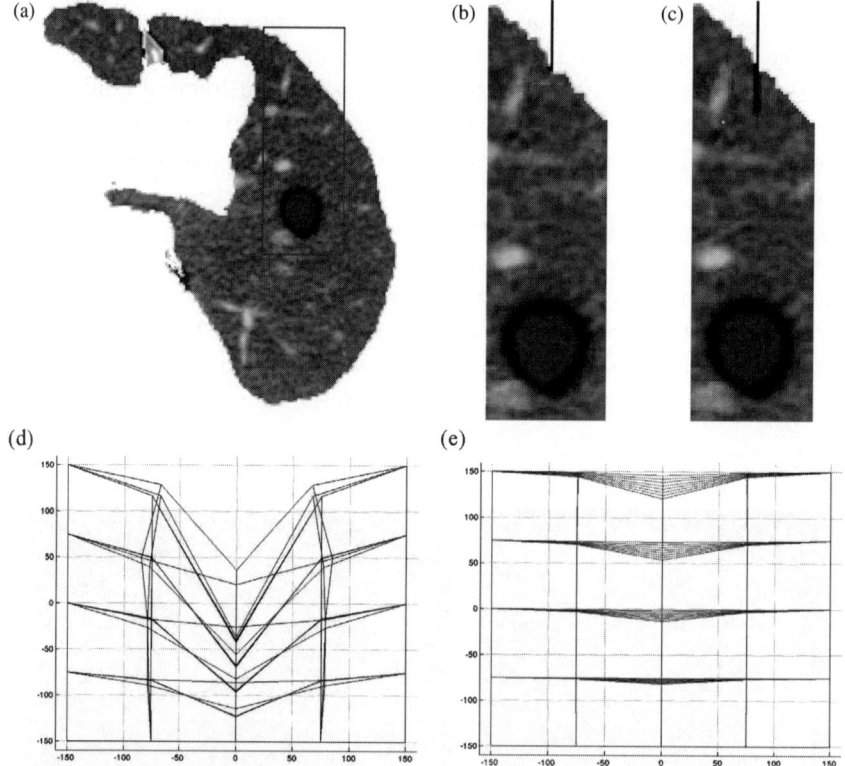

Fig. 19.   Finite element simulation of liver deformation due to needle insertion: (a) planar view of a human liver with a synthesized tumor; (b) deformation of liver surface due to insertion of needle; (c) deformation and subsequent cutting of liver tissue during needle insertion; (d) view of the deformation sequence using multi-linear model; (e) view of the deformation sequence using linear elastic model.

than the break stress of liver during compression $(2.313 \times 10^5 \text{ Pa})$. In Fig. 19(b), the liver surface was first deformed by the introduction of a needle. The deformation of the liver continues until the maximum stress of the liver tissue reached in Fig. 19(c). Figures 19(d) and 19(e) compares the deformation sequence from the multi-linear model and that of the linear elastic model a constant Young's modulus at 625 kPa (see Sec. 4). The former agrees with the nonlinear force–displacement behavior of liver tissue during deformation and is clearly closer to the deformation observed during surgery.

7. Concluding Remarks

An experimental approach can be adopted in the study of biomechanical modeling for computer aided surgical simulation. The approach involves deriving the theoretical models based on experimental results from customary designed experiments, and validating surgical simulation that are based on these models using experiments. The focus of this study is on liver organ.

Understanding the biomechanics of liver is important in virtual reality based surgical simulation as well as actual surgical intervention and medical image registration.[59-61] Various methods on measuring and modeling of tissue for computer aided surgery have been reported in the literature. These include simple poking interaction using biological or phantom tissue, e.g.[62,63] viscoelastic characterization of tissue, e.g.[64] as well as uniaxial loading and indentation experiments with porcine liver.[19,20,25,26] To validate the biomechanical model, Howe and colleagues developed a phantom known as "Truth Cube".[65] However, the truth cube does not consider tissue probing and cutting which are among the most common surgical tasks. Recent study[66] has attempted to compare human and porcine kidney tissues. It is generally believe that the mechanical properties of human and porcine liver tissues are similar.

Validation of computer aided surgical application is itself a challenging problem. In order to have adequate validation of, e.g. needle insertion, we need to track the needle path possibly using some imaging modalities, among the many practical issues to be considered. Although we are confident of the clinical viability of the biomechanical model and simulation, there remain some challenging research issues that warrant further investigation.

7.1. *Methods of experiment*

There are limitations with the uniaxial elongation or compression experiments in this study. The alternative multi-axial tests will subject the tissue sample to tremor such as extensive cutting and possibly freezing. We have conducted independent experiments and found that freezing will cause significant changes to the mechanical properties of liver tissue. Hence, we are of the view that uniaxial test is a feasible and preferred approach in this context. Given that the standard deviation of the experimental stress–strain data was high, it is important to improve the accuracy of subsequent numeric computations in analysis. A possible statistical method is normalization which is a process of scaling the numbers in a data set. A way to normalize the stress–strain data is to center the strain data at zero mean and scale it to unit standard deviation. The "goodness" of fit could be improved with the normalized stress–strain curve. The standard errors in curve fitting should be smaller.

To relate the general multi-axial state in 3D deformation with the stress–strain relation from uniaxial test, the concept of equivalent stress and strain could be used as the intermediate layer. The mechanical properties of liver tissue can possibly be defined upon the lower level liver lobules. The work on measuring and modeling the mechanical properties of liver lobules is on going. Relating tissue at macro and micro scales were previously investigated by Vawter et al.[67] for lung.

An interesting topic for our future pursuit in experimental biomechanics is to measure the mechanical properties of liver cells and investigate their relationship with the liver lobule and the liver tissue. Preparation of the liver cell sample and the associated engineering issues such as micromanipulator control are problems that we have faced in our attempted investigation beyond liver lobule.

7.2. *Viscoelastic properties of liver tissue and constitutive modeling*

The fact that there is considerable difference in stress response to loading and unloading implies that the history of strain affects the stress, and hence, liver tissue is a viscoelastic material. As first approximation, the viscoelastic properties are assumed to be negligible. This assumption is supported by the observation that the liver tissue is relatively strain rate independent. The contribution of linear viscoelasticity is small relative to overall mechanical properties, particularly for computer aided surgical simulation when the strain rate has less variation and is only moderate quantitatively. Nevertheless, by incorporating the viscoelastic properties of liver tissue into the study will inevitably improve the proposed model.

From our experiments, the average relaxation times for constant strain and stress after compression and elongation are 6.9 s, 51.2 s and 17.5 s, 24.0 s respectively. The corresponding relaxation modulus for compression and elongation are 45.9 N/m and 101.1 N/m respectively with a standard linear solid (or Kelvin model). The resultant stress–strain relationship can barely represent up to 10% of the strain. The study reveals that a linear viscoelastic model is possibly not adequate. Liver is a highly nonlinear viscoelastic material. A nonlinear viscoelastic model which is very computational intensive is required for high accuracy.

The viscoelastic properties and shear forces of soft biological tissue were considered in some recent studies on constitutive equations for liver tissues, e.g. Refs. 68 and 69. There were more studies on viscoelastic properties of brain tissues, e.g. Refs. 70 and 71 since brain tissue is more viscous. Viscoelastic behaviors of liver tissue sample had also been detected in our relaxation and creeping tests, and were reported in Ref. 26. We are in the process of introducing a strain rate dependent component into the combined energy constitutive model. This effort to include the nonlinear viscoelastic effect of liver tissue will be done keeping the computation cost as low as possible so that the model remains feasible for computer aided surgical simulation.

7.3. *Hepatic blood flow and biphasic poroelastic constitutive modeling*

Load testing with an extremely vascular organ such as liver (0.4–1 L of blood, 80% of mass is from cells) under *ex vivo* conditions could produce elastic and viscous behaviors that are different from *in vivo* conditions.[72,73] Liver is very unique in its microanatomy relative to hepatic arterial, portal venous (unique dual input supply) and hepatic venous blood with interconnecting lobular sinusoidal anatomy. Other organs will behave differently when distended with blood under normal vascular pressures.

A living liver is porous, and possibly a biphasic poroelastic model may better represent the experimental data if liver tissues are submerged in circulating Ringer's solution during experiment. To our best knowledge, poroelastic model has not been applied to represent liver's mechanical properties. In addition to its complexity, the poroelastic model has its limitation in biological application — unlike engineering materials such as porous rock, the fluid flow through tiny vessels in the case of liver tissue. These micro-vessels known as capillaries have tangible walls that have different mechanical properties compared to that of liver tissue comprising mainly liver cells. Furthermore, the vascular system is a closed system. Blood perfusing tissue produces an internal pressure or tension that is different from that produced by just perfusing the tissue and letting the perfusate exit through exposed and open vessels as will always be the case when biopsy like samples are tested. In order to approach what occurs in the living body, experiments on a whole intact liver will have to be conducted. Nevertheless, the boundary conditions will be extensive and meaningful data analysis may not be possible.

7.4. *Biomechanics of hepatic vessel*

An alternative will be to separately consider the biomechanics of liver tissue and the vessels in which the blood flow. Modeling of the extensive micro-vessels that flow out from the primary hepatic vascular network is the next step for vascular network modeling. To handle the small sizes and highly irregular shapes of these vessels, statistically geometrical modeling technique is possibly a good approach compared to conventional techniques.

In Conclusion, much work has been accomplished and yet much work remains to be done. Computer aided surgery is a young field — this term originated in the early 1980s. In recent years, scientists and engineers have paid much attention to applying the physical principles and engineering methods to the behavior of parts of human body, considering it as both a structure and a machine, particularly in computer aided surgical simulation. However, it soon become apparent that what have be taken for granted in conventional engineering no longer necessarily applies.

The passive material properties of biological tissues are not linearly elastic. As is shown here, the liver tissue is non-homogeneous, possibly incompressible, highly nonlinear, largely nonlinear viscoelastic and transversely isotropic. The liver tissue is rather porous and the interstitium is filled with fluid. When all of these factors are coupled, the problem of how to describe the mechanical properties of liver tissue in a simple and accurate mathematical form for computer aided surgery becomes quite acute. Furthermore, as a living organism, liver tissue responses to stress and strain biologically as well as mechanically. The complexity of modeling will increase when considering diseased organs where the technology will find most useful application. Surgeons do not operate on normal organs so future work needs to consider how conditions such as cirrhosis/fibrosis, inflammation, infection or lesions such as tumors or cysts need to be eventually incorporated into the biomechanical modeling process. This is a difficult task and will require diseased human fresh autopsy or experimental animal tissue samples. It is only natural to start on normal tissue, but eventually, disease processes need to be considered, especially when considering the interactions of instruments and the tissue.

Knowledge of anatomy and physiology is as important as the engineering principles in biomechanics. The various constitutive equations described here, with hypothesis ranging from linear elastic, hyperelastic, multi-linear, viscoelastic to porous materials, represent only a modest effort in this challenging field. The various sophisticated approaches in biomechanics for engineering analysis may not be done at interactive speeds demanded by typical computer aided surgical application, but it is often desirable to interact with the simulation as it happens to steer the computation so as to improve treatment outcomes. Advancement in computational techniques coupled with the advancement in computing hardware may remedy the often conflicting requirement of accuracy and interactivity. This will contribute to the further integration of biomechanics with computer simulation in computer aided surgery.

Acknowledgments

This work is partially supported by "Research for the Future Program (JSPS-RFTF 99I00904)" funded by Japan Society for the Promotion of Science and "Research on medical devices for analyzing, supporting and substituting the function of human body" funded by Ministry of Health, Labor and Welfare. We would like to acknowledge the following individuals in University of Tokyo for their contributions to this ongoing scientific endeavor: Dr. Etsuko Kobayashi, A/Prof.

Xien Chen, Prof. Toshiaki Hisada, Mr. Yosuke Nishimura and Mr. Kengo Mayumi. Valuable comments on the drafts from Prof. James H. Anderson, Johns Hopkins University School of Medicine, Dr. Chee-Cheon Chui, Defence Science Organization, Singapore and Prof. Teoh Swee Hin, National University of Singapore, Singapore were appreciated.

References

1. R. B. Metson, M. J. Cosenza and M. J. Cunningham, Physician experience with an optical image guidance system for sinus surgery, *Laryngoscope* **110**(6) (1995) 972–976.
2. G. Burdea, *Force and Touch Feedback for Virtual Reality* (Wiley, New York, 1996).
3. P. N. Brett, C. A. Fraser, M. Henningan, M. V. Griffiths and Y. Kamel, Automated surgical tools for penetrating flexible tissue, *IEEE Eng. Med. Biol.* (1997) 264–270.
4. J. M. Rolfe and K. J. Staples, *Flight Simulators* (Cambridge University Press, England, 1986), pp. 232–249.
5. J. Wachtel, The future of nuclear plant simulation in the United States, in *Simulation for Nuclear Reactor Technology*, D. G. Walton, ed. (Cambridge University Press, England, 1985), p. 339–349.
6. J. H. Anderson, C. Chui, Y. Cai, Y. Wang, Z. Li, X. Ma, W. L. Nowinski, M. Solaiyappan, K. Murphy, P. Gailloud and A. Venbrux, Virtual reality training in interventional radiology — the Johns Hopkins and Kent Ridge Digital Laboratory experience, *Semin. Interven. Radiol.* **19**(2) (2002), 179–185.
7. C. Chui, J. H. Anderson and W. L. Nowinski, A simulation system to design and evaluate patient-specific interventional radiology medical devices, in *Business Briefing: Medical Device Manufacturing and Technology* (World Markets Research Centre, United Kingdom, 2002).
8. Y. Cai, C. Chui, X. Ye, J. H. Anderson, K. M. Liew and I. Sakuma, Simulation-based virtual prototyping of customized catheterization devices, *ASME J. Comput. Inform. Sci. Eng.* **4** (2004) 132–139.
9. K. Miller and K. Chinzei, Modeling of soft tissues deformation, *J. Comput. Aided Surg.* 1(Suppl.) (1995) 62–63.
10. I. Sakuma, T. Awao, K. Masamune, T. Nakagori, T. Asano, H. Inada and T. Dohi, Passive navigation system for precise positioning of a needle electrode in radio frequency ablation, *Proc. Comput. Assisted Radiol. Surg.* (2000), p. 978.
11. D. Sorid and S. K. Moore, The virtual surgeon, *IEEE Spectrum* (2000), pp. 26–31.
12. D. L. G. Hill, C. R. Maurer, R. J. Maciunas, J. A. Barwise, J. M. Fitzpatrick and M. Y. Wang, Measurement of intraoperative brain surface deformation under a craniotomy, *Neurosurgery* **43**(2) (1998) 514–526.
13. F. J. Carter, T. G. Frank, P. J. Davies, D. McLean and A. Cuschieri, Biomechanical testing of intra-abdominal soft tissue, *Med. Image Anal.* **5** (2001) 231–236.
14. R. Muthupillai, D. J. Lomas, P. J. Rossman, J. F. Greenleaf, A. Manduca and R. L. Ehman, Magnetic resonance elastography by direct visualization of propagating acoustic strain waves, *Science* **269**(99) (1995) 1854–1857.
15. A. P. Pathak, M. B. Silver-Thorn, C. A. Thierfelder and T. E. Prieto, A rate-controlled indentor for *in vivo* analysis of residual limb tissues, *IEEE Trans. Rehabilitation Eng.* **6**(1) (1998) 12–20.
16. S. K. Kyriacou, C. Schwab and J. D. Humphrey, Finite element analysis of nonlinear orthotropic hyperelastic membranes, *Comput. Mech.* **18** (1996) 269–278.

17. M. Kauer, V. Vuskovic, J. Dual, G. Szekely and M. Bajka, Inverse finite element characterization of soft tissue, *Proc. MICCAI 2001, LNCS 2208* (Springer–Verlag, New York, 2001), pp. 128–136.

18. P. J. Davies, F. J. Carter and A. Cuschieri, Mathematical modelling for keyhole surgery simulation: A biomechanical model for spleen tissue, *IMA J. Appl. Math.* **67** (2002) 41–67.

19. H. Tie and J. P. Desai, A biomechanical model of the liver for reality-based haptic feedback, *MICCAI(1) 2003, LNCS 2878* (Springer–Verlag, New York, 2003), pp. 75–82.

20. K. Onodera, X. Chen, T. Hisada, Identification of biomechanical material properties of soft tissues, *Proc. Jpn. Comput. Eng. Soc. Ann. Conf.* 2001 (Tokyo, Japan, 2001), (in Japanese).

21. J. Kim and M. A. Srinivasan, Characterization of viscoelastic soft tissue properties from *In vivo* animal experiments and inverse FE parameter estimation, in *Proceedings MICCAI 2005, LNCS 3750*, J. Duncan and G. Gerig, eds. (Springer–Verlag, New York, 2005), pp. 599–606.

22. Y. Fung, *Biomechanics — Mechanical Properties of Living Tissues*, Second Edition (Springer–Verlag, New York, 1993).

23. H. Yamada, *Strength of Biological Materials* (Williams & Wilkins, Baltimore, USA, 1970).

24. K. Miller and K. Chinzei, Constitutive modelling of brain tissue: Experiment and theory, *J. Biomech.* **30**(11/12) (1997) 1115–1121.

25. C. Chui, E. Kobayashi, X. Chen, T. Hisada and I. Sakuma, Combined compression and elongation experiments and nonlinear constitutive modeling of liver tissue for surgical simulation, *IFMBE J. Med. Biolog. Eng. Comput.* **42**(6) (2004) 787–798.

26. I. Sakuma, Y. Nishimura, C. Chui, E. Kobayashi, H. Inada, X. Chen and T. Hisada, *In vitro* measurement of mechanical properties of liver tissue under compression and elongation using a new test piece holding method with surgical glue, in *Surgical Simulation and Soft Tissue Modeling, LNCS 2673*, N. Ayache and H. Delingette, eds. (Springer–Verlag, New York, 2003), pp. 284–292.

27. K. Hayashi, N. Stergiopulos, J.-J. Meister, S. E. Greenwald and A. Rachev, Techniques in the determination of the mechanical properties and constitutive laws of arterial walls, in *Cardiovascular Techniques*, C. Leondes, ed. (CRC Press, 2001), Chapter 6.

28. C. Bruyns and M. Ottensmeyer, Measuring soft-tissue mechanical properties to support development of a physically based virtual animal model, in *MICCAI 2002, LNCS 2488*, T. Dohi and R. Kikinis, eds. (Springer–Verlag, New York, 2002), pp. 283–289.

29. G. J. Tortora, *Principles of Human Anatomy*, 9th Edition (John Wiley & Sons, 2002).

30. D. Haemmerich, I. dos Santos, D. J. Schutt, J. G. Webster and D. M. Mahvi, *In vitro* measurements of temperature-dependent specific heat of liver tissue, *Med. Eng. Phys.* **28**(2) (2006) 194–197.

31. K. J. Chua, S. K. Chou and J. C. Ho, An analytical study on the thermal effects of cryosurgery on selective cell destruction, *J. Biomech.* **40**(1) (2006) 100–116.

32. C. Chui, Y. Nishimura, E. Kobayashi, H. Inada and I. Sakuma, A medical simulation system with unified multilevel biomechanical model, *Proc. 5th Asian Pacific Cong. Med. Biolog. Eng.* 2002 (CDROM).

33. J. Vossoughi, Constitutive modelling of biological materials, in *The Biomedical Engineering Handbook*, J. D. Bronzino, ed. (CRC Press, 1995), pp. 263–272.

34. P. J. Davies, F. J. Carter, D. G. Roxburgh and A. Cuschieri, Mathematical modelling for keyhole surgery simulations: Spleen capsule as an elastic membrane, *J. Theoret. Med.* **1** (1999) 247–262.
35. K. Miller, Constitutive modelling of abdominal organs, *J. Biomech.* **33** (2000) 367–373.
36. J. W. Melvin, R. L. Stalnaker and V. L. Roberts, Impact injury mechanisms in abdominal organs, *SAE Trans.* **730968** (1973) 115–126.
37. T. T. Tanaka and Y. C. Fung, Elastic and inelastic properties of the canine aorta and their variation along the aortic tree, *J. Biomech.* **7**(4) (1974) 357–370.
38. Y. Fung, Elasticity of soft tissues in simple elongation, *Am. J. Physiol.* **213** (1967) 1532–1544.
39. R. M. Kenedi, T. Gibson and C. H. Daly, Bioengineering studies of human skin: the effects of unidirectional tension, in *Structure and Function of Connective and Skeletal Tissue*, S. F. Jackson, S. M. Harkness and G. R. Tristram, eds. (Scientific Committee, St. Andrews, Scotland, 1964), pp. 388–395.
40. M. D. Ridge and V. Wright, The description of skin stiffness, *Biorheology* **2** (1964) 67–74.
41. F. R. Schmidlin, M. Thomason, D. Oller, W. Meredith, J. Moylan, T. Clancy, P. Cunningham and C. Baker, Force transmission and stress distribution in a computer simulated model of the kidney: An analysis of the injury mechanisms in renal trauma, *J. Trauma* **40** (1996) 791–796.
42. M. Farshad, M. Barbezat, F. Schmidlin, L. Bidaut, P. Niederer and P. Graber, Material characterization and mathematical modeling of the pig kidney in relation with biomechanical analysis of renal trauma, *Proc. North Am. Cong. Biomech.* (Waterloo, Ontario, Canada, 1998).
43. M. Mooney, A theory of large elastic deformation, *J. Appl. Phys.* **11** (1940) 582–592.
44. D. R. Veronda and R. A. Westmann, Mechanical characterizations of skin-finite deformations, *J. Biomech.* **3**(1) (1970) 111–124.
45. K. Takamizawa and K. Hayashi, Strain energy density function and uniform strain hypothesis for arterial mechanics, *J. Biomech.* **20**(1) (1987) 7–17.
46. K. Hayashi, Experimental approaches on measuring the mechanical properties and constitutive laws of arterial walls, *ASME J. Biomech. Eng.* **115** (1993) 481–487.
47. J. Xie, J. Zhou and Y. Fung, Bending of blood vessel wall: Stress–strain laws of the intima-media and adventitial layers, *ASME J. Biomech. Eng.* **117** (1995) 136–145.
48. T. Hisada and H. Noguchi, *Principle and Application of Non Linear Finite Element Methods* (Maruzen, Tokyo, Japan, 1995) (in Japanese).
49. M. E. Zobitz, Z. Luo and K. An, Determination of the compressive material properties of the supraspinatus tendon, *ASME J. Biomech. Eng.* **123** (2001) 47–51.
50. D. Bogen, Strain energy description of biological swelling I single fluid compartment models, *ASME J. Biomech. Eng.* **109** (1987) 252–256.
51. Y. Fung, S. Liu and J. Zhou, Remodeling of the constitutive equation while a blood vessel remodels itself under stress, *ASME J. Biomech. Eng.* **115** (1993) 453–459.
52. Y. Fung, Biorheology of soft tissue, *Biorheology* **10** (1973) 139–155.
53. Y. Ling, Uniaxial true stress–strain after necking, *AMP J. Technol.* **5** (1996) 37–48.
54. H. Demiray, A note of the elasticity of soft biological tissues, *J. Biomech.* **5**(3) (1972) 309–311.
55. D. Terzopoulos and K. Fleischer, Deformable models, *The Visual Comput.* **4** (1988) 306–331.
56. S. Cotin, H. Delingette and N. Ayache, Real-time volumetric deformable models for surgical simulation using finite elements and condensation, in *Proc. Eurograph. 96* (Springer–Verlag, New York, 1996), pp. 57–66.

57. G. Szekely, C. Brechbuehler, R. Hutter, A. Rhomberg, N. Ironmonger and P. Schmid, Modeling of soft tissue deformation for laparoscopic surgery simulation, *Med. Image Anal.* **4** (2000) 57–66.

58. S. K. Kyriacou and D. Davatzikos, A biomechanical model of soft tissue deformation with applications to non-rigid registration of brain images with tumor pathology, in *Proc. MICCAI 98, LNCS 1496* (Springer–Verlag, New York, 1998), pp. 531–538.

59. J. B. A. Mainz and M. A. Viergever, A surgery of medical image registration, *Med. Image Analy.* **2**(1) (1998) 1–36.

60. D. J. Hawks, P. J. Ewards, D. Barratt, J. M. Blackall, G. P. Penney and C. Tanner, Measuring and modeling soft tissue deformation for image guided interventions, in *Surgical Simulation and Soft Tissue Modeling, LNCS 2673*, N. Ayache and H. Delingette, eds. (Springer–Verlag, New York, 2003), pp. 1–14.

61. H. F. Reinhart, CT-guided real-time stereotaxy, *Acta Neurochir. Suppl.* **46** (1989) 107–108.

62. D. Aulignac, R. Balaniuk and C. Laugier, A haptic interface for a virtual exam of the human thigh, *Proc. IEEE Int. Conf. Robotics Automat.* (2000), pp. 2452–2456.

63. I. Brouwer, Measuring *in vivo* animal soft tissue properties for haptic modeling in surgical simulation, in *Proc. Med. Meets Virtual Reality* (IOS Press, 2001), pp. 69–74.

64. S. Doko, J. J. LeGrice and B. H. Smaill, A triaxial-measurement shear-test device for soft biological tissues, *J. Biomech. Eng.* **122** (2000) 471–478.

65. A. E. Kerdok, Soft tissue characterization: mechanical property determination from biopsies to whole organs, *Whitaker Foundation Biomedical Research Conference*, 2001.

66. J. G. Snedeker, M. Barbezat, P. Niederer, F. R. Schmidlin and M. Farshad, Strain energy as a rupture criterion for the kidney: Impact tests on porcine organs, finite element simulation, and a baseline comparison between human and porcine tissues, *J. Biomech.* **38** (2005) 993–1001.

67. D. L. Vawter, Y. C. Fung and J. B. West, Constitutive equation of lung tissue elasticity, *ASME J. Biomech. Eng.* **101** (1980) 38–45.

68. Z. Liu and L. Bilston, On the viscoelastic character of liver tissue: Experiments and modeling of linear behavior, *Biorheology* **37**(3) (2002) 191–201.

69. Z. Liu and L. Bilston, Large deformation shear properties of liver tissue, *Biorheology* **39**(6) (2000) 735–742.

70. D. W. A. Brands, G. W. M. Peters and P. H. M. Bovendeerd, Design and numerical implementation of a 3D nonlinear viscoelastic constitutive model for brain tissue during impact, *J. Biomech.* **37** (2004) 127–134.

71. L. Bilson, Z. Liu and N. Phan-Tien, Large strain behavior of brain tissue in shear — Some experimental data and differential constitutive model, *Biorheology* **38** (2001) 335–345.

72. J. D. Brown, J. Rosen, Y. S. Kim, L. Chang, M. N. Sinanan and B. Hannaford, *In vivo* and *in situ* compressive properties of porcine abdominal soft tissues, in *Proc. Med. Meets Virtual Reality* (IOS Press, 2003), pp. 26–32.

73. A. E. Kerdok, M. P. Ottensmeyer and R. D. Howe, The effects of perfusion on the viscoelastic characteristics of liver, *J. Biomech.* (2005) In Press.

74. C. Chui, E. Kobayashi, X. Chen, T. Hisada and I. Sakuma, Tranversely isotropic properties of porcine liver tissue: Experiments and constitutive modeling, *Med. Biol. Eng. Comput.* **45**(1) (2007) 99–106.

CHAPTER 8

ULTRASOUND MEASUREMENT OF SWELLING BEHAVIORS OF ARTICULAR CARTILAGE *IN SITU*

QING WANG and YONG-PING ZHENG*

Department of Health Technology and Informatics
The Hong Kong Polytechnic University
Kowloon, Hong Kong, China
* ypzheng@ieee.org

1. Introduction

1.1. *Articular cartilage*

Articular cartilage is the thin white layer of soft connective tissue that covers the articulating bony ends in diarthrodial joints, such as the end surfaces of the tibia and femur, and the posterior surface of the patella inside the knee joint. Although articular cartilage is a tiny tissue in the body, it provides joints with excellent lubrication and wearing characteristics, and maintains a smooth efficient force-bearing system. It is hard to imagine how the skeleton to bear the weight of the body and conduct the movement without articular cartilage. It has been found that the exact compositions and structure of articular cartilage depend greatly on anatomy location, depth, and age, as well as the pathological state of the tissue.[1-3] The complex hydrated-charged nature and magic functions of articular cartilage have attracted tremendous research interests.

1.1.1. *Negative charged proteoglycan-collagen matrix*

Chondrocytes, proteoglycans (PGs), collagens and water are the major components of articular cartilage. Therefore, articular cartilage is usually regarded to consist of chondrocytes and extracellular matrix (ECM, 95% of the total wet weight).[1] The ECM is primarily composed of water (75% of wet weight), collagen fibrils (mainly type II) (20%), PGs (5%), and other components, such as enzymes, growth factors, lipids, and adhesives.[1]

PGs and collagens interact with each other to form the porous solid matrix swollen with water. PGs are bio-macromolecules, produced by chondrocytes and secreted into the matrix. A single PG aggregan molecule consists of a protein core to which numerous glycosaminoglycan (GAG) chains are bounded by sugar bonds. The aggregated PGs are strongly electronegative due to the negatively charged groups of SO_3^- and COO^-, which are quantified as the fixed charge density (FCD).[4,5] Therefore, the matrix is negatively charged and has a swelling behavior.

While the charged-hydrated soft tissue is bathing in NaCl solution, the ions freely move with the interstitial fluid by convection or shift through the interstitial fluid by diffusion.[4] The cations are attracted by the negative charges of PGs by the virtue of the electro-neutrality law, creating a substantial Donnan osmotic pressure. The ionic strains were gained in the continuum theory.[6] With the development of the theory, ions are regarded as the third phase of articular cartilage in the triphasic theory.[4] In 1997, a quadriphasic theory, an extension of triphasic theory, proposed that the ion phase is divided into two independent phases, i.e. cation phase and anion phase.[7] However, this theory has not been widely applied yet.

1.1.2. Layered structure and mechanical properties

The layered structure is determined by the morphology of the components and important to the functions and properties of articular cartilage. The tissue can be roughly divided into three layers, i.e. surface, middle, and deep layer occupying approximately 10–20%, 40–60% and 30% of the total tissue thickness, respectively, (Fig. 1).[1] Each layer contributes individually to the properties of intact articular cartilage.

1.1.2.1. Surface layer (or superficial zone)

The surface layer is the thinnest layer but forms smooth surface. In this layer, PG content is lower while collagen and water contents are highest.[1,8,9] Collagen fibrils orientate tangential to the surface and form a dense network. Consequently, cells enmeshed in this zone are in an elliptic shape with the long axial parallel to the

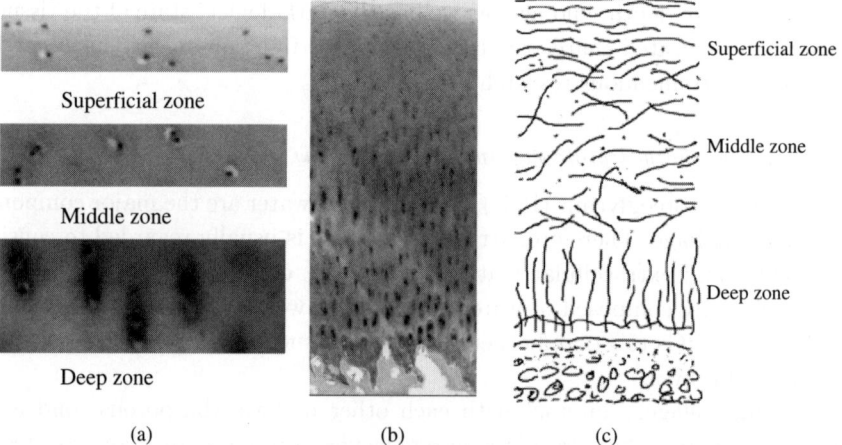

Fig. 1.   (a–b) Histology of articular cartilage stained with Safranin O and fast green; (a) shows the enlarged images at different layers in (b); (c) schematic of the layered structure of articular cartilage.

surface. The surface layer can resist shear stresses during the joint motions[10] and limits the swelling stress.[4,5,11,12]

1.1.2.2. Middle layer (or transitional zone)

The middle layer occupies more than half of the whole cartilage layer. It plays an important role in mechanical function (transform the tensile force to compressive force).[1] In this area, chondrocytes tend to be round. Collagen fibers are randomly arranged with a lower density but attached with the high concentration of PGs, which plays a vital role in swelling of cartilage.[4,5,13]

1.1.2.3. Deep layer (or radial zone)

The deep layer contains a high content of collagen and PGs but a low content of water. This zone distributes loads and resists compression. Collagen fibers of the deep zone are bundled together, orientated vertically to the interface between cartilage and the calcified cartilage, and tightly attached to the underlying bone tissue.[2,14] The changes in the cellular shape correspond to the orientation of collagen fibres. Chondrocytes appear to arrange in lines perpendicular to the cartilage-bone interface. It has been found that this layer is stiffer than the upper layers.[13,15] There is a special layer beneath the deep layer called calcified zone. Its stiffness ranges between the stiffness of cartilage and bone.[16] It provides a tight junction between the cartilage layer and the bone tissue and thus resists the stresses.[14] It has been demonstrated that there is a difference between the *ex situ* behaviors and properties and the *in situ* ones.[17–19]

The composition-structure relationship determines the mechanical properties of articular cartilage. The interesting orientation of collagen fibrils is greatly responsible for the mechanical properties of articular cartilage. The size, structural rigidity, and complicated molecular conformation of the negative charged matrix contribute to the electrochemical mechanical behavior of articular cartilage.[1]

In short, the inhomogeneous distribution and anisotropic orientation of the cartilage matrix significantly contribute to the biochemical, mechanical properties of articular cartilage.

1.1.3. *Inhomogeneity and anisotropy of mechanical properties*

The mechanical properties (including tension, compression, shear, viscoelasticity, and swelling) of articular cartilage are determined by its compositions and structure and described by material parameters, such as Young's modulus, the aggregate modulus, shear modulus and Poisson's ratio. These parameters are measured at equilibrium using creep or stress-relaxation test (confined or unconfined compression test, and indentation test), constant-strain-rate tensile test, and shear test. To determine the deformation of the tissuestress and strain are necessary to be measured. Although the results depend on specimen species, size, anatomy location and the protocol and objectives of the experiments, previous studies have found that these parameters are inhomogeneous, depth-dependent and closely relative to composition and structure.

The zonal variations of the mechanical properties of articular cartilage have been measured in tension[20–23] and in compression[15,24] using carefully excised tissue slides at different depths. It should be noted that the overall integrity of articular cartilage could not be protected during these measurements. The nonhomogeneous deformation distribution within the full-thickness cartilage layer was theoretically predicted.[25–27] In the 1990s, the inhomogeneity of the mechanical properties of articular cartilage was directly measured using a confocal microscope[28] and a video microscope.[29,30] A new optical method was developed for the investigation of the nonuniform strain distribution with the cartilage layer during free-swelling induced by varying the concentration of the bathing saline solution.[13,31] These optical methods demonstrated that the strain distribution of cartilage was significantly depth-dependent. However, the strain map was measured along one side of the excised specimen. It is not clear whether the depth-dependent material properties of articular cartilage obtained in such a "destructive" way would be the same as those in its natural intact state. Associated with compression or indentation, ultrasound has been used to facilitate the direct measurement of the depth-dependent mechanical properties of articular cartilage, such as the transient Poisson's ratio,[32] and the compressive strain.[33] Cohn *et al.*[34,35] extended the elastography technique[36,37] to an elastic ultrasound microscope system. A 2D ultrasound elastomicroscopy system was developed to map deformations of articular cartilage.[38] During the recent years, the inhomogeneous swelling of cartilage was investigated using osmotic loading combined with optical imaging[31] and ultrasound.[39]

In addition, the degeneration of articular cartilage induced changes in compositions and structure of the cartilage layer. As a result, the mechanical properties must be affected. It was discovered that the mechanical parameters of the PG-degraded tissue including shear modulus,[40] compressive modulus[41,42] and aggregate modulus in swelling[13,43] greatly reduced, while superficial swelling strain increased.[13,43]

1.2. Swelling behavior of articular cartilage

Swelling is a special property of articular cartilage, which plays an important role in weight bearing and movement of joints. Ultrasound provides a unique approach to investigate the cartilage swelling.

1.2.1. Origin of swelling

As a result of the physicochemical forces, swelling is often defined as the ability of articular cartilage to alter (gain or lose) in dimension, weight and hydration when an osmotic load exerts on the tissue.[44] During the past three decades, the mechanism of swelling and the development of methods to quantify swelling have been of great interests.

The swelling behavior of articular cartilage is considered as an electro-chemomechanical coupling phenomenon of cartilage, which is attributed to the interactions between the fixed negative charges and mobile ions.[4] Mainly, two force resources give rise to a swelling pressure within cartilage.[1,4] One is the imbalance of ions caused by negative fixed charges, which attract counter-ions to create a substantial pressure in the interstitium higher than the ambient pressure in the bath solution. This part of swelling pressure is known as the Donnan osmotic pressure (π), which is related to the fixed charge density (c^F) of PGs and the electrolyte concentration (c^*) of the external bathing solution and thereby adjusted by the ion concentration of the bathing solution. The other is the charge-to-charge repulse force generated by the charged groups fixed along GAG chains, known as the chemical-expansion pressure. This swelling pressure balances with the collagen tension, so no swollen behavior can be detected under normal conditions.[4,5,11,12] The pre-swollen state of cartilage plays an essential role in the biomechanical functions.[8,18] When external forces are exerted on cartilage, the swollen cartilage carries forces like a cushion.[44]

When the cartilage tissue is bathed in a hypertonic salt solution (with a high concentration of salt ions), the difference of the ion concentration between the cartilage matrix and the bathing solution decreases. In other words, the Donnan osmotic pressure reduced. As a result, the tissue shrinks and loses water. In contrast, when the cartilage tissue is bathed in a hypotonic salt solution (with a low concentration of salt ions), the difference of the ion concentration increases. The tissue swells and gains water. The variations in dimension and hydration can be measured during these procedures.[1,4,6,45] It has been reported that the swelling strain distribution is inhomogeneous throughout the thickness of articular cartilage.[4,5,31,39,46]

According to the origin of swelling, the swelling behavior of articular cartilage reflects the changes in the PG concentration, FCD, water volume fraction, and the intrinsic mechanical properties of the cartilage solid matrix.[4,5,10,11,31,40,47–52] It is noted that the effects of osmotic pressure loading within the ECM are different from the effects produced types of practical mechanical loading conditions achieved in the laboratory.[53] Therefore, the study on cartilage swelling induced by osmotic load is useful to provide the insight understanding of articular cartilage.

1.2.2. *Osmosis-induced swelling behavior*

Osmotic loading technique by varying the concentration of the bathing saline solution is a simple and useful method to induce and investigate mechanical-combined swelling[6,8,11,17,22,48,54] and free-swelling behavior of articular cartilage.[18,31,39] Generally, the concentration of NaCl solution is altered at 2 M, 0.15 M, and 0.015 M. The solution containing 0.15 M NaCl is taken to represent a physiological saline. The $0.015\,M$ NaCl is regarded as hypotonic solution; the $2\,M$ saline is considered as hypertonic solution. The transient osmosis-induced swelling and shrinkage strains were obtained using ultrasound in a recent study.[39] In the early studies, the water gains of different zones of articular cartilage were weighted to indirectly qualify the swelling behavior while the *ex situ* samples were at equilibrium in hypotonic saline.[5,12,17] The equilibrium swelling strain of the full-thickness was optically measured and the averaged unaxial modulus H_A was predicted.[18] Using osmotic stress, collagen network was found to play an important role in limiting hydration and containing PG content.[55] The osmosis-induced mechanical properties of cartilage were characterized in tension[22,54] and in confined/unconfined compression.[11,17,48] In these studies, the isometric swelling phenomena in cartilage strips strains with a fixed length were examined at very low applied tensile or compression. The changes in the forces induced by changing the bath ionic concentration were recorded.

To study swelling, the state equilibrating in $2\,M$ saline solution is usually regarded as the reference state. The reference inhomogeneous distribution of water volume fraction ϕ_0^w and PG-associated negative FCD (c_0^F) are generally required by the estimation of swelling pressure.[4] They can be measured by using the weighting method to calculate the weight of cartilage slices and the dry weight after lyophilized,[13,31,49,56] mechanical method[8] or by using MRI.[9] Triphasic theory is developed based on the achievements of previous studies, especially on the biphasic theory. Articular cartilage is modelled as a triphasic material, composed of solid phase (PG-collagen matrix), fluid phase (water) and ion phase.[4] With regarding of the ion concentration and electrical potential effects, triphasic theory provides the thermodynamic foundation and the complex mechanical chemical electrokinetic mechanism for cartilage swelling, deformation, and viscoelasticity. Therefore, triphasic theory can describe the electrochemomechanism of swelling more comprehensively than any other former theories.

The heterogeneous composition and micro-structural organization of cartilage tissue determine the intrinsic inhomogeneity of the swelling behavior. This property is important to the functions of articular cartilage because the gradient of swelling pressure from the surface to the deep well protects the fatigue of articular cartilage.[5] Since the early 1980s, it has been discovered that the cartilage tissue dimensionally swell when the concentration of the external solution was changed. In Myer's study,[6] the dimensional swelling measured by stereomicroscope and tension device showed that the osmosis-induced contractions of the superficial, middle and deep zone varied and the largest contraction occurred at the deep zone of the cartilage layer. However, the cartilage layer had to be cut into slices in these studies and thereby lost the integrity of the full-thickness cartilage layer.

Recently, with the decrease of ion concentration, the swelling of the intact cartilage layer separated from the underlying bone layer using a surgical chisel was studied by the measurements of a geometric parameter curvature and two swelling parameters including stretch and area change.[18] A matrix-dependent anisotropy in controlling the swelling-induced residual strains with sample orientation was found and the collageneous surface zone was proved to be a structurally important element in swelling procedure.[18] Using a high-resolution optical system and computer-based image acquisition system, 2D swelling-induced residual strains in the cut surface of the cartilage-bone samples were measured.[13,31] The nonuniformity of the swelling strains at different zones was also observed. It was noted that the deep zone had compressive strains while the tensile strains were observed in the middle and superficial zones.[13,31] These experimental results demonstrated that the limitation of the surface layer and the subchondral bone layer were both important for the anisotropic and inhomogeneous swelling behavior of articular cartilage. When articular cartilage was degenerated, the OA cartilage showed a considerable increase in water content of the middle zone and a responsible slight increase in the superficial and deep zones when the sliced samples were soaked into a hypotonic saline (0.015 M NaCl).[5] In contrast, few changes of equilibrium hydration happened in the normal cartilage.[5]

Many previous studies investigated the equilibrated swelling of articular cartilage, but did not have a capability of monitoring the transient swelling and progressive degeneration in real time. After Tepic *et al.*[57] first probed the hydration process of the dehydrated cartilage using ultrasound, no further insight studies were carried out. Until recently, to *in situ* study the transient swelling of articular cartilage, an ultrasound approach was developed to monitor the depth-dependent swelling.[39,58] It has been demonstrated that it is feasible to use high-frequency ultrasound to monitor and qualify the transient behavior of articular cartilage during the free swelling or shrinkage process induced by the concentration change of the bathing saline solution as well as the progressive enzyme digestion.[39,58]

In this paper, ultrasound characterizations of swelling behavior of articular cartilage were introduced. The first part briefly introduced background and literature review on cartilage swelling. Specimen preparation, experiment protocols of ultrasound-measured swelling were described in the method section. Followed by the conclusion part, the recent results of parametric extraction of swelling behavior of articular cartilage were introduced and discussed.

2. Methods

2.1. *Specimen preparation*

Cylindrical cartilage-bone plugs approximately 3 mm thick were cored from fresh mature bovine patellae without obvious lesions using a metal punch with a diameter of 6.35 mm. Specimens were wrapped in wet gauze soaked with physiological saline, and stored in a refrigerator at $-20°C$ until testing. It has been previously reported that cryopreservation, freezing and thawing of the specimen may not affect its biomechanical and acoustic properties.[59-64] The specimens were removed from the

−20°C condition to the 3°C condition at night before testing day and thawed in physiological saline for one hour before testing.[18,39,58]

2.2. *Ultrasound swelling measurement system (USMS)*

In this paper, two non-contact 3D ultrasound swelling measurement systems (3D USMS) were introduced. One was a manually-controlled 3D USMS, which was designed to monitor the swelling behavior of articular cartilage at one observation site. The other was a motor-controlled 3D USMS, also called as ultrasound-elastomicroscopy system. The transducer can scan along the diameter direction to form ultrasound biomicroscopy (UBM) image (B-mode image with a micron order of high resolution). Figure 2 shows the block diagram of the experiment setup.

2.2.1. *Manually-controlled 3D ultrasound system*

A manually-controlled 3D USMS was built to monitor the deformation of cartilage specimen under osmotic loading in a non-contact and non-destructive way. An ultrasound pulser/receiver (Model 5601A, Panametrics, Waltham, MA, USA) was used to drive a nominal 50 MHz focused broadband polymer (PVDF) ultrasound transducer with a focal length of 12.7 mm, a −6 dB focal zone diameter of 0.1 mm and a focal zone depth of 0.95 mm (Panametrics, Waltham, MA, USA). The focal point of the transducer was placed approximately at the middle portion of the specimen thickness by adjusting the position of the transducer to maximize the ultrasound signals reflected from the specimen. The axial and lateral resolutions of the focused ultrasound beam were approximately 100 μm and 50 μm, respectively. The center frequency of this transducer was 35 MHz, and its −6 dB bandwidth ranged from 24 to 46 MHz. Ultrasound waves radiated via the saline solution and propagated through the tissue. A-mode ultrasound radio frequency (RF) signals reflected or scattered within artilage cartilage were received and amplified by the

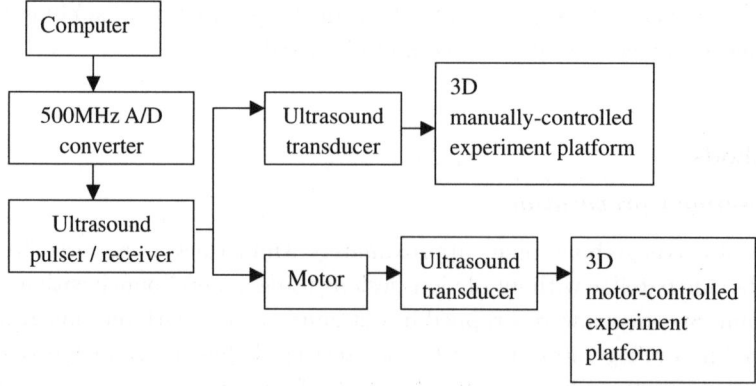

Fig. 2.   Block diagram of the experiment setups.

ultrasound pulser/receiver. The bandwidth of the receiver was set to 5 to 75 MHz. The maximum gain of the pulser/receiver was used in this study to acquire the sufficient amplitude of the ultrasound echoes. The attenuation (unit in dB) of the pulser/receiver was set at zero to obtain the saturated RF signals or at a certain dB value to achieve the unsaturated RF signals with maximum amplitude. The received ultrasound signals were digitized by an 8-bit A/D converter card with a sampling rate of 500 MHz (Model CompuScope 82GPCI, Gage, Canada) installed in the computer. The A/D converter was triggered by the trigger signal out of the pulser/receiver. A-mode RF ultrasound signals reflected from the wire, the cartilage surface and the cartilage-bone interface were continuously recorded at a sampling rate of approximately one frame per 0.6 s. The ultrasound RF signals were displayed on the monitor in real time and automatically saved into the hard disk for offline data analysis. Meanwhile, the M-mode image constructed by A-mode signals demonstrates the shifts of the ultrasound echoes from the cartilage tissues at different depths during the shrinkage and swelling processes. The brightness or color in the M-mode image represents the amplitude of the ultrasound RF signals.

During the test, the cartilage-bone plug was fixed on the bottom of the container, surrounded by rubber gel (Blu-Tack, Australia), and submerged in the saline solution. The outer ring of the surface of the cartilage disc with a width of approximately 0.6 mm was gently covered by the rubber gel. Therefore, the diffusion of ions and water was not allowed from the sides of the specimen and the free swelling in the central portion of the specimen could be treated as an *in-situ* condition. A 3D translating stage with micrometers (Model R301MMX/2201MMXY, Ball Slide Positioning Stages, Deltron Precision Inc.) was designed to align the focused ultrasound beam into the cartilage specimen. One low-profile micrometer was attached to the ultrasound transducer in the z direction to vertically move the ultrasound beam and the other two were fixed in the x and y directions respectively to horizontally translate the specimen. Using this stage, the ultrasound transducer could be manually moved to the position over the central portion of the cartilage specimen with the focal zone of ultrasound beam located inside the cartilage layer to obtain the maximum echo amplitude. The temperature of the bathing solution was detected using a digital thermometer with a stainless steel probe (CheckTemp 1, EUROTRONIK, German). The room temperature and humidity were detected using a digital thermo-hygrometer (Model #411, OMEGA Engineering Inc., Stamford, CT, USA).

2.2.2. *Motor-controlled 3D ultrasound system*

A motor-controlled 3D scanning USMS was built to investigate the inner section of cartilage specimen during swelling and shrinkage progresses in a non-contact and non-destructive way. In this system, the computer and the ultrasound pulser/receiver were as same as the ones mentioned in the 3D manually-controlled

USMS. The 3D translating device (Parker Hannifin Corporation, Irvine, CA, USA) consisted of a compumotor controller and a 3D translating frame. A smaller sized focal ultrasound transducer with a center frequency of 42 MHz and a focal length of 12 mm was fixed at the end of the mechanical arm, the movement of which was controlled by the computer-controlled stepper-motor. After the position of the transducer was adjusted along the z direction to maximize the ultrasound signals reflected from the specimen, the transducer could be automatically translated along the diameter of the specimen in the x direction or the y direction to obtain B-mode ultrasound image. The vertical and horizontal precisions of the 3D translating device were up to 1 μm. The resolution for the flight-time measurement was 2 ns in this study, with 500 MHz sampling rate. Using the assumed average ultrasound velocity in articular cartilage of 1675 m/s,[65] the corresponding displacement resolution in the tissue could approach to approximately 1.7 μm. Therefore, this method using high frequency ultrasound is so called ultrasound biomicroscopy (UBM) imaging. The scanning speed was set using the custom-designed program. Ultrasound biomicroscopic image reconstructed by A-mode signals demonstrates the ultrasound echoes from one section of the cartilage tissues at different depths during the shrinkage and swelling processes. One frame of UBM image shows the B-mode image of depth-dependent deformation of the cartilage specimen along one section. The brightness or color in the UBM image represents the amplitude of the ultrasound RF signals.

With functions such as the automatic segmentation and 2D tracking method,[38] the custom-designed program was used for 1D and 2D data collection, signal processing and display. A region of interest (ROI) could be outlined by a rectangle in the B-mode image to analyze the distribution of the movement of the interstitial tissue at different depths. The tissue displacement images and corresponding elastographs could be acquired during the different periods.

2.3. Experiment protocols of swelling behavior

2.3.1. Dimension-dependence of swelling behavior

The specimen was removed from the $-20°$C condition to the 3$°$C condition at night before the test day. In the test day, the specimen was removed from the refrigerator and marked in the horizontal and vertical directions. The specimen ($\phi = 6.35$ mm) was installed onto the container bottom and fixed with rubber gel, which was correspondingly marked to match the markers on the specimen (Fig. 3). Then the specimen was submerged in the physiological saline solution. It was thawed for one hour to approach equilibrium. The concentration of the bath solution was increased from 0.15 to 2 M in the shrinkage phase and decreased back to 0.15 M in the swelling phase. Each phase lasted for one hour. The deformation of the cartilage specimen induced by the osmotic pressure was recorded using USMS.

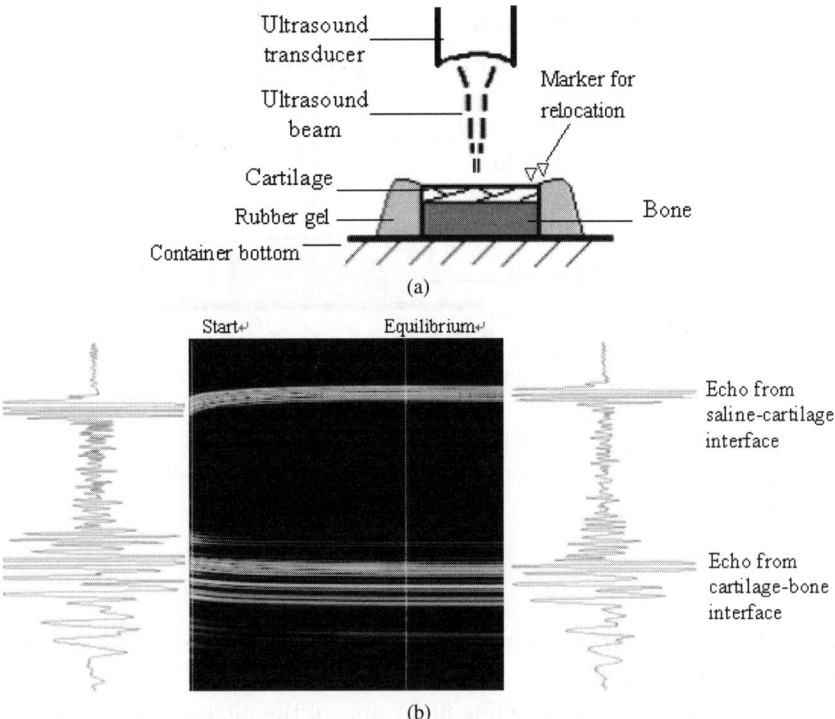

(a)

(b)

Fig. 3. (a) An enlarged schematic of in*situ* ultrasound monitoring. Cylindrical specimen was fixed using rubber gel. Two triangles represent the locations for markers on the specimen and rubber gel. (b) M-mode ultrasound image and the A-mode echoes collected at start and equilibrium states.

After one round of the shrinkage-swelling test, the specimen was removed from the bottom of the container and its dimension was reduced using a surgical scalpel to remove full-thick cartilage tissues from two sides symmetrically. The cylindrical cartilage-bone specimens were cut into slim cartilage-bone specimens with a width of 4 mm. Then the specimen with the smaller dimension was reinstalled back to the container. Careful attention was paid to keep the markers on the cartilage well matched to the markers on the rubber gel (Fig. 4). Therefore, the specimen could be observed at the approximately same observation point. After the second round of the shrinkage-swelling test was finished, the specimen was taken out and its width was reduced to approximately 3 mm. Then the specimen was put back for monitoring. The same protocol was followed for the specimen reduced the dimension to 2 mm × 6 mm (width × length) and 2 mm × 4 mm.

Two quantitative parameters were extracted from the transient swelling and shrinkage behaviors. They were the maximum strain (ε_{max}) of the transient strain (ε) of the cartilage layer (Eq. (1)) and the slope (k) of the logarithm of the normalized time shift of the cartilage-bone interface.[57] The slope (k) was used to describe the diffusion speed of ions and water between cartilage and the bathing

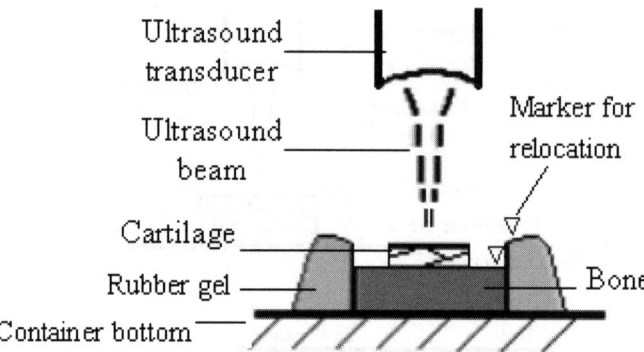

Fig. 4.   Specimen with a smaller dimension was installed on the bottom of the container as same as in Fig. 3.

saline. The logarithm of the normalized time shift $(y(n))$ of the cartilage-bone interface is defined as Eq. (2).

$$\varepsilon = \frac{d}{h}, \tag{1}$$

where h is the thickness of the cartilage layer, d is the displacement of the cartilage layer, which is given by $d = c_s \times T/2$, c_s is the sound speed in the saline and T denotes the shift of the corresponding flight time of the ultrasound echoes from the saline-cartilage interface during shrinkage or swelling phase. This value could be achieved using cross-correlation algorithm.

$$y(n) = \log((x_{\max} - x(n))/x_{\max}), \tag{2}$$

where $x(n)$ is the data of the time shift of the superficial cartilage layer measured using cross-correlation algorithm. $x_{\max}$ presents the maximum value of $x(n)$. Then, k can be acquired from the linear fitting of the linearly descending part of $y(n)$ from the start of changing the saline solution to the time approaching 50% of the $x_{\max}$.

2.3.2. In situ measurement compared with ex situ measurement

After the cartilage-bone plug with a cartilage size of $2\,\mathrm{mm} \times 4\,\mathrm{mm}$ was monitored during the shrinkage and swelling processes, the full-thickness cartilage layer was separated from the bone by the scalpel. The cartilage slice without bone was also monitored at the proximal central point according to the same protocol of the shrinkage and swelling tests using a specially designed container to mount the cartilage layer (Fig. 5). The ex situ measured parameters were compared with those in situ.

2.3.3. Shrinkage-swelling test

As mentioned before, the thawed specimen plug was installed onto the container bottom (Fig. 3(a)) and submerged in the physiological saline solution for one hour.

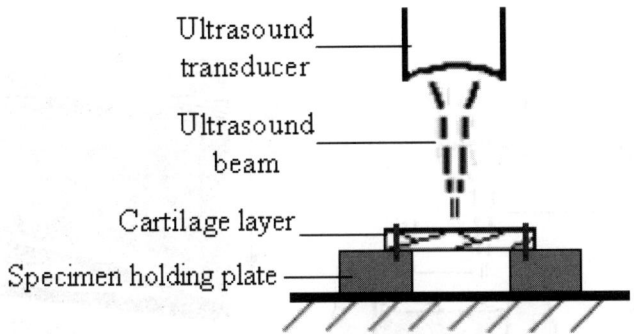

Fig. 5. An enlarged schematic of *ex situ* ultrasound monitoring. Two ends of the rectangle cartilage layer were fixed on a plate using two strings.

The ultrasound signals were collected at equilibrium. Then, the saline was removed using an injection syringe and the container was filled with the 2 M saline. The whole procedure of changing the saline was completed within 30 s. Under this condition, the ion concentration inside the cartilage matrix was lower than that of the external bathing solution. This imbalance resulted in a Donnan osmotic loading on the cartilage. With the diffusion of the ions and water, the interstitial swelling pressure generated by negative charges along PGs decreased. The dynamic contraction of the cartilage layer at different depths could be observed in the ultrasound signals. The cartilage sample was allowed to equilibrate for approximately one hour. After the new equilibrium was reached, the bathing saline was quickly changed back to 0.15 M NaCl within 30 s. Under this condition, the ionic concentration inside the cartilage tissue was higher in comparison with the concentration of the bathing solution. Consequently, the Donnan osmotic pressure with an opposite direction against that during the shrinkage phase caused cartilage swelling. The interstitial swelling pressure generated by negative charges along PGs increased. The swelling process was monitored for another hour.

Every ∼0.6 second one frame of A-mode signals was sampled during the shrinkage and swelling phases. In real time, M-mode image was reconstructed by A-mode signals (Fig. 3(b)). Two quantitative parameters were extracted from the transient swelling and shrinkage behaviors. They were the maximum strain ($\varepsilon_{\max}$) of the transient strain (ε) of the cartilage layer, which was calculated using Eq. (1), and the time to reach the peak value, named as duration.

2.3.4. *Monitoring swelling behavior using ultrasound elastomicroscopy*

Following the same protocol, the thawed cartilage-bone plug was fixed on the bottom of the container and equilibrated for one hour in physiological saline solution (0.15 M NaCl), and then the solution was immediately replaced by the hypertonic saline (2 M NaCl). The deformation of cartilage under the osmotic loading was scanned by the ultrasound biomicroscopy imaging system (3D motor-controlled

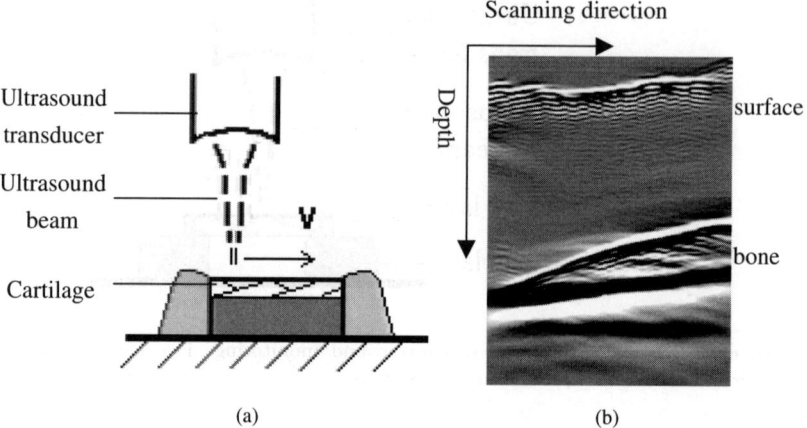

Fig. 6. An enlarged schematic of the ultrasound scanning part. Specimen was installed on the bottom of the container. Ultrasound transducer was automatically moved with a speed of v, which is controlled by the computer. (b) UBM image of the specimen.

USMS). Through the control of the compumotor, the transducer was moved from one side of the specimen to the other side along the diameter direction with a speed (Fig. 6(a)). The UBM image was formed with 164 A-mode lines (Fig. 6(b)). The central section with a length of ∼4 mm was monitored and the depth of the image was ∼3 mm. The transducer translated from the left side (set as starting point) to the right side (end point) and then returned to the starting point with a fast speed to begin another scanning trip. In this study, it took approximately 0.3 s to collect one frame of A-mode signal and the rate of ultrasonic biomicroscopy imaging was approximately 48 s per frame of UBM image.

2.4. *Data analysis*

The results were presented in the form of mean ± SD. Paired t-test was used to test the significance of the difference between the parameters in the shrinkage and swelling phases. One-Way ANOVA was used to test the significance of the difference among the parameters of specimens with different dimensions. The statistical analysis software SPSS (V11.5, SPSS Inc., Chicago, USA) was used for data analysis.

3. Results and Discussions

3.1. *Transient swelling strain*

Not only the swelling strains but also the shrinkage strains (or de-swelling strain) were measured. It was found that the cartilage surface tended to deform rapidly and then moved upwards or downwards gradually close to the equilibrium state in approximately one hour after changing the concentration of the saline solution. This interesting phenomenon demonstrated that the cartilage specimen might experience

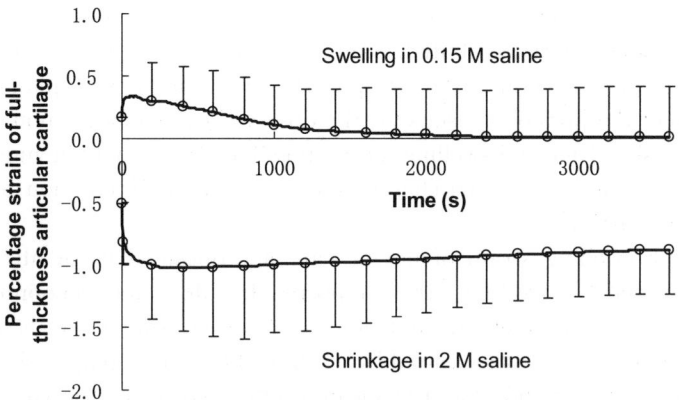

Fig. 7. The shrinkage strain and the swelling strain versus the measurement time. The error bars represent standard deviations of the results of the 20 specimens.

a "relaxation" state after reaching its maximum shrinkage or swelling amplitude (Fig. 7), i.e. the surface moved back towards the original state. The absolute peak value of the shrinkage strain $(1.01 \pm 0.62\%)$ was significantly larger than that of the swelling strain $(0.40 \pm 0.33\%)$ $(p < 0.05$, paired t-test). The shrinkage duration $(1194 \pm 1129\,\text{s})$ was also significantly $(p < 0.05$, paired t-test) larger than the swelling duration $(302 \pm 717\,\text{s})$. It was noted that the peak swelling strain correlated with the peak shrinkage strain $(R^2 = 0.586, p < 0.05)$, while such a correlation did not exist between the shrinkage duration and the swelling duration. This phenomenon might be caused by the anisotropic mechanical properties and ion diffusion rates of articular cartilage at different depths. Further explanation to this finding requires more theoretical and experimental studies.

The shrinkage and swelling behaviors of cartilage showed an "overshoot-relaxation" phenomenon similar to a monotonically decreased "salt-induced stress relaxation" behavior of cartilage has been earlier observed using a confined configuration.[48] One possible reason may be the interactions between the PG matrix and the collagen fibres in the cartilage surface zone. According to the conventional theories, the Donnan osmotic pressure plays a dominant role in the free swelling behavior of cartilage.[4,12,13] With the decreased saline concentration, swelling stress in cartilage increased and the sample was allowed to swell. However, it was soon balanced with the constraining force of the stretched collagen network, particularly the reinforced collagen fibrils in the cartilage superficial zone. The cartilage sample had a tendency to be compressed back to its initial state. In contrast, swelling stress in cartilage decreased when the saline concentration was increased. The total pressure squeezed on the cartilage and allowed the cartilage to shrink. Also balanced by the tensile force of collagen fibres and their interaction with the proteoglycan matrix, the cartilage surface moved backwards after the strain reached the peak. Another possible reason for the phenomenon is related to ion redistribution. During the shrinkage (de-swelling) process, the cartilage tissue at certain depths might absorb more ions than those required for balancing the fixed charges at that region.

This may cause a temporary overshoot of the shrinkage followed by a relaxation phase as the ions are redistributed. Similar explanation could also be applied for the overshoot phenomenon of the swelling. However, the above explanations might only be two of the possible reasons for the observed overshoot phenomenon during the transient shrinkage and swelling. Other possible causes could include the depth-dependent distribution of fixed charge density[13] and the interaction between ions and collagen matrix.[48]

The peak swelling strain of bovine cartilage obtained using ultrasound was smaller than the 3% swelling strain reported by Mow and Schoonbeck[17] using the water-weight-gain method, but appeared to be similar to Eisenberg and Grodzinsky's result ($<1\%$) measured by a uniaxial confined compression method.[11] Narmoneva *et al.*[56] found that the mean swelling strain of the canine cartilage strips was approximately 1%. The inconsistency of the reported swelling strains could be due to individual variations of the specimen location, joint, species, age, degeneration status, specimen configuration, and measurement technique.

3.2. *Transient changes in ultrasound speed*

It was demonstrated that the sound speed in cartilage gradually increased when the concentration of the bathing solution was increased from 0.15 to 2 M. It increased by $4.4 \pm 2.1\%$ after one hour. When the concentration of the saline solution was changed back to 0.15 M, the sound speed gradually decreased by up to $5.6 \pm 1.6\%$. The magnitudes of these two changes were significantly different ($p < 0.05$, paired t-test). The percentage change of the sound speed in cartilage during the shrinkage and the swelling processes both exponentially depends on the measurement time ($R^2 = 0.9957$, $R^2 = 0.9988$, respectively) (Fig. 8).

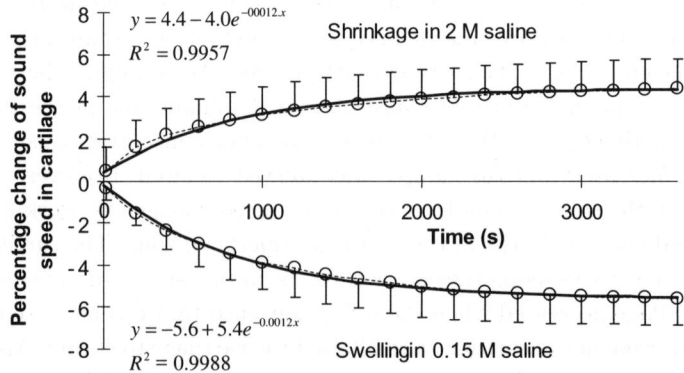

Fig. 8. Ultrasound speed in cartilage increases during the shrinkage process. In contrast, sound speed decreases during the swelling process. Experimental data (dashed lines and marks) can be well fitted by exponential functions (solid lines). The error bars represent standard deviations of the results of 20 specimens.

Ultrasound speed related to the interstitial condition of cartilage is of major importance in the quantitative measurement of the tissue. The averaged transient change of ultrasound speed in the cartilage layer reflected the alterations of the tissue during shrinkage or swelling process, including the tissue density, ion movement and water diffusion. In a recent study, the digestion process was successfully tracked using ultrasound.[58]

In many pervious studies, the speed at equilibrium in cartilage was assumed to be different constant values,[33,42,66-72] which ranged from 1654 m/s to 1765 m/s. Due to the layered structure of articular cartilage, the depth-dependence and inhomogeneity of sound speed in the tissue were investigated.[60,65,73] Since ultrasound. speed depends on many factors, not only the properties of the tissue but other factors such as temperature and intensity of pressure, some researchers proposed their concerns about the validity of results measured using ultrasound.[73,74] Although the uncertainty of ultrasound velocity in cartilage is still in controversy, the validity or reproducibility studies of ultrasonic measurement have confirmed that the ultrasonic method is acceptable[39,66,68,75-78] with the wide use of ultrasound technique in research on articular cartilage. Nieminen *et al.*[51] believed that a constant ultrasound speed could be accepted in the measurement of the cartilage thickness based on their results that there was mild difference in the averaged sound speed in the full-thickness cartilage.

3.3. *Effect of specimen dimension on swelling measurement*

In pairwise comparison of the peak strains of cartilage samples with different dimensions, the statistical analysis of LSD Post Hoc Tests of One-Way ANOVA showed that there were significant differences ($p < 0.05$) in the peak shrinkage strains between the small samples (2 mm × 6.35 mm) and the larger samples (ϕ=6.35 mm and 4 mm × 6.35 mm). However, no significant differences ($p > 0.05$) among the peak swelling strains were found for the cartilage-bone specimens with various sizes. The absolute slope values calculated from the logarithm of the normalized time shift of the cartilage-bone interface (or the bottom surface for the cartilage samples without bone). From the statistical results of LSD Post Hoc Tests of One-Way ANOVA, the slope values for the cylindrical samples with a diameter of 6.35 mm and the larger slim specimens with a width of 4 mm and 3 mm were significantly ($p < 0.05$) lower than those of the specimens with smaller dimensions (2 mm × 6.35 mm and 2 mm × 4 mm) and the cartilage specimens without bone. It was reflected that the ions permeated into or moved out of the cartilage tissue faster with the decrease of specimen dimension (Fig. 9).

However, there are few studies on the dimension-dependence of cartilage swelling. The present study expected to demonstrate that whether the dimension of the specimen would affect the cartilage swelling. It is well known that high frequency ultrasound has a high resolution and it has been applied to monitor a

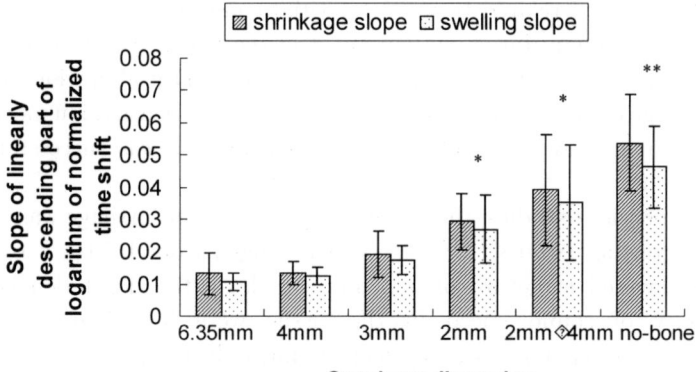

Specimen dimension

Fig. 9.   The absolute values of the slope calculated from the logarithm of the normalized time shift of the cartilage-bone interface or the bottom surface for the cartilage samples without bone. The error bar represents the standard deviations of the results of 10 specimens. "6.35 mm" represents the specimens with a diameter of 6.35 mm; "4 mm", "3 mm", and "2 mm" represent the specimens with a width of 4 mm, 3 mm, and 2 mm, respectively. "2 mm × 4 mm" represents the rectangular specimens with a width of 2 mm and a length of 4 mm. "no-bone" represents the "2 mm × 4 mm" cartilage layers separated from the bone. * Significant difference ($p < 0.05$ by LSD Post Hoc Tests of One-Way ANOVA). ** Significant difference ($p < 0.05$ by One-Way ANOVA) between the cartilage specimens attached to the bone without the bone tissue.

relative small specimen.[72,79] In the present study, the focal zone diameter of 50 MHz focused ultrasound transducer reached 0.1 mm. The results of our experiments suggested that the width of the specimen should not be too small (not < 2 mm) when ultrasound was used to detect the swelling behaviors of articular cartilage. From the results, it is believed that the geometry of the specimen should be taken into account in the studies on the biomechanical properties of articular cartilage as well as in other materials.

3.4. Differences between in situ and ex situ measurements

The peak strains (shrinkage -0.0131 ± 0.0105; swelling 0.0118 ± 0.0042) of the 2 mm × 4 mm cartilage specimens without bone were measured significantly ($p < 0.05$) larger than the strains of the corresponding cartilage-bone specimens (shrinkage -0.0046 ± 0.0027; swelling 0.0075 ± 0.0024). And the *ex situ* strains of the cartilage layer were significantly ($p < 0.05$) larger than the *in situ* strains of the cartilage-bone specimens with larger dimensions.

In addition, the absolute permeation slopes (shrinkage 0.0538 ± 0.0148; swelling 0.0464 ± 0.0128) of the full-thickness cartilage layer without the bone tissue increased significantly ($p < 0.05$) in compared with those (shrinkage 0.0392 ± 0.0173; swelling 0.0352 ± 0.0180) of the corresponding 2 mm × 4 mm samples with bone (Fig. 9).

In the study, since cartilage samples were attached to the bone tissue, the obtained results reflected the swelling behavior and the material properties of the cartilage *in situ*. The separation of the cartilage layer from the bone made the specimen lose its *in situ* properties. The statistical results of the pairwise comparison showed that the absolute peak shrinkage and swelling strains of the cartilage samples without bone were significantly larger than those of the cartilage-bone specimens. It was consistent with the result of Mow and Schoonbeck's study.[17] Setton's study[18] demonstrated that the cartilage layer without the support or limitation of the bone behaved in curling and swelling. It indirectly provided evidence for the difference between cartilage specimens in *in-situ* and *ex-situ* conditions. This study provided evidence that the cartilage disc detached from the subchondral bone tended to swell more in comparison with *in-situ* intact condition.

3.5. *Depth-dependence of swelling behavior*

The shift of the ultrasound echoes at different depths from the articular cartilage represented the spatial change of the articular cartilage tissue. The averaged values ($n = 14$) of the equilibrium swelling strains for deep (30% of the total thickness), middle (55%), and surface (15%) zones were successfully measured using ultrasound (Fig. 10). The nonuniformity of the swelling strains at different zones was observed. It was noted that the deep zone had compressive strains while the tensile strains were observed in the middle and superficial zones. The strain of the middle zone was larger than that of the superficial zone. We compensated the change of the sound speed in the strain calculation assuming the change of the sound speed as a linear function of depth. Based on triphasic theory,[4,13] the aggregate moduli at different zones were predicted using the ultrasound-measured strain data. It was found that the region near the bone had a relatively higher modulus (24.5 ± 11.1 MPa) than the middle zone and the surface layer (7.0 ± 7.4 MPa and 3.0 ± 3.2 MPa, respectively).

Figure 11 shows the result of a type 2D scanning during the shrinkage process of the cartilage induced by the change of saline from 0.15 to 2 M. To analyze the distribution of the movement of the interstitial tissue at different depth, a region of

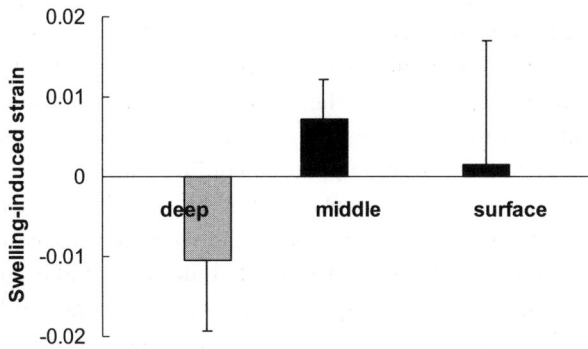

Fig. 10. Nonuniform swelling-induced strains in cartilage grouped into three zones; the swelling-induced strains were compressive in the deep zone and tensile in the middle and surface zones.

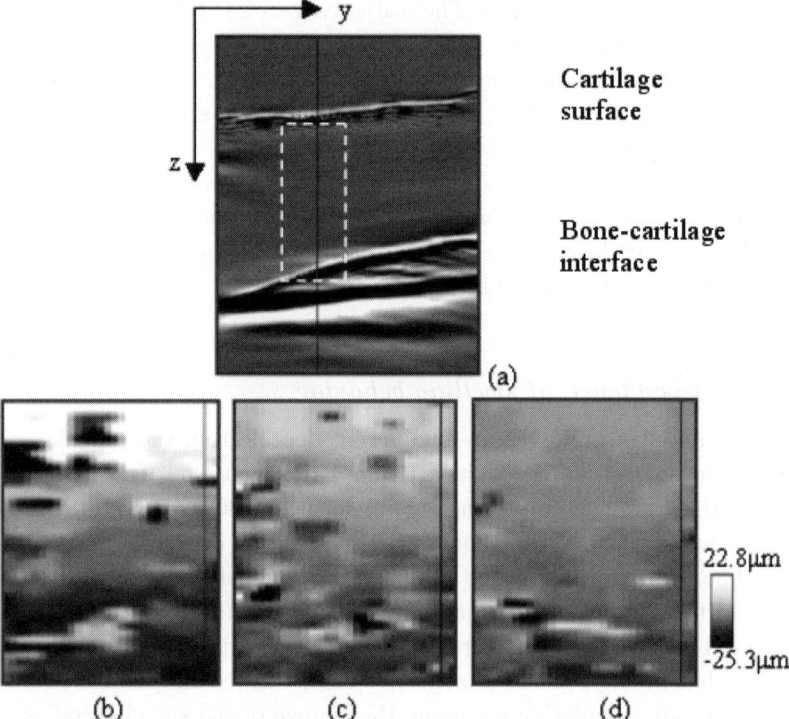

Fig. 11.   (a) An UBM image of the cartilage cross-section. The grey levels of the image linearly represent the amplitude of the RF signals. The images were sampled at a rate of approximately 48 s per frame. The image of displacement distribution of the region of interest indicated by the dashed rectangle (divided into 15 × 40 segments) in (a) are calculated using the 2D a cross-correlation tracking method. The displacement distribution of articular cartilage extracted from the 2D images obtained at (a) 2.5 min and 4.2 min, (b) 5.8 min and 7.5 min, and (d) 10.8 min and 12.5 min. The grey levels of images (b–c) represent the displacement value of the segments at two moments during the shrinkage phase.

interest is outlined by the dashed rectangle in the B-mode image shown in Fig. 11(a). The tissue displacement images during the different periods are formed using the automatic segmentation and 2D tracking method.[38] Figures 11(b)–(d) show the changes in the distribution of the displacement of the tissue at different moments. They indicate that the movement of the tissue is large during the beginning phase of the swelling and shrinkage processes. As time going, the movements of tissues inside cartilage tend to be zero and approach equilibrium.

Our results of the depth-dependent swelling strain of bovine articular cartilage were similar to the results of the canine and human cadaver cartilage.[13,31] It has been known that most of the PGs are located in the middle zone of articular cartilage and the fixed negative charges on the PGs play a primary role in swelling.[1,5] Therefore, the swollen middle layer may cause a compressive stress on the deep zone. In addition, the *in situ* configuration that the deep zone was attached to the bone might give a rigid support to place the cartilage matrix in a state of compression.

It is also known that collagen fibre organization in cartilage is highly nonuniform and anisotropic. Fibres are oriented tangential to the surface at the superficial zone to confine the swelling stress.[4,11,12] This may explain why the tensile strain of the surface layer is lower than that of the middle zone.

4. Conclusions

This paper introduced our studies on the ultrasonic characterization of swelling behavior of articular cartilage *in situ*. The ultrasound-swelling and ultrasound-elastomicroscopy systems have potentials for the investigation of the transient deformations of articular cartilage at different depths during swelling and shrinkage procedures. Ultrasound approaches can inherently provide non-destructive and *in-situ* assessment of articular cartilage.

Acknowledgments

This work was partially supported by the Research Grants Council of Hong Kong (PolyU 5199/02E, PolyU 5245/03E) and The Hong Kong Polytechnic University.

References

1. V. C. Mow, W. Y. Gu and F. H. Chen, Structure and function of articular cartilage and meniscus, in *Basic Orthopaedic Biomechanics and Mechano-Biology*, 3rd edition. V. C. Mow and R. Huiskes eds., (Lippincott Williams & Wilkins, Philadelphia, PA, USA, 2005), pp. 181–258.
2. V. C. Mow and C. T. Hung, Biomechanics of articular cartilage, in *Basic Biomechanics of the Musculoskeletal System*, 3rd edition. M. Nordin and V. H. Frankel eds., (Lea & Feviger Philadelphia, London, 2001), pp. 60–101.
3. Y. C. Fung, Bone and Cartilage, in *Biomechanics Mechanical Properties of Living Tissues*, 2nd edition, (Springer-Verlag, New York Inc., 1993), pp. 500–544.
4. W. M. Lai, J. S. Hou and V. C. Mow, A triphasic theory for the swelling and deformation behaviors of articular cartilage, *J. Biomech. Eng.* **113** (1991) 245–258.
5. A. Maroudas, Balance between swelling pressure and collagen tension in normal and degenerate cartilage, *Nature* **260** (1976a) 808–809.
6. E. R. Myers, W. M. Lai and V. C. Mow, A continuum theory and an experiment for the ion -induced swelling behavior of articular cartilage, *J. Biomech. Eng.* **106** (1984) 151–158.
7. J. M. Huyghe and J. D. Janssen, Quadriphasic mechanics of swelling incompressible porous media, *Int. J. Eng. Sci.* **35**(8) (1997) 793–802.
8. C. C.-B. Wang, X. E. Guo, D. N. Sun, V. C. Mow, G. A. Ateshian and C. T. Hung, The functional environment of chondrocytes within cartilage subjected to compressive loading: A theoretical and experimental approach, *Biorheology* **39** (2002) 11–25.
9. E. M. Shapiro, A. Borthakur, J. H. Kaufman, J. S. Leigh and R. Reddy, Water distribution patterns inside bovine articular cartilage as visualized by ^{1}H magnetic resonance imaging, *Osteoarthr. Cartilage* **9** (2001) 533–538.

10. V. C. Mow and X. E. Guo, Mechano-electrochemical properties of articular cartilage: their inhomogeneities and anisotropies, *Ann. Rev. Biomed. Eng.* **4** (2002) 175–209.

11. S. R. Eisenberg and A. J. Grodzinsky, Swelling of articular cartilage and other connective tissues: Electromechanochemical forces, *J. Ortho. Res.* **3** (1985) 148–159.

12. A. Maroudas, J. Mizrahi, E. P. Katz, E. J. Wachtel and M. Soudry, Physicochemical properties and functional behavior of normal and osteoarthritic human cartilage, in *Articular Cartilage Biochemistry.* K. E. Kuettner, R. Schleyerbach and V. C. Hascall eds., (Raven Press, New York, 1986), pp. 311–329.

13. D. A. Narmoneva, J. Y. Wang and L. A. Setton, A noncontacting method for material property determination for articular cartilage from osmotic loading, *Biophys. J.* **81** (2001) 3066–3076.

14. E. B. Hunziker, M. Michel and D. Studer, Ultrastructure of adult human cartilage matrix after cryotechnical processing, *Microsc. Res. Technol.* **37** (1997) 271–284.

15. A. C. Chen, W. C. Bae, R. M. Schinagl and R. L. Sah, Depth- and strain-dependent mechanical and electromechanical properties of full-thickness bovine articular cartilage in confined compression, *J. Biomech.* **34**(1) (2001) 1–12.

16. P. L. Mente and J. L. Lewis, Elastic modulus of calcified cartilage is an order of magnitude less than that of subchondral bone, *J. Orthop. Res.* **12**(5) (1994) 637–647.

17. V. C. Mow and J. M. Schoonbeck, Contribution of Donnan osmotic pressure towards the biphasic compressive modulus of articular cartilage, in *Transaction of the 30th Annual Orthopaedic Research Society*, Vol. 9 (Altanta, Georgia, 1984), p. 262.

18. L. A. Setton, H. Tohyama and V. C. Mow, Swelling and curling behaviors of articular cartilage, *J. Biomech. Eng.-T. ASME.* **120** (1998) 355–361.

19. D. L. Skaggs, W. H. Warden and V. C. Mow, Radial tie fibers influence the tensile properties of the bovine medial meniscus, *J. Orthop. Res.* **12**(2) (1994) 176–185.

20. S. L. Y. Woo, W. H. Akeson and G. F. Jemmott, Measurements of nonhomogeneous, directionalmechanical properties of articular cartilage in tension, *J. Biomech.* **9** (1976) 785.

21. V. Roth and V. C. Mow, The intrinsic tensile behavior of the matrix of bovine articular cartilage and its variation with age, *J. Bone Jt. Surg.* **62** (1980) 1102–1117.

22. F. Guilak, A. Ratcliffe, N. Lane, M. P. Rosenwasser and V. C. Mow, Mechanical and biochemical changes in the superficial zone of articular cartilage in canine experimental osteoarthritis, *J. Orthop. Res.* **12** (1994) 474–484.

23. A. Verteramo and B. B. Seedhom, Zonal and directional variations in tensile properties of bovine articular cartilage with special reference to strain rate variation, *Biorheology* **41**(3–4) (2004) 203–213.

24. L. A. Setton, V. C. Mow, F. J. Muller, J. C. Pita and D. S. Howell, Mechanical properties of canine articular cartilage are significantly altered following transection of the anterior cruciate ligament, *J. Orthop. Res.* **12**(4) (1994) 451–463.

25. L. A. Setton, W. Gu, M. W. Lai and V. C. Mow, Predictions of swelling-induced pre-stress in articular cartilage, in *Mechanics of Poroelastic Media*, A. P. S. Selvadurai ed., (Kluwer Academic Publishers, Dordrecht, 1995), pp. 299–320.

26. V. C. Mow, S. C. Kuer, W. M. Lai and C. G. Armstrong, Biphasic creep and stress relaxation of articular cartilage in compression: Theory and experiments, *J. Biomech. Eng.* **102** (1980) 73–84.

27. C. C.-B. Wang, C. T. Hung and V. C. Mow, An analysis of the effects of depth-dependent aggregate modulus on articular cartilage stress-relaxation behavior in compression, *J. Biomech.* **34** (2001) 75–84.

28. F. Guilak, A. Ratcliffe and V. C. Mow, Chondrocyte deformation and local tissue strain in articular cartilage: A confocal microscopy study, *J. Orthop. Res.* **13** (1995) 410–421.

29. R. M. Schinagl, M. K. Ting, J. H. Price and R. L. Sah, Video microscopy to quantitate the inhomogeneous equilibrium strain within articular cartilage during confined compression, *Ann. Biomed. Eng.* **24** (1996) 500–512.

30. R. M. Schinagl, D. Gurskis, A. C. Chen and R. L. Sah, Depth-dependent confined compression modulus of fullthickness bovine articular cartilage, *J. Orthop. Res.* **15** (1997) 499–506.

31. D. A. Narmoneva, J. Y. Wang and L. A. Setton, Nonuniform swelling-induced residual strains in articular cartilage, *J. Biomech.* **32** (1999) 401–408.

32. M. Fortin, J. Soulhat, A. Shirazi-Adl, E. B. Hunziker and M. D. Buschmann, Unconfined compression of articular cartilage: Nonlinear behavior and comparison with a fibril-reinforced biphasic model, *J. Biomech. Eng.* **122**(2) (2000) 189–95.

33. Y. P. Zheng, A. F. T. Mak, K. P. Lau and L. Qin, An ultrasonic measurement for *in vitro* depth-dependent equilibrium strains of articular cartilage in compression, *Phys. Med. Biol.* **7** (2002) 3165–3180.

34. N. A. Cohn, S. Y. Emelianov, M. A. Lubinski and M. O'Donnell, An elasticity microscope: Part I. Methods, *IEEE Trans. Ultrason. Ferroelectr. Freq. Control* **44** (1997a) 1304–1319.

35. N. A. Cohn, S. Y. Emelianov and M. O'Donnell, An elasticity microscope: Part II. Experimental results, *IEEE Trans. Ultrason. Ferroelectr. Freq. Control* **44** (1997b) 1320–1331.

36. J. Ophir, I. Cespedes, H. Ponnekanti, Y. Yazdi and X. Li, Elastography: A quantitative method for imaging the elasticity of biological tissues, *Ultrason. Imaging* **13** (1991) 111–134.

37. J. Ophir, S. K. Alam, B. Garra, F. Kallel, E. Konofagou, T. Krouskop and T. Varghese, Elastography: Ultrasonic estimation and imaging of the elastic properties of tissues, *Proc. Inst. Mech. Eng.* **213** (1999) 203–233.

38. Y. P. Zheng, S. L. Bridal, J. Shi, A. Saied, M. H. Lu, B. Jaffre, A. F. T. Mak and P. Laugier, High resolution ultrasound elastomicroscopy imaging of soft tissues: System development and feasibility, *Phys. Med. Biol.* **49** (2004b) 3925–3938.

39. Q. Wang and Y. P. Zheng, Non-contact evaluation of osmosis-induced shrinkage and swelling behavior of articular cartilage *in situ* using high-frequency ultrasound, *Instrument. Sci. Technol.* **34**(3) (2006) 317–334.

40. W. Zhu, V. C. Mow, T. J. Koob and D. R. Eyre, Viscoelastic shear properties of articular cartilage and the effects of glycosidase treatments, *J. Orthop. Res.* **11**(6) (1993) 771–781.

41. L. Qin, Y. Zheng, C. Leung, A. Mak, W. Choy and K. Chan, Ultrasound detection of trypsin-treated articular cartilage: Its association with cartilaginous proteoglycans assessed by histological and biochemical methods, *J. Bone Miner. Metab.* **20**(5) (2002) 281–287.

42. Y. P. Zheng, C. X. Ding, J. Bai, A. F. T. Mak and L. Qin, Measurement of the layered compressive properties of trypsin-treated articular cartilage: An ultrasound investigation, *Med. Biol. Eng. Comput.* **39** (2001) 534–541.

43. C. M. Flahiff, V. B. Kraus, J. L. Huebner and L. A. Setton, Cartilage mechanics in the guinea pig model of osteoarthritis studied with an osmotic loading method, *Osteoarthr. Cartilage* **12** (2004) 383–388.

44. H. J. Mankin, V. C. Mow, J. A. Buckwalter, J. P. Iannotti and A. Ratcliffe, Form and function of articular cartilage, in *Orthopaedic Basic Science*. S. R. Simnon, ed., (American Academy Orthopaedic Surgeons, 1994), pp. 2–44.

45. D. N. Sun, W. Y. Gu, X. E. Guo, W. M. Lai and V. C. Mow, A mixed finite element formulation of triphasic mechano-electrochemical theory for charged, hydrated biological soft tissues, *Int. J. Num. Methods Eng.* **45** (1999) 1375–1402.

46. A. Maroudas, Transport of solutes through cartilage – permeability to large molecules, *J. Anat.* **122** (1976b) 335–347.

47. M. R. DiSilvestro and J. K. Suh, Biphasic poroviscoelastic characteristics of proteoglycan-depleted articular cartilage: simulation of degeneration, *Ann. Biomed. Eng.* **30**(6) (2002) 792–800.

48. S. R. Eisenberg and A. J. Grodzinsky, The kinetics of chemically induced nonequilibrium swelling of articular cartilage and corneal stroma, *J. Biomech. Eng.* **109** (1987) 79–89.

49. C. M. Flahiff, D. A. Narmoneva, J. L. Huebner, V. B. Kraus, F. Guilak and L. A. Setton, Osmotic loading to determine the intrinsic material properties of guinea pig knee cartilage, *J. Biomech.* **35** (2002) 1285–1290.

50. V. C. Mow, A. Ratcliffe and S. L. Y. Woo, Part II Cartilage biomechanics, in *Biomechanics of Diarthrodial Joints*, Vol. I (Springer-Verlag, New York Inc., 1990), pp. 215–451.

51. H. J. Nieminen, J. Toyras, J. Rieppo, M. T. Nieminen, J. Hirvonen, R. Korhonen and J. S. Jurvelin, Real-time ultrasound analysis of articular cartilage degradation *in vitro*, *Ultrasound Med. Biol.* **28**(4) (2002) 519–525.

52. J. Toyras, J. Rieppo, M. T. Nieminen, H. J. Helminen and J. S. Jurvelin, Characterization of enzymatically induced degradation of articular cartilage using high frequency ultrasound, *Phys. Med. Biol.* **44** (1999) 2723–2733.

53. V. C. Mow, C. C. Wang and C. T. Hung, The extracellular matrix, interstitial fluid and ions as a mechanical signal transducer in articular cartilage, *Osteoarthritis Cartilage* **7**(1) (1999) 41–58.

54. A. J. Grodzinsky, V. Roth, E. Myers, W. D. Grossman and V. C. Mow, The significance of electromechanical and osmotic forces in the nonequilibrium swelling behavior of articular cartilage in tension, *J. Biomech. Eng.* **103** (1981) 221–231.

55. P. J. Basser, R. Schneiderman, R. A. Bank, E. Wachtel and A. Maroudas, Mechanical properties of the collagen network in human articular cartilage as measured by osmotic stress technique, *Arch. Biochem. Biophys.* **351**(2) (1998) 207–219.

56. D. A. Narmoneva, H. S. Cheung, J. Y. Wang, D. S. Howell and L. A. Setton, Altered swelling behavior of femoral cartilage following joint immobilization in a canine model, *J. Orthop. Res.* **20** (2002) 83–91.

57. S. Tepic, T. Macirowski and R. W. Mann, Mechanical properties of articular cartilage elucidated by osmotic loading and ultrasound, in *Biophysics, Proc. Nat. Acad. Sci.* Vol. 80 (June, USA, 1983), pp. 3331–3333.

58. Y. P. Zheng, J. Shi, L. Qin, S. G. Patil, V. C. Mow and K. Y. Zhou, Dynamic depth-dependent osmotic swelling and solute diffusion in articular in articular cartilage monitored using real-time ultrasound, *Ultrasound Med. Biol.* **30** (2004a) 841–849.

59. G. N. Kiefer, K. Sundby, D. McAllister, N. G. Shrive, C. B. Frank, T. Lam and N. S. Schachar, The effect of cryopreservation on the biomechanical behavior of bovine articular cartilage, *J. Orthop. Res.* **7** (1989) 494–501.

60. D. H. Agemura, W. D. Jr., O'Brien, J. E. Olerud, L. E. Chun and D. E. Eyre, Ultrasonic propagation properties of articular cartilage at 100 MHz, *J. Acoust. Soc. Am.* **87**(4) (1990) 1786–1791.

61. F. T. D'Astous and F. S. Foster, Frequency dependence of ultrasound attenuation and backscatter in breast tissue, *Ultrasound Med. Biol.* **12** (1986) 795–808.

62. N. Dhillon, E. C. Bass and J. C. Lotz, Effect of frozen storage on the creep behavior of human intervertebral discs, *Spine* **26** (2001) 883–888.

63. H. K. W. Kim, P. S. Babyn, K. A. Harasiewicz, H. K. Gahunia, K. P. H. Pritzker and F. S. Foster, Imaging of immature articular cartilage using ultrasound backscatter microscopy at 50 MHz, *J. Orthop. Res.* **13** (1995) 963–970.

64. M. K. Kwan, S. A. Hacker, S. L. Y. Woo and J. S. Wayne, The effect of storage on the biomechanical behavior of articular cartilage – A large strain study, *J. Biomech. Eng-T. ASME.* **114** (1992) 149–153.

65. S. G. Patil, Y. P. Zheng, J. Y. Wu and J. Shi, Measurement of depth-dependency and anisotropy of ultrasound speed of bovine articular cartilage *in vitro*, *Ultrasound Med. Biol.* **30**(7) (2004) 953–963.

66. V. E. Modest, M. C. Murphy and R. W. Mann, Optical verification of a technique for *in situ* ultrasonic measurement of articular cartilage thickness, *J. Biomech.* **22** (1989) 171–176.

67. G. A. Joiner, E. R. Bogoch, K. P. Pritzker, M. D. Buschmann, A. Chevrier and F. S. Foster, High frequency acoustic parameters of human and bovine articular cartilage following experimentally-induced matrix degradation, *Ultrason. Imaging* **23** (2001) 106–116.

68. J. S. Jurvelin, T. Rasanen, P. Kolmonen and T. Lyyra, Comparison of optical, needle probe and ultrasonic techniques for the measurement of articular cartilage thickness, *J. Biomech.* **28**(2) (1995) 231–235.

69. S. L. Myers, K. Dines, D. A. Brandt, K. D. Brandt and M. E. Albrecht, Experimental assessment by high frequency ultrasound of aticular cartilage thickness and osteoarthritic changes, *J. Rheumatol.* **22** (1995) 109–116.

70. J. Toyras, H. J. Nieminen, M. S. Laasanen, M. T. Nieminen, R. K. Korhonen, J. Rieppo, J. Hirvonen, H. J. Helminen and J. S. Jurvelin, Ultrasonic characterization of articular cartilage, *Biorheology* **39**(1–2) (2002) 161–169.

71. M. S. Laasanen, S. Saarakkala, J. Toyras, J. Hirvonen, J. Rieppo, R. K. Korhonen and J. S. Jurvelin, Ultrasound indentation of bovine knee articular cartilage *in situ*, *J. Biomech.* **36** (2003) 1259–1267.

72. M. Fortin, M. D. Buschmann, M. J. Bertrand, F. S. Foster and J. Ophir, Dynamic measurement of internal solid displacement in articular cartilage using ultrasound backscatter, *J. Biomech.* **36** (2003) 443–447.

73. J. Q. Yao and B. B. Seedhom, Ultrasonic measurement of the thickness of human articular cartilage *in situ*, *Rheumatol.* **38** (1999) 1269–1271.

74. D. Lee and J. A. Bouffard, Ultrasound of the knee, *Eur. J. Ultrasound* **14**(1) (2001) 57–71.

75. C. Adam, F. Eckstein, S. Milz and R. Putz, The distribution of cartilage thickness in the knee-joints of old-aged individuals-measurement by A-mode ultrasound, *Clin. Biomech.* **13** (1998) 1–10.

76. D. G. Disler, E. Raymond, D. A. May, J. S. Wayne and T. R. McCauley, Articular cartilage defects: *In vitro* evaluation of accuracy and interobserver reliability for detection and grading with US, *Radiology* **215** (2000) 846–851.

77. R. W. Mann, Comment on 'Ultrasonic measurement of the thickness of human articular cartilage *in situ*' by Yao and Seekhom, *Rheumatology* **40** (2001) 829–831.

78. M. S. Laasanen, J. Toyras, J. Hirvonen, S. Saarakkala, R. K. Korhonen, M. T. Nieminen, I. Kiviranta and J. S. Jurvilin, Novel mechano–acoustic technique and instrument for diagnosis of cartilage degeneration, *Physiol. Meas.* **23** (2002) 491–503.

79. Q. Wang and Y. P. Zheng, Evaluation of osmosis-induced deformation of articular cartilage using ultrasound biomicroscopy imaging, in *Proc. ISB XXth Congr. – ASB 29th Ann. Meet.* (Cleveland, Ohio, USA, July 31 – August 5, 2005), p. 440.

CHAPTER 9

NON-LINEAR ANALYSIS OF THE RESPIRATORY PATTERN

P. CAMINAL*, B. GIRALDO†, M. VALLVERDÚ‡ and L. DOMINGO

Biomedical Engineering Research Centre (CREB)
Departament ESAII, Technical University of Catalonia, Barcelona, Spain
* *pere.caminal@upc.edu*
† *beatriz.giraldo@upc.edu*
‡ *montserrat.vallverdu@upc.edu*

S. BENITO

Dep. Intensive Care Medicine
Hospital de la Santa Creu i Sant Pau, Barcelona, Spain
SBenito@santpau.es

D. KAPLAN

Dep. Mathematics and Computer Science
Macalester College, St. Paul, Minnesota, USA
kaplan@macalester.edu

A. VOSS

Dep. Medical Engineering and Biotechnology
University of Applied Sciences Jena, Germany
voss@fh-jena.de

Traditional time domain techniques of data analysis are often not sufficient to characterize the complex dynamics of respiration. In this study the respiratory pattern variability is analyzed using symbolic dynamics. A group of 20 patients on weaning trials from mechanical ventilation are studied at two different pressure support ventilation levels, in order to obtain respiratory volume signals with different variability. Time series of inspiratory time, expiratory time, breathing duration, fractional inspiratory time, tidal volume and mean inspiratory flow are analyzed. Two different symbol alphabets, with three and four symbols, are considered to characterize the respiratory pattern variability. Assessment of the method is made using the 40 respiratory volume signals classified using clinical criteria into two classes: Low (LV) or high (HV) variability. A discriminant analysis using single indices from symbolic dynamics has been able to classify the respiratory volume signals with an out-of-sample accuracy of 100%.

1. Introduction

The analysis of respiratory pattern variability provides a new tool to study the action of chemoreflexes without application of external stimuli.[1] Determination of the variability of the respiratory volume also enables to know the ability of patients to control the mean tidal volume in response to alterations in respiratory demand.[2] Recently, it has been described that respiratory variability was reduced in patients with restrictive lung disease, compared with that of healthy subjects.[3] One of the most challenging problems in intensive care[4] is the process of discontinuing mechanical ventilation, termed weaning. It has been hypothesized that the variability of the respiratory pattern could be a convenient weaning criteria to reduce the number of patients not successfully weaned.[5]

The possible causes of breath-to-breath variability in the pattern of breathing have been discussed.[6–10] This variability may be explained either by a central neural mechanism or by instability in the chemical feedback loops.[11] Some studies are related to an elevated controller gain, coupled with the presence of delays and response lags in the chemoreflex loops, that may lead to instability in feedback control and give rise to periodic breathing.[12] On the other hand, the nonlinear behavior of the central neural mechanisms together with the muscle activities and the lung function may introduce non-stochastic variability in the respiratory system. In this way, variations in the pattern of breathing may occur as uncorrelated random variations, correlated random changes, or as one of two types of non-random variations: Periodic oscillations or non-random non-periodic fluctuations.[13,14]

The traditional techniques of data analysis in the time and frequency domains are often not sufficient to characterize the complex dynamics of respiration. Various attempts have been reported to apply the concept of nonlinear dynamics to the analysis of complex physiological systems[15–17] and to distinguish between variations that are random and those that are deterministic. Several methods describing the nonlinear deterministic variability of physiological time series have been proposed: Correlation dimension, Lyapunov exponents, Kolmogorov-Sinai entropy, etc.[6,18,19] Schreiber and Schmitz[20] showed that nonlinear prediction is an excellent method for detecting nonlinearity in signals where determinism has not been established previously. Other approaches may present limitations according to the fractal nature of the time series[21–23] or even can lead to misinterpretations of the data.[18] Cardiorespiratory synchronization in humans and nonlinear analysis of heart rate and respiratory dynamics have also been analyzed using a prediction framework.[24–26]

In this work, we introduce nonlinear analyses of respiratory dynamics that may enable an automatic classification of the underlying physiological processes. The object of the investigation is the quantitative analysis of the nonlinear behavior of the respiratory dynamics with regard to its complex organization. This analysis could be of importance to find a set of indices that characterize the variability of the respiratory volume. In this way, we apply symbolic dynamics analysis[27] and non-linear prediction methods.[28] Since respiratory volume can be measured non-invasively, these indices may be advantageous in future automatic diagnostic of patients.

2. Analyzed Data

A group of twenty patients on weaning trials from mechanical ventilation were studied. These patients were recorded in the Department of Intensive Care Medicine at Santa Creu i Sant Pau Hospital, according to a protocol approved by the local ethic committee and with an informed consent obtained. The respiratory volume signals were obtained by means of a respiratory inductive plethismograph (Respitrace Model 150). The signals were recorded with a National Instruments board (PCI 1200) and using Labview software, which sampled the data at 250 Hz.

Each patient was underwent two different levels of pressure support ventilation (PSV), classified as low PSV and high PSV. In this way, the database contains respiratory volume signals with different variability, mainly due to the fact that changes in pressure support are often associated with changes in variability. The first step in the protocol was the selection of a high PSV for each patient, followed by a relaxing period of 15 min before the initiation of the first data recording for 30 min. Then, a low PSV was selected for each patient, followed by a relaxing period of 15 min before the initiation of the second data recording for 30 min. The two different levels of pressure support ventilation in the 20 patients were 5 ± 2 cm H_2O for low PSV and 18 ± 2 cm H_2O for high PSV. The 40 recordings of 30 min were classified by the medical doctors into two classes, low (LV) or high (HV) variability, using clinical criteria based on three variables: Respiratory rate, minute ventilation and rapid shallow breathing index (respiratory rate/tidal volume).[29] When the decrease of PSV produced a statistical significant change ($p < 0.05$) of at least two of the three variables presented, the clinical criteria assigned a change from HV to LV. If the decrease of PSV did not produce a statistical significant change in at least two of the three variables, the clinical criteria assigned the same variability level. In this last case the variability was assigned as HV when the respiratory rate was lower than 25 breaths/min, and LV when respiratory rate was higher than 25 breaths/min. This clinical variability criteria classified the 40 recordings as 24 LV and 16 HV.

The time series considered in this study were: Inspiratory time T_I, expiratory time T_E, duration of the respiratory cycle $T_{Tot} = T_I + T_E$, fractional inspiration time T_I/T_{Tot}, tidal volume V_T, and mean inspiratory flow V_T/T_I (Fig. 1). To obtain the values of these time series a signal processing of the respiratory volume was applied, based on the identification of the inspiratory and expiratory periods.

This work proposes the automatic classification of the volume signals in high or low variability. For out-of-sample evaluation, the 40 volume recordings were organized into two sets: a training set and a testing set. The training set includes patients presenting both LV and HV levels when changing the PSV (nine patients and 18 volume recordings) and the testing set includes the other 22 volume recordings.

3. Methods

3.1. *Symbolic dynamics*

Figure 2 shows, as an example, the T_{Tot} time series obtained from two respiratory volume signals classified as LV and HV, respectively. The concept of Symbolic

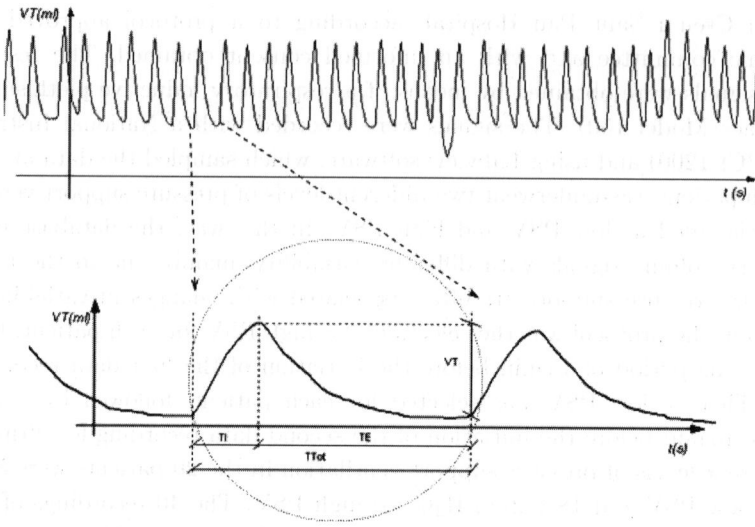

Fig. 1. Inspiratory time T_I, expiratory time T_E, duration of the respiratory cycle $T_{Tot} = T_I + T_E$, and tidal volume V_T.

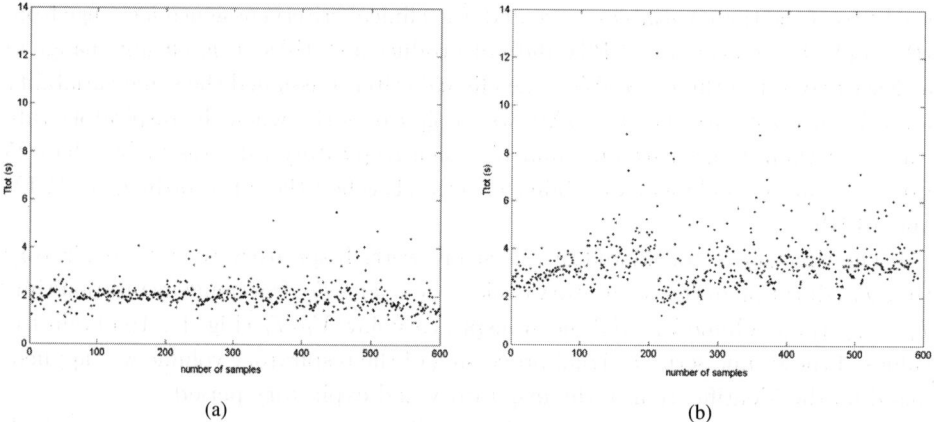

Fig. 2. Recordings of the T_{Tot} time series from the same patient submitted to two different levels of PSV: (a) low variability behavior; (b) high variability behavior.

Dynamics is based on the elimination of detailed information, in order to keep the robust properties of the dynamics by a coarse-graining of the measurements.[27,30] In this way, the time series is transformed into a symbol sequence from an alphabet.

In this study, two alphabets were considered, $\Theta = \{0, 1, 2\}$ and $\Omega = \{0, 1, 2, 3\}$, and their effect on the transformed series compared. These transformations (Eqs. (1) and (2)) were based on the mean value μ of each analyzed time series and also based on a non-dimensional parameter α^{27} that characterizes the ranges where the symbols

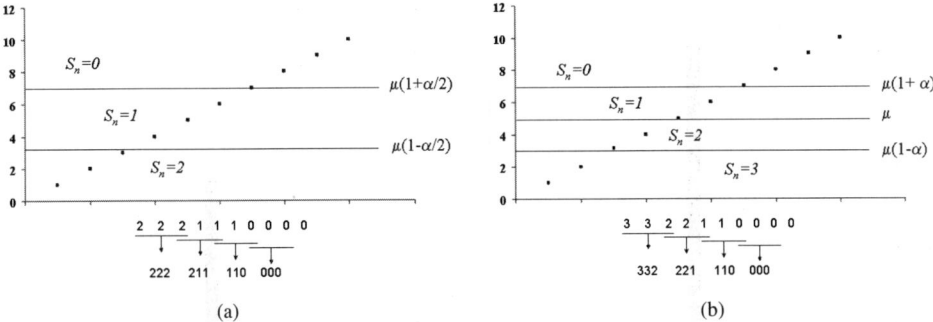

(a) (b)

Fig. 3. Description of the basic principle of symbolic dynamics, the symbol extraction from a time series and the construction of words: (a) considering the symbol alphabet $\Theta = \{0, 1, 2\}$; (b) considering the symbol alphabet $\Omega = \{0, 1, 2, 3\}$.

are defined (Fig. 3).

$$
S_n = \begin{cases} 0 & \text{if } b_n > (1 + \alpha/2)\,\mu \\ 1 & \text{if } (1 - \alpha/2)\,\mu < b_n \le (1 + \alpha/2)\,\mu \\ 2 & \text{if } b_n \le (1 - \alpha/2)\,\mu \end{cases} \tag{1}
$$

$$
S_n = \begin{cases} 0 & \text{if } b_n > (1 + \alpha)\mu \\ 1 & \text{if } \mu < b_n \le (1 + \alpha)\mu \\ 2 & \text{if } (1 - \alpha)\mu < b_n \le \mu \\ 3 & \text{if } b_n \le (1 - \alpha)\mu \end{cases} \tag{2}
$$

with $n = 1, 2, 3, \ldots, N$, where N is the common length of 400 samples and b_n are the values of the time series. Figures 3(a) and 3(b) present examples of these transformations produced by both alphabets, Θ and Ω, respectively.

In order to characterize the symbol strings, obtained by transforming the time series to S_n (Eqs. (1) or (2)), in this study, we analyzed the probability distribution of words with length $\ell = 3$ (Fig. 3). The words consisted of three symbols either if the considered alphabet was Θ or Ω, obtaining a total of 3^ℓ and 4^ℓ different possible word types, respectively.

The histograms of the probability occurrence of each word type for the time series $T_I, T_E, T_{Tot}, T_I/T_{Tot}$, V_T, and V_T/T_I were obtained. Figure 4 (three symbols of Θ) and 5 (four symbols of Ω alphabet) show the histograms of the probability occurrence of each word type obtained from T_{Tot} series of the same patient with low (Fig. 4(a) and Fig. 5(a)) and high (Fig. 4(b) and Fig. 5(b)) variability.

Different parameters were involved in this process, and their values had to be suitably selected. These parameters were: Parameter α, number of overlapped symbols in consecutive words τ, and probability threshold p_{TH} of the word occurrences.

In order to obtain the optimal parameter values that characterize the variability, each parameter was studied by fixing the remaining parameters to specific values. The parameter values that obtained the highest statistical difference, when

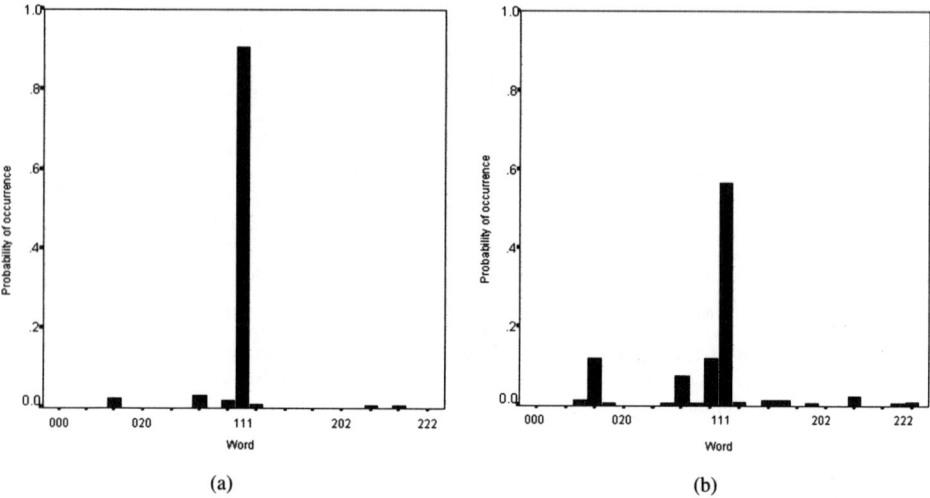

Fig. 4. Histograms obtained from T_{Tot} time series of the same patient submitted to two different levels of PSV: (a) low variability behavior; (b) high variability behavior. Considering the symbol alphabet $\Theta = \{0, 1, 2\}$ and the word length of $\ell = 3$.

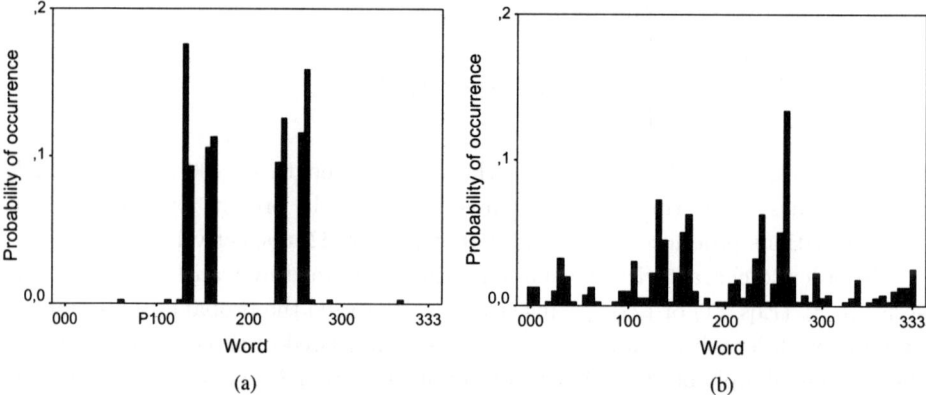

Fig. 5. Histograms obtained from T_{Tot} time series of the same patient submitted to two levels of PSV: (a) low variability behavior; (b) high variability behavior. Considering the symbol alphabet $\Omega = \{0, 1, 2, 3\}$ and the word length of $\ell = 3$.

comparing both groups of patients, were considered the optimal values. A nonparametric Mann–Whitney test was applied to differentiate between the groups.

Several indices were proposed in order to differentiate low variability and high variability:

- probability of occurrence $p(w_{ijk})$ of each word type w_{ijk}. The histograms shown in Figs. 4 (three symbols) and 5 (four symbols) present the probability of occurrence of each word type obtained from T_{Tot} series of the same patient with low (a) and high (b) variability,

- number of words w p_{TH} whose probability of occurrence is higher than a probability threshold p_{TH}, considering different p_{TH} values. For example, in Fig. 4(a) and 4(b) the number of words whose probability of occurrence is higher than the probability threshold $p_{TH} = 6\%$ is $w_6 = 1$ and $w_6 = 4$, respectively,

- number of forbidden words fw whose probability of occurrence is lower than 0.1%. This threshold has been selected according to.[31] This index fw calculates the number of words which seldom or never occur.

One of the most influential parameter in the process was α. Therefore, this parameter was carefully studied, and a range of values from 0.01 to 0.6 was considered. For fixed α values, the most characteristic τ values were determined from the three possible values (0, 1 and 2). In order to define the most suitable probability threshold p_{TH}, a range of values from 1% to 10% was considered.

From the histograms of the probability of occurrence of each word type a simple complexity measure was also evaluated using the Shannon entropy Sh.[32]

3.2. Non-linear prediction

Figure 6 shows LV and HV volume signals. The HV signal in this case is at a slower frequency and, qualitatively displays greater irregularity both in the waveform of a single cycle and the spacing of cycles. The amplitude range of the signals is approximately the same. We sought to quantify this irregularity by measuring the auto-regressive predictability of the signal. The time series is used to construct a model of the dynamics; the model is then used to predict other signal segments. The resulting prediction error quantifies irregularity.

There are different ways to construct dynamical models from data. Since all of the state variables of the systems are not directly measured or even known, we used the lag embedding technique to represent the system's state variables. By embedding the scalar time series D_t, the following vector sequence is created:

$$\mathbf{D}_t = (D_t, D_{t-1}, \ldots, D_{t-(m-1)}), \tag{3}$$

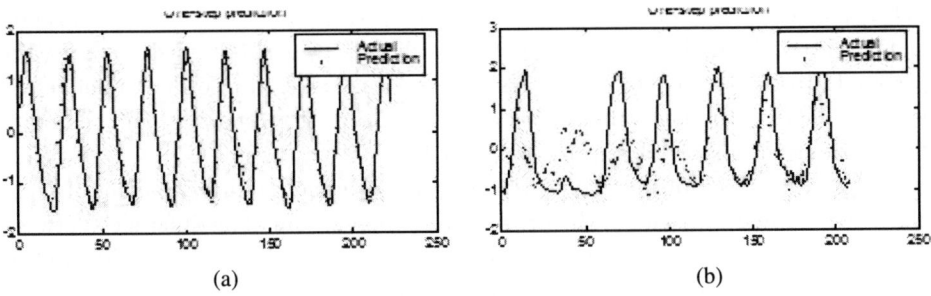

(a) (b)

Fig. 6. (a) Low and (b) high variabilities. Mean respiratory period has been selected as prediction horizon. (-) Actual measurement and (.) one-step prediction of respiratory volume of patients with clinically labeled.

where m is the embedding dimension. Each $\mathbf{D}_t$ is a point in the m-dimensional embedding space, and the embedded time series can be regarded as a sequence of points, one point at each time t. Each point represents the state of the system at that time where m is the embedding dimension. Each $\mathbf{D}_t$ is a point in the m-dimensional embedding space, and the embedded time series can be regarded as a sequence of points, one point at each time t. Each point represents the state of the system at that time.

A deterministic data set sampled at discrete times can be described by a discrete-time map

$$\mathbf{D}_{t+1} = F(\mathbf{D}_t) \tag{4}$$

which is, however, immediately applicable only if the mapping $\mathbf{F}$ is known. With $\mathbf{F}$ unknown some assumptions about its properties have to be made. With the minimal assumption that the mapping $\mathbf{F}$ is continuous the following prediction scheme can be constructed.[28,33] This method implements a nonlinear regression model by stitching smoothly together a large number of locally linear models. The method works as follows: In order to predict the future state $\mathbf{D}_{t+1}$ given the present one $\mathbf{D}_t$, the state that is closest to $\mathbf{D}_t$ with respect to some norm is searched. Let us say that this closest point has time index a. The definition of determinism is that future events are set causally by the past events. $\mathbf{D}_t$ describes the past events to D_{t+1}. Similarly $\mathbf{D}_a$ describes the past events to the measurement D_{a+1}. If $\mathbf{D}_t$ is close to $\mathbf{D}_a$, and if the system is deterministic, then it is expected that D_{a+1}, will also be close to D_{t+1}. In the same way D_{a+h} will be used as a predictor of D_{t+h} and it will be called P_{t+h}.

Every measurement of a continuous quantity is only valid up to some finite resolution and this fact has to be taken into account. The finite resolution implies that looking for the single closest state is no longer the best can be done since interpoint distances are contaminated with an uncertainty. All points within a close region in phase space have to be considered to be equally good predictions a priori. Then the proposed prediction algorithm to be used forms a neighborhood $U(\mathbf{D}_t)$ around the point $\mathbf{D}_t$. For all points $\mathbf{D}_{ai} \in U(\mathbf{D}_t)$, that is, all points close to $\mathbf{D}_t$ look up the individual predictions $\mathbf{D}_{a+h}$. Then the matrix $\mathbf{H}$ of the application $\{\mathbf{D}_{a+h}\} = \mathbf{H}\{\mathbf{D}_{ai}\}$ is obtained, that transforms the points of the neighborhood $U(\mathbf{D}_t)$ into their predictions. Finally, the prediction p_{TH} is obtained applying the matrix $\mathbf{H}$ to the vector $\mathbf{D}_t$. Two ways have been considered in order to define the neighborhood: i) the neighbors inside an hypersphere of radius ε around the point $\mathbf{D}_t$; ii) the K neighbors closest to the point $\mathbf{D}_t$.

Given a method for making a prediction P_{t+h}, an actual measurement of D_{t+h} is needed in order to decide if the prediction is good or bad. The difference between P_{t+h} and D_{t+h} is the prediction error, which informs about the quality of the prediction. As a single prediction might be good or bad just by chance, in order to give a more meaningful indication of the determinism in the data an average of many prediction errors should be taken.

Two different ways have been considered in order to define this indication of determinism: i) Cross-prediction; ii) Leave-one-out auto-prediction. In the cross-prediction approach the time series is broken into M segments. For each of the M segments, one at a time, the model is fit and then residuals are calculated on each of the other segments. The residuals are summarized by one number, the mean absolute value. The result is a $M \times M$ matrix of cross-predictabilities. In this study the respiratory volume data set at each PSV level that contains 18000 samples has been divided in $M = 3$ segments of 6000 samples. In this case the 3×3 matrix has six entries (the diagonal elements that correspond to self prediction are not computed) and their mean value is computed in each patient for each PSV level.

In the leave-one-out auto-prediction the time series of length N is modelled N different times: For each model, a single data point is left out when fitting the model and the residual for the model is computed only for the left-out data point. The result is a set of residuals one for each point, that provide an estimate of the prediction error of a model. In this study the respiratory volume data set at each PSV level has been divided in nine subsets of $N = 2000$ samples. In this way the mean prediction error related to each patient for each PSV level corresponds to the mean absolute value of the prediction errors in the nine subsets.

A preprocessing step has been applied to each respiratory volume data set in order to improve the analysis of the results. Each respiratory volume signal has been normalized by substracting by its mean value and dividing by its standard deviation. Figures 6(a) and 6(b) shows the actual measurements and predictions for the respiratory volume of a patient with clinically labelled low and high variabilities (LV and HV), respectively. The different quality of the prediction is shown comparing LV and HV.

3.2.1. Parameter setting

The first analysis related with the nonlinear prediction was done in order to select between auto-prediction or cross-prediction methodologies. Three patients (CRR, MMX and SAT) that clinically present two different variability levels (LV and HV) when changing the PSV were randomly selected for the analysis. An embedding dimension $m = 2$ was considered. Two kinds of neighborhoods were analyzed: The neighbors inside an hypersphere of radius $\varepsilon = 0.2$ and the $K = 20$ closest neighbors. Tables 1 and 2 present as an example the values obtained in patient CRR using the neighbors inside an hypersphere and the K closest neighbors, respectively. In the three analyzed patients the auto-prediction methodology presented the best statistical significant differences (p-value) when comparing LV and HV signals. Then this methodology has been selected for the next steps.

In order to decide the best kind of neighborhood to discriminate the different irregularity of the respiratory volume, in low and high variabilities, the following neighborhoods were considered: the neighbors inside hyperspheres of radius $\varepsilon = 0.1, 0.2, 0.3$ and $K = 20$ closest neighbors. The same three patients were analyzed

Table 1. Mean ± standard deviation for the mean prediction error of the patient CRR with $m = 2$, $\varepsilon = 0.20$, when considering leave-one-out auto-prediction and nonlinear cross-prediction. Statistical significance (p-value) when comparing low and high variability levels.

	LV	HV	p-value
Leave-one-out auto-prediction	0.41 ± 0.06	0.82 ± 0.11	0.008
Nonlinear cross-prediction	0.45 ± 0.04	0.90 ± 0.06	0.028

Table 2. Mean ± standard deviation for the mean prediction error of the patient CRR with $m = 2$, $K = 20$, when considering leave-one-out auto-prediction and nonlinear cross-prediction.

	LV	HV	p-value
Leave-one-out auto-prediction	0.36 ± 0.05	0.76 ± 0.09	0.008
Nonlinear cross-prediction	0.43 ± 0.03	0.88 ± 0.06	0.027

and an embedding dimension $m = 2$ was considered. Table 3 presents as an example the values obtained in patient CRR. In the three analyzed patients the statistical significance (p-value) obtained when comparing LV and HV signal were found not dependent of the different neighborhood methodology. Then, as the radius of the hyperspheres could be dependent of the embedding dimension, the K closest neighbors methodology has been selected for the next steps.

The next analysis has been done to select the best prediction horizon h. For each patient and for each PSV level the mean respiratory period has been calculated. This mean respiratory period translated to sample units is called h_{Ttot}. Three prediction horizons have been considered: $0.5h_{Ttot}$, h_{Ttot} and $2h_{Ttot}$. The three patients were analyzed and the embedding dimension $m = 2$ was considered. Table 4 presents as an example the values obtained in patient CRR using the different prediction horizons. In the three analyzed patients the statistical significance (p-value) obtained when comparing LV and HV signals were found not dependent

Table 3. Mean ± standard deviation for the mean prediction error of the patient CRR with $m = 2$ when considering different radius ε of the hyperspheres and the $K = 20$ closest neighbors.

	LV	HV	p-value
$\varepsilon = 0.1$	0.41 ± 0.05	0.81 ± 0.09	0.008
$\varepsilon = 0.2$	0.41 ± 0.06	0.82 ± 0.11	0.008
$\varepsilon = 0.3$	0.38 ± 0.06	0.81 ± 0.11	0.008
K neighbors	0.36 ± 0.05	0.76 ± 0.09	0.008

Table 4. Mean ± standard deviation for the mean prediction error of the patient CRR with $m = 2$ when considering different prediction horizons h.

	LV	HV	p-value
$0.5h_{Ttot}$	0.34 ± 0.07	0.67 ± 0.09	0.008
h_{Ttot}	0.36 ± 0.05	0.76 ± 0.09	0.008
$2h_{Ttot}$	0.55 ± 0.07	0.81 ± 0.09	0.008

of the considered h value. A prediction horizon of h_{Ttot} has been selected for the next steps.

3.2.2. *Non-linear determinism in the respiratory volume signal*

The typically slower frequency of the HV signals suggests that a frequency domain analysis using, e.g. power spectrum analysis, might be effective at performing the discrimination. In order to assess to what extent our non-linear prediction method processes information not accessible to linear method, we used the method of surrogate data.[34] This method involves generating synthetic volume signals, called surrogate data, with the same Fourier spectra, mean, standard deviation, and other percentiles as the original data. All of the information that could be accessed by a linear power spectrum analysis, whatever form that analysis might take, is contained in the surrogate data. The algorithm to generate this surrogate data is based on the null hypothesis that the data comes from a stationary linear process with Gaussian white noise inputs.

A set of surrogate data is generated for each volume signal tested. For all the signals (original data and surrogate data) a non-linear index is computed. Then, a statistical test is applied between the set of surrogate data and the original data.

If the null hypothesis is rejected, this suggests that the original data are due to a non-linear deterministic process and/or non-Gaussian inputs or non-stationarity. In the case of the signals analyzed in this study, 10 series of surrogate data have been generated for each of the volume signals of the three patients CRR, MMX and SAT. The non-linear index selected has been the mean prediction error.

3.3. *Discriminant analysis*

A discriminant analysis was applied to obtain a discriminant function that would enable the automatic classification of the volume signals as high (HV) or low (LV) variability. To know the best variables to be introduced in the discriminant analysis, a previous non-parametric analysis of variance test (Mann–Whitney) was used to analyze statistically the differences between the respiratory volume signals with LV and HV. Different variables from the classical time-domain analysis and from the symbolic dynamics and non-linear prediction methods were considered.

From the respiratory volume signals training set, different discriminant functions were obtained and subsequently validated with the testing set. The validation was performed by comparing the results obtained from the discriminant functions with the classification made by medical doctors.

4. Results

Time domain analysis of the time series was previously done. Table 5 shows the results obtained with the mean values $\bar{x}$, standard deviations $SD(x)$ and interquartile ranges $IQR(x)$ of T_I, T_E, T_{Tot}, T_I/T_{Tot}, V_T and V_T/T_I when comparing low and high variability levels, defined using clinical criteria. $\bar{T}_E$, $SD(T_E)$, $IQR(T_E)$, $\overline{T_{Tot}}$, $SD(T_{Tot})$, $IQR(T_{Tot})$ and $\overline{T_I/T_{Tot}}$ presented the best significant differences.

4.1. Symbolic dynamics

The first study, based on the symbolic dynamics analysis, was carried out and analyzed in order to select the parameter values that characterize the physiological process. The first parameter to be determined was α, considering all other

Table 5.   Mean, standard deviation $sd(x)$, and interquartile range $IQR(x)$ when comparing low and high variability levels.

	Low variability	High variability	p-value
$\overline{T_I}$	0.87 ± 0.10	1.07 ± 0.22	0.038
$SD(T_I)$	0.15 ± 0.06	0.29 ± 0.19	0.024
$IQR(T_I)$	0.16 ± 0.09	0.22 ± 0.11	n.s.
$\overline{T_E}$	1.43 ± 0.19	1.62 ± 0.67	<0.0005
$SD(T_E)$	0.30 ± 0.14	1.43 ± 0.63	<0.0005
$IQR(T_E)$	0.25 ± 0.12	1.14 ± 0.67	<0.0005
$\overline{T_{Tot}}$	2.30 ± 0.27	3.96 ± 0.80	<0.0005
$SD(T_{Tot})$	0.34 ± 0.16	1.49 ± 0.64	<0.0005
$IQR(T_{Tot})$	0.29 ± 0.13	1.22 ± 0.71	<0.0005
$\overline{T_I/T_{Tot}}$	0.38 ± 0.024	0.29 ± 0.039	<0.0005
$SD(T_I/T_{Tot})$	0.057 ± 0.024	0.091 ± 0.018	0.012
$IQR(T_I/T_{Tot})$	0.061 ± 0.046	0.092 ± 0.030	n.s.
$\overline{V_T}$	438.0 ± 174.0	599.07 ± 202.8	n.s.
$SD(V_T)$	104.23 ± 57.70	131.88 ± 67.85	n.s.
$IQR(V_T)$	76.36 ± 33.87	90.4 ± 34.79	n.s.
$\overline{V_T/T_I}$	513.9 ± 205.1	584.3 ± 181.1	n.s.
$SD(V_T/T_I)$	146.40 ± 90.78	168.53 ± 95.20	n.s.
$IQR(V_T/T_I)$	111.75 ± 55.61	130.49 ± 94.09	n.s.

parameters with fixed values, no overlapped symbols in consecutive words and $p_{TH} = 0\%$. Table 6 shows the number of words whose probability of occurrence differentiated significantly between low and high variability, when considering the three symbol alphabet Θ applied to the T_{Tot} and T_I/T_{Tot} series.[35] Table 7 shows the results obtained when the four symbol alphabet Ω was applied. Those tables present the results obtained with the best α parameters for different levels of statistical significance $p < 0.05$, $p < 0.01$ and $p < 0.005$. The best α parameters were those that gave the highest number of significant words. Similar analysis were done considering the time series T_I, T_E, V_T and V_T/T_I.

Studying the influence of the different overlapping τ values, Tables 8 and 9 present the results obtained for different τ values when the T_{Tot} and T_I/T_{Tot} series were analyzed. In Table 8 it can be seen that the highest number of significant words in T_{Tot} series was obtained when τ was 1 or 2, and $\alpha = 0.5$. The results obtained with both values, $\tau = 1$ and $\tau = 2$, were similar. It seemed more reasonable to choose $\tau = 1$ because of the reduced computing time. However, when the alphabet was

Table 6. Number of significant words of T_{Tot} and T_I/T_{Tot} series for different α parameters, considering the alphabet Θ and $\tau = 0$.

Number of words	T_{Tot}				T_I/T_{Tot}			
	$\alpha = 0.475$	$\alpha = 0.5$	$\alpha = 0.525$	$\alpha = 0.55$	$\alpha = 0.125$	$\alpha = 0.15$	$\alpha = 0.4$	$\alpha = 0.425$
$p < 0.05$	14	15	15	14	11	11	12	10
$p < 0.01$	8	10	12	9	3	6	6	4
$p < 0.005$	6	7	8	8	3	2	4	3

Table 7. Number of significant words of T_{Tot} and T_I/T_{Tot} series for different α parameters, considering the alphabet Ω and $\tau = 0$.

Number of words	T_{Tot}			T_I/T_{Tot}		
	$\alpha = 0.1$	$\alpha = 0.25$	$\alpha = 0.5$	$\alpha = 0.1$	$\alpha = 0.2$	$\alpha = 0.5$
$p < 0.05$	21	18	9	8	8	0
$p < 0.01$	9	11	2	0	0	0
$p < 0.005$	6	8	1	0	0	0

Table 8. Number of significant words of T_{Tot} and T_I/T_{Tot} series for different τ parameters, considering the alphabet Θ.

Number of words	T_{Tot}									T_I/T_{Tot}					
	$\alpha = 0.475$			$\alpha = 0.5$			$\alpha = 0.525$			$\alpha = 0.15$			$\alpha = 0.4$		
τ	0	1	2	0	1	2	0	1	2	0	1	2	0	1	2
$p < 0.05$	14	17	18	15	15	19	15	16	18	11	12	15	12	17	18
$p < 0.01$	8	13	12	10	14	14	12	12	15	6	5	6	6	7	9
$p < 0.005$	6	9	10	7	12	13	8	11	11	2	4	5	4	3	9

Table 9. Number of significant words of T_{Tot} and T_I/T_{Tot} series for different τ parameters, considering the alphabet Ω.

Number of words	T_{Tot}			T_I/T_{Tot}		
	$\alpha = 0.25$			$\alpha = 0.2$		
τ	0	1	2	0	1	2
$p < 0.05$	18	24	37	8	6	8
$p < 0.01$	11	15	21	0	1	0
$p < 0.005$	8	11	14	0	0	0

Table 10. Words whose probability occurrences (mean $\pm$ sd) in T_{Tot} and T_I/T_{Tot} series presented the most significant differences between both groups, considering the alphabet Θ.

	Probability	Low variability	High variability	p-value
T_{Tot}	$p(w_{110})$	0.019 ± 0.016	0.064 ± 0.029	0.0001
$\alpha = 0.5, \tau = 1$	$p(w_{111})$	0.846 ± 0.182	0.451 ± 0.242	0.0005
	$p(w_{221})$	0.005 ± 0.011	0.032 ± 0.022	0.001
T_I/T_{Tot}	$p(w_{001})$	0.008 ± 0.012	0.029 ± 0.015	0.002
$\alpha = 0.4, \tau = 2$	$p(w_{011})$	0.019 ± 0.014	0.035 ± 0.011	0.003
	$p(w_{112})$	0.031 ± 0.021	0.067 ± 0.032	0.001
	$p(w_{211})$	0.029 ± 0.018	0.058 ± 0.028	0.002

Table 11. Words whose probability occurrences (mean $\pm$ sd) in T_{Tot} and T_I/T_{Tot} series presented the most significant differences between both groups, considering the alphabet Ω.

	Probability	Low variability	High variability	p-value
T_{Tot}	$p(w_{000})$	0.003 ± 0.005	0.024 ± 0.044	0.04
$\alpha = 0.25, \tau = 2$	$p(w_{122})$	0.070 ± 0.041	0.028 ± 0.020	0.024
	$p(w_{211})$	0.071 ± 0.031	0.021 ± 0.015	0.001
	$p(w_{221})$	0.072 ± 0.041	0.029 ± 0.023	0.019
	$p(w_{233})$	0.004 ± 0.006	0.028 ± 0.016	0.0001
	$p(w_{332})$	0.005 ± 0.006	0.031 ± 0.020	0.003
T_I/T_{Tot}	$p(w_{100})$	0.004 ± 0.006	0.015 ± 0.009	0.019
$\alpha = 0.2, \tau = 2$	$p(w_{121})$	0.062 ± 0.031	0.027 ± 0.022	0.011
	$p(w_{312})$	0.003 ± 0.004	0.009 ± 0.005	0.024

composed of four symbols (Ω) the highest number of significant words was obtained with $\tau = 2$ and $\alpha = 0.25$ (Table 9). When the T_I/T_{Tot} series were analyzed the parameters that achieved the best statistical significant differences between groups were $\alpha = 0.4$ when using the three symbol alphabet (Table 8) and $\alpha = 0.2$ using the four symbol alphabet (Table 9), furthermore, they both required $\tau = 2$ symbols.

Tables 10 and 11 show the words whose probability occurrence in T_{Tot} and in T_I/T_{Tot} series presented the most significant differences when comparing low and high variability. These tables present the mean and the standard deviation (mean ± sd) of the probability of occurrence and the statistical significant level (p-value). These results were obtained using the parameters α and τ selected previously. However, the statistical significant levels were lower when considering the time series T_I, T_E, V_T and V_T/T_I.

The study of the number of words whose probability of occurrence was higher than a probability threshold is presented in Tables 12 and 13, considering different probability thresholds. The tables show a selection of the most promising results. The study of the T_{Tot} and in T_I/T_{Tot} series showed that the best statistical significant levels p <0.005 were obtained taking into account the probability threshold from 1% to 6%. The number of forbidden words (words with a low probability of occurrence) allowed to obtain a statistically significant difference between groups when the alphabet Θ was used, with $p = 0.002$ for T_{Tot} series and $p = 0.014$ for T_I/T_{Tot} series (Table 14). However, lower statistical differences were obtained when the alphabet Ω was used (Table 14). The differences were

Table 12. Number of words wp$_{th}$ whose probability occurrence is higher than a probability threshold p_{TH} in T_{Tot} and T_I/T_{Tot} series considering the alphabet Θ.

	Probability threshold	Low variability mean ± sd	High variability mean ± sd	p-value
T_{Tot}	$p_{TH} = 2\%$	$w2 = 6.5 \pm 5.5$	$w2 = 14.5 \pm 4.2$	0.001
$\alpha = 0.5, \tau = 1$	$p_{TH} = 5\%$	$w5 = 1.6 \pm 1.5$	$w5 = 5.2 \pm 2.7$	0.0014
	$p_{TH} = 6\%$	$w6 = 1.2 \pm 0.6$	$w6 = 4.0 \pm 1.8$	0.0005
T_I/T_{Tot}	$p_{TH} = 1\%$	$w1 = 9.0 \pm 6.5$	$w1 = 18 \pm 6.4$	0.004
$\alpha = 0.4, \tau = 2$	$p_{TH} = 2\%$	$w2 = 6.1 \pm 4.9$	$w2 = 12.8 \pm 11.5$	0.004

Table 13. Number of words wp$_{th}$ whose probability occurrence is higher than a probability threshold p_{TH} in T_{Tot} and T_I/T_{Tot} series considering the alphabet Ω.

	Probability threshold	Low variability mean ± sd	High variability mean ± sd	p-value
T_{Tot}	$p_{TH} = 1\%$	$w1 = 14.1 \pm 6.0$	$w1 = 27.2 \pm 6.7$	0.0005
$\alpha = 0.25, \tau = 2$	$p_{TH} = 2\%$	$w2 = 8.9 \pm 1.9$	$w2 = 14.0 \pm 3.4$	0.001
	$p_{TH} = 5\%$	$w5 = 6.3 \pm 1.94$	$w5 = 4.11 \pm 2.3$	0.04
T_I/T_{Tot}	$p_{TH} = 2\%$	$w2 = 10.4 \pm 4.7$	$w2 = 14.7 \pm 3.9$	0.04
$\alpha = 0.2, \tau = 2$	$p_{TH} = 5\%$	$w5 = 6.4 \pm 2.5$	$w5 = 3.9 \pm 2.3$	0.04

Table 14. Number of forbidden words: number of words whose probability occurrence is lower than $p_{TH} = 0.1\%$.

mean ± sd	T_{Tot}		T_I/T_{Tot}	
	Low variability	High variability	Low variability	High variability
alphabet Θ	16.9 ± 6.8 p-value = 0.002	8.1 ± 4.7	11.5 ± 7.6 p-value = 0.014	4.0 ± 5.3
alphabet Ω	32.5 ± 14.7 p-value = 0.02	10.0 ± 5.5	26.4 ± 18.8 p-value = n.s.	15.2 ± 17.4

Table 15.   Shannon entropy.

mean ± sd	T_{Tot}		T_I/T_{Tot}	
	Low variability	High variability	Low variability	High variability
alphabet Θ	0.76 ± 0.64 p-value < 0.0005	3.18 ± 0.58	1.49 ± 1.15 p-value $= 0.001$	3.69 ± 0.60
alphabet Ω	3.59 ± 0.70 p-value $= 0.001$	4.82 ± 0.38	3.98 ± 0.93 p-value $=$ n.s.	4.66 ± 0.96

also lower when considering the time series T_I, T_E, V_T and V_T/T_I. The Shannon entropy allowed to obtain a statistically significant difference between groups when the alphabet Θ was used, with $p < 0.0005$ for T_{Tot} series and $p = 0.001$ for T_I/T_{Tot} series (Table 15), and when the alphabet Ω was used a statistically significant difference was obtained ($p = 0.001$) for T_{Tot} series. The differences were lower when considering the time series T_I, T_E, V_T and V_T/T_I.

4.2. Non-linear prediction

Table 16 shows the results obtained when surrogate data method was applied to the respiratory volume signals of LV and HV in the three selected patients CRR, MMX and SAT who had both LV and HV recordings.[36] The mean prediction error (mpe) of the original signal (Q_D), and the mean ± sd of the mpe of the surrogate data ($\mu_H \pm \sigma_H$) are presented. For both low and high variability recordings of the three patients the respiratory volume signals of the patients analyzed have significant differences with respect to surrogate data generated, and so the null hypothesis can be rejected.

In order to analyze the level of irregularity in the respiratory volume signals related to high variability in comparison with the low variability, Table 17 shows the mean prediction errors (mpe) obtained for $m = 2$ when considering all the patients. The results show a statistically significant difference ($p < 0.0005$) between both groups.

The role of the embedding dimension m on the prediction errors has been analyzed in all the patients for each one of the PSV levels. Figure 7 shows as

Table 16.   Values of mean prediction error for volume signals and surrogate data with statistical significance.

	Q_D	$\mu_H \pm \sigma_H$	p-value
CRR-LV	0.36	0.49 ± 0.01	< 0.0005
CRR-HV	0.72	0.75 ± 0.01	< 0.0005
MMX-LV	0.24	0.31 ± 0.01	< 0.0005
MMX-HV	0.33	0.39 ± 0.01	< 0.0005
SAT-LV	0.31	0.40 ± 0.01	< 0.0005
SAT-HV	0.70	0.79 ± 0.01	< 0.0005

Table 17. Mean $\pm$ sd of the mean prediction errors (*mpe*) and the embedding dimensions (*m*) needed to model the dynamics of the patients with a reduced mean prediction error (*e*) of 0.35, 0.40 and 0.45 (*me35*, *me40* and *me45*, respectively).

	Low variability	High variability	*p*-value
mpe	0.35 ± 0.09	0.63 ± 0.08	<0.0005
me35	3.3 ± 2.0	6.8 ± 1.7	<0.0005
me40	2.4 ± 0.7	5.9 ± 1.5	<0.0005
me45	2.1 ± 0.3	5.1 ± 1.4	<0.0005

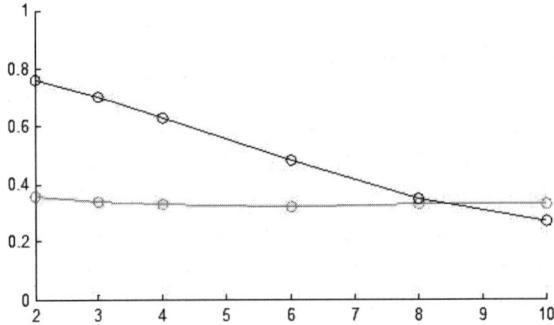

Fig. 7. Prediction errors obtained as a function of the embedding dimension for the patient CRR. The line on the top belongs to the HV signal.

an example the relation between the mean prediction error and the embedding dimension for the patient CRR. Line labelled as CRR20 belongs to the HV signal and CRR06 to the LV signal.

Another way to characterize predictability involves finding embedding dimension needed to model the dynamics of the patients with a low prediction error. For example in patient CRR (Fig. 7) an embedding dimension $m = 8$ is needed to get a *mpe* below 0.4 when analyzing the HV signal, while a $m = 2$ is enough to get the same prediction error for the LV signal. The values of the embedding dimension (*m*) needed to model the dynamics of the signals with a prediction error (*e*) of 0.35, 0.40, 0.45 (*me35*, *me40* and *me45*, respectively) have been calculated. Table 17 shows the values of the *me35*, *me40* and *me45* when analyzing all the patients. The embedding dimension needed to model the dynamics of the patients with a low prediction error show a statistical significant difference ($p < 0.0005$) between both low and high variability signals.

4.3. *Discriminant analysis*

The aim of the last part of this study was to obtain discriminant functions able to discriminate low and high respiratory pattern variability. From the time series

Table 18. Discriminant functions using variables from the
time-domain analysis: LV, low variability; HV, high variability.

	False LV	False HV	Accuracy
$SD(T_{Tot})$	2	1	86%
$IQR(T_{Tot})$	2	0	91%
$IQR(T_E)$	2	0	91%
$IQR(T_{Tot}), IQR(T_E)$	2	0	91%
$IQR(T_{Tot}), SD(T_{Tot})$	1	1	91%
$IQR(T_E), SD(T_{Tot})$	1	1	91%
$IQR(T_E), SD(T_E)$	1	1	91%

of the training set different discriminant functions of one or two variables were
constructed using the most significant parameters from the time-domain analysis
and the symbolic dynamic analysis. Table 18 presents a summary of the results
achieved using the variables from the time-domain analysis, during the evaluation
process with the 22 respiratory volume signals of the testing set. In this process
a signal was considered False HV when the discriminant function classified it as
high variability when it was considered by the medical doctor as low variability.
A signal was considered as False LV when the discriminant function classified it as
low variability when it was considered by the medical doctor as high variability.
Accuracy is the percentage of volume signals correctly classified.

The variables obtained with the symbolic dynamics analysis (Table 19)
presented better discriminant results than the best variables proposed from the
time-domain analysis (Table 18). The time domain analysis parameters were not
able to get a complete correct classification of the 22 testing set recordings, even
when two indices were combined. However, the evaluation process using single
variables of the alphabet Θ with the 22 recordings of the T_{Tot} time series of the
testing set achieved a complete correct classification (Table 19) when considering
the indices: Probability of occurrence of the word type 111, $p(w_{111})$, probability of
occurrence of the word type 221, $p(w_{221})$, number of words whose probability
of occurrence is higher than 2%, $w2$, and number of words whose probability of
occurrence is higher than 5%, $w5$. Taking the alphabet Ω into account, a correct
classification could only be obtained combining two variables. The entropies do not
obtain the best results in the discriminant analysis.

From the T_I/T_{Tot} series of the training set, different discriminant functions
were constructed with each single index (Table 19). As it is shown in this table, the
evaluation process with the 22 recordings of the T_I/T_{Tot} series of the testing set
achieved the best results when considering the number of words whose probability
of occurrence is higher than 2% ($w2$), with an accuracy of 95% using the alphabet
Θ. However, when the study was done using the alphabet Ω the maximum accuracy
obtained with the T_I/T_{Tot} series was 91%.

The variables obtained with the nonlinear prediction methodology presented
better discriminant results than the best variable proposed from the time-domain

Table 19. Discriminant functions using variables from the symbolic dynamics analysis: LV, low variability; HV, high variability.

		Alphabet Θ				Alphabet Ω		
		False LV	False HV	Accuracy (%)		False LV	False HV	Accuracy (%)
T_{Tot}	$p(w_{111})$	0	0	100	$p(w_{122})$	2	0	91
	$p(w_{221})$	0	0	100	$p(w_{221})$	2	0	91
	$w2$	0	0	100	Sh	1	1	91
	$w5$	0	0	100	$p(w_{000}), w1$	0	0	100
	$w6$	1	0	95	$p(w_{233}), w1$	0	0	100
	fw	2	0	91	$p(w_{233}), fw$	0	0	100
	Sh	1	0	95	$p(w_{332}), fw$	0	0	100
T_I/T_{Tot}	$p(w_{001})$	2	0	91	$w2$	1	1	91
	$p(w_{011})$	2	0	91				
	$w1$	2	0	91				
	$w2$	1	0	95				
	fw	2	0	91				
	Sh	2	0	91				

Table 20. Discriminant functions using variables from the nonlinear prediction analysis: LV, low variability; HV, high variability.

	False LV	False HV	Accuracy (%)
mpe	0	1	95
$me35$	2	0	91
$me40$	1	1	91
$me45$	1	3	82
$mpe, me35$	1	2	86
$mpe, me40$	1	0	95
$mpe, me45$	1	0	95

analysis. Table 20 shows the results obtained using discriminant functions of one and two variables. The mpe and the mpe combined with the embedding dimension needed to get a mpe of 0.40 or 0.45 achieved an accuracy of 95%.

5. Discussion and Conclusions

The main objective of this work is to develop methodologies able to characterize the different respiratory pattern variabilities contained in the volume signals. The respiratory pattern variability of 20 patients is studied by analyzing the nonlinear dynamics of the respiratory system. The symbolic dynamics analysis and the nonlinear prediction method are considered. In this way, from each respiratory volume recording the T_I, T_E, T_{Tot}, T_I/T_{Tot}, V_T and V_T/T_I series are obtained and their complex behavior represented by symbolic dynamics. For this purpose two time series transformations based on symbolic dynamics are performed and a methodology is developed in order to characterize the different respiratory pattern variability.

The differences between the complex behaviors involved in high and low variability can clearly be seen by observing the histograms obtained after the symbolic transformation of the time series. Figures 5(a) and 5(b) show the histograms constructed from the same patient where it is observed that the high variability behavior presents more dynamical complexity than the low variability.

The symbolic dynamics methodology involves analyzing the effect of the parameters that are utilized in the proposed symbolic dynamic analysis: The parameter α, the number of the overlapped symbols in consecutive words τ and the probability threshold p_{TH} of the word occurrences. The more suitable parameter values are selected for the analysis of both symbol transformations. The results show that the probability of occurrences of the words obtained from both transformations is higher in the high variability class than in the low variability class, if the words contain the symbols 0 or 2 for the three symbol alphabet or the symbols 0 or 3 for the four symbol alphabet, as it is observed in Tables 10 and 11.

Analyzing the different probability thresholds p_{TH}, T_{Tot} series presents better statistical significant levels than T_I/T_{Tot}, as can bee seen in Tables 12 and 13. Using the three symbol alphabet transformation (Table 12), T_{Tot} series are better characterized ($p < 0.0005$) by the occurrence probabilities higher than $p_{TH} = 6\%$ when high and low variability classes are compared. The high variability behavior is characterized by a higher number of words (4.0 ± 1.8) than the low variability behavior (1.2 ± 0.6). The four symbol alphabet transformation produces a similar behavior when the occurrence probabilities of the words is higher than $p_{TH} = 1\%$ (Table 13). The occurrence probability is concentrated on 14 words for low variability behavior and on 27 words for high variability behavior. Furthermore, Table 14 shows the forbidden words fw whose probability occurrence is lower than $p_{TH} = 0.1\%$. In both transformations the number of fw is higher in low variability class than in high variability class. The best results are obtained when considering the time series T_{Tot} and T_I/T_{Tot} rather than the volume related time series V_T and V_T/T_I. Respiratory center responds mainly with tachyapnea in front of acute respiratory failure. This fact may justify that the time intervals of respiratory pattern obtain more significant results than the volume of breath.

In the non-linear prediction method the volume time series have been used to construct a model of the respiratory system dynamics and the accuracy of the predictions made from the model have been analyzed. Two different ways have been considered in order to define the indication of determinism: Cross-prediction and leave-one-out auto-prediction. Two kinds of neighborhoods have been analyzed: The neighbors inside a hypersphere of radius ε and the K neighbors closed to a point in the phase space. The incidence of different prediction horizons has also been considered. The analysis of the prediction error as a function of the embedding dimension has been used to propose a new index to discriminate different respiratory pattern variability levels. Highly statistically significant differences have been obtained when comparing the mean prediction error of the volume signals clinically classified as low variability in relation with high variability signals ($p < 0.0005$).

The results obtained using the method of surrogate data means that the nonlinear prediction method is detecting signs of nonlinearity, nonstationarity or non-gaussianity in the signals. But note that the prediction errors for the surrogate data in the different classes of HV and LV signals follow roughly the same pattern of variability as for the original data. That is, there is lower nonlinear prediction error for surrogates from LV signals than for surrogates from HV signals. Since the surrogate data has, by construction, no statistically identifiable non-linear, non-stationary, or non-Gaussian components, this suggests that it might be possible to find some linear analysis method that can perform a discrimination between LV and HV similar to the one using non-linear prediction. This does not necessarily mean, however, that the physiological mechanisms generating the linear structures are themselves linear.

All analyzes are performed using a training set of time series. Discriminant functions of one or two variables are constructed using this training set and validated on 22 time series of a testing set. The discriminant analysis carried out, when using the non-linear prediction, obtained discriminant functions able to classify with an accuracy of 95% the testing respiratory volume signals, while the discriminant analysis using classical time–domain variables presented lower accuracy (91%). The discriminant analysis carried out using symbolic dynamics obtained discriminant functions able to classify correctly all the testing set series using single variables obtained from the symbolic dynamic analysis. The results show that the symbol alphabet is appropriate for our purpose since it can better characterize the respiratory pattern variability involved in the investigated process. It means that the symbol alphabet keeps the robust properties and the global information of the main system.

The clinical relevance of such a method of discriminating respiratory volume variability is related with the study of the action of chemoreflexes without application of external stimuli, and the analysis of the ability of patients to control the mean tidal volume in response to alterations in respiratory demand. Furthermore, this method could be a convenient weaning criteria to reduce the number of patients not successfully weaned.

The analysis of the respiratory time series by non-linear dynamics leads to a significantly improved identification of two variability levels, low and high, in comparison with the linear analysis in the time domain. Furthermore, it is presumed that the irregular time courses of the respiratory time series can be characterized more adequately by the methodology based on the three symbol alphabet. The results obtained in this work show that words containing three symbols are convenient to characterize the variability of the respiratory time series. It seems that the proposed methodology could allow an automatic classification of the volume signals in high or low variability. However, these results should be validated by a larger number of patients, especially to prove the ability of this discriminant function approach.

Acknowledgments

This work was partially supported by grant CICYT TEC2004-02274 from the Spanish government.

References

1. J. G. Van den Aardweg and J. M. Karemaker, *Am. J. Respir. Crit. Care Med.* **165** (2002) 1041–1047.
2. H. Wrigge, W. Golisch, J. Zinserling, M. Sydow, G. Almeling and H. Burchardi, *Intensive Care Med.* **25** (1999) 790–798.
3. T. Brack, A. Jubran and M. J. Tobin, *Am. J. Respir. Crit. Care Med.* **165** (2002) 1260–1264.
4. M. J. Tobin, *New Engl. J. Med.* **344** (2001) 1986–1996.
5. N. del Rosario, C. S. Sassoon, K. G. Chetty, S. E. Gruer and C. K. Mahutte, *Eur. Respir. J.* **10**(11) (1997) 2560–2565.
6. E. N. Bruce and J. A. Daubenspeck, in *Control of Breathing* (Marcel Dekker, 1995), pp. 285–314.
7. F. L. Eldridge, *Chest* **73** (1978) 256–258.
8. H. Gautier, *Clin. Sci.* **58** (1980) 343–348.
9. S. A. Sahn, C. W. Zwillich and N. Dick, *J. Appl. Physiol.* **43** (1977) 1019–1025.
10. R. B. Schoene, *Respir. Care* **34** (1989) 500–509.
11. G. Benchetrit, *Respir. Physiol.* **122** (2000) 123–129.
12. M. C. Khoo, *Respir. Physiol.* **122** (2000) 167–182.
13. E. N. Bruce, *J. Appl. Physiol.* **80** (1996) 1079–1087.
14. A. Jubran and M. J. Tobin, *Am. J. Respir. Crit. Care Med.* **162** (2000) 1202–1209.
15. D. R. Rigney, W. C. Ocasio, K. P. Clark, J. Y. Wei and A. L. Goldberger, *Circulation* (1992) 651–659.
16. R. G. Turcott and M. C. Teich, *Ann. Biomed. Eng.* **24** (1996) 269–293.
17. P. Achermann, R. Hartmann, A. Gunziger, W. Guggenbuhl and A. Brobely, *Electroencephalogr. Clin. Neurophisiol.* **90** (1994) 384–387.
18. M. Small, K. Judd, M. Lowe, M and S. Stick, *J. Appl. Physiol.* **86** (1999) 359–376.
19. M. Akay, T. Lipping, K. Moodie and P. J. Hoopes, *Early Human Develop.* **70** (2002) 55–71.
20. T. Schreiber and A. Schmitz, *Phys. Rev. E* **55** (1997) 5443–5447.
21. M. Sammon, J. R. Romaniuk and E. Bruce, *J. Appl. Physiol.* **75** (1993) 887–901.
22. N. Wessel, U. Meyerfeldt, A. Schirdewan, J. Kurths and A. Voss, *Ann. Conf. IEEE Eng. Med. Biol. Soc.* **20**(1) (1998) 326–329.
23. J. M. Tapanainen, M. D. Seppänen, R. Laukkanen, A. Loimaala and H. V. Huikuri, *Ann. Noninvasive Electrocardiol.* **4**(1) (1999) 10–18.
24. D. Hoyer, D. T. Kaplan, F. Shaaf and M. Eiselt, *IEEE Eng. Med. Biol.* **17** (1998) 26–31.

25. D. Hoyer, U. Leder, H. Hoyer, B. Pompe, M. Sommer and U. Zwiener, *Med. Eng. Phys.* **24** (2002) 33–43.

26. F. Censi, G. Calcagnini, S. Lino, S. R. Seydnejad, R. I. Kitney and S. Cerutti, *Med. Biolog. Eng. Comput.* **38** (2000) 416–426.

27. A. Voss, J. Kurths, H. J. Kleiner, A. Witt, N. Wessel, P. Saparin, K. J. Osterziel, R. Schurath and R. Dietz, *Cardiovasc. Res.* **31** (1996) 419–433.

28. H. Kantz and T. Schreiber, in *Nonlinear Time Series Analysis* (Cambridge University Press, 2000), pp. 42–57.

29. X. Capdevila, P. F. Perrigault, M. Ramonatxo, J. P. Roustan, P. Peray, A. Francoise and C. Prefaut, *Crit. Care Med.* **26** (1998) 79–87.

30. M. Baumert, T. Walther, J. Hopfe, H. Stepan, R. Faber and A. Voss, *Med. Biolog. Eng. Comput.* **40** (2002) 241–245.

31. J. Kurths, A. Voss, P. Saparin, A. Witt, H. J. Kleiner and N. Wessel, *Chaos* **5**(1) (1995) 88–104.

32. H. Kantz and T. Schreiber, *Nonlinear Time Series Analysis* (Cambridge University Press, 1997).

33. D. Kaplan and L. Glass, in *Understanding Nonlinear Dynamics* (Springer-Verlag, 1995), pp. 314–338.

34. J. Theiler, S. E. Eubank, A. Longtin, B. Galdrikian and D. Farmer, *Phys. D* **58** (1992) 77–94.

35. P. Caminal, M. Vallverdú, B. Giraldo, S. Benito and A. Voss A., *IEEE Trans. Biomed. Eng.* **52**(11) (2005) 1832–1839.

36. P. Caminal, L. Domingo, B. Giraldo, M. Vallverdú, S. Benito, G. Vázquez and D. Kaplan, *Med. Biolog. Eng. Comput.* **42**(1) (2004) 86–91.